Sonography Scanning

PRINCIPLES AND PROTOCOLS

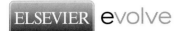
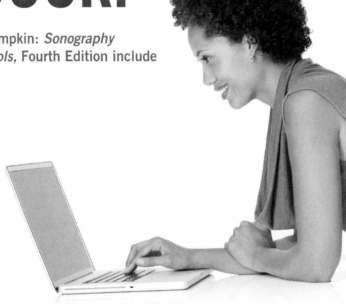

Sonography Scanning

PRINCIPLES AND PROTOCOLS

FOURTH EDITION

BETTY BATES TEMPKIN, BA, RT(R), RDMS
Ultrasound Consultant
Formerly Clinical Director of the Diagnostic
  Medical Sonography Program
Hillsborough Community College
Tampa, Florida

ELSEVIER
SAUNDERS

ELSEVIER
SAUNDERS

3251 Riverport Lane
St. Louis, Missouri 63043

SONOGRAPHY SCANNING: PRINCIPLES AND PROTOCOLS,
FOURTH EDITION   ISBN: 978-1-4557-7321-3
Copyright 2015, 2009, 1999, 1993 by Saunders, an imprint of Elsevier Inc.

Notices

Executive Content Strategist: Sonya Seigafuse
Content Development Specialist: Laurie Gower
Content Coordinator: John Tomedi
Marketing Manager: Jaime Augustine
Publishing Services Manager: Jeff Patterson
Project Manager: Mary Stueck
Text Designer: Renée Duenow

Working together
to grow libraries in
developing countries

www.elsevier.com • www.bookaid.org

Printed in the United States of America

Last digit is the print number: 9 8 7 6 5

To Max
"Remarkable, Soulful, Honorable"
and
To David
"Exceptional, Insightful, Generous"

Contributors

Peggy Ann Malzi Bizjak, MBA, RDMS, RT(R)(M), CRA
Radiology Manager–Ultrasound
Radiology and Medical Imaging Department
University of Virginia Health System;
Adjunct Faculty
Diagnostic Medical Sonography Program
Piedmont Virginia Community College
Charlottesville, Virginia

Amy T. Dela Cruz, MS, RDMS, RVT
Medical Sonography Program Director
South Piedmont Community College
Monroe, North Carolina
*Musculoskeletal Scanning Protocol for Rotator Cuff, Carpal Tunnel,
    and Achilles Tendon*

Kristin Dykstra Downey, AS, RT(R), RDMS
Echovascular Sonographer
Allied Mobile Imaging
Ooltewah, Tennessee
Neonatal Brain Scanning Protocol

Wayne C. Leonhardt, BA, RT(R), RVT, RDMS
Faculty
Foothill College of Ultrasound
Los Altos, California;
Staff Sonographer, Technical Director, and Continuing
    Education Director
Summit Medical Center
Oakland, California
Thyroid and Parathyroid Glands Scanning Protocol

Maureen E. McDonald, BS, RDMS, RDCS
Staff Echocardiographer
Adult Echocardiography Instructor and Lecturer
Thomas Jefferson University Hospital
Philadelphia, Pennsylvania
Adult Echocardiography Scanning Protocol
Pediatric Echocardiography Scanning Protocol

Marsha M. Neumyer, BS, RVT, FSVU, FAIUM, ASDMS
International Director
Vascular Diagnostic Educational Services
Vascular Resource Associates
Harrisburg, Pennsylvania
Abdominal Doppler and Color Flow Imaging
Cerebrovascular Duplex Scanning Protocol
Peripheral Arterial and Venous Duplex Scanning Protocols

Betty Bates Tempkin, BA, RT(R), RDMS
Ultrasound Consultant
Formerly Clinical Director of the Diagnostic Medical Sonography
    Program
Hillsborough Community College
Tampa, Florida
Guidelines; Scanning Planes and Scanning Methods; Scanning Protocol
    for Abnormal Findings and Pathology; Abdominal Aorta Scanning
    Protocol; Inferior Vena Cava Scanning Protocol; Liver Scanning Protocol;
    Gallbladder and Biliary Tract Scanning Protocol; Pancreas Scanning
    Protocol; Renal Scanning Protocol; Spleen Scanning Protocol; Female Pelvis
    Scanning Protocol; Transvaginal Scanning Protocol for the Female Pelvis;
    Obstetrical Scanning Protocol For First, Second, And Third Trimesters;
    Male Pelvis Scanning Protocol for the Prostate Gland, Scrotum, and Penis;
    Thyroid and Parathyroid Glands Scanning Protocol; Breast Scanning
    Protocol; Neonatal Brain Scanning Protocol

Editorial Review Board

Preface

Sonography Scanning: Principles and Protocols came about as a result of my teaching, as well as practical scanning experience. During my 22 years as a sonographer—most of which I have spent as a clinical director and teaching in scanning labs as well as the hospital setting—I realized that sonographers needed a basic approach to the performance of scans, a pattern as well as a benchmark for their work. My purpose in writing this text is to provide a step-by-step method for scanning and image documentation for physician diagnostic interpretation. I hope this "how to" scanning approach takes the struggle out of scanning and ensures thoroughness and accuracy. The enumeration of scanning steps and required images for each examination promotes the establishment of standards and improves examination quality. The structure of this text should make it easy to read, simple to follow, and practical to use. The text begins with an introductory chapter that includes topics such as guidelines for the general use of the text, professional standards, clinical standards, case presentation, scanning prerequisites, image quality and labeling, and methods by which sonographic findings are described.

Subsequent sections cover technical parameters, including scanning planes and their anatomical interpretations and scanning methods, followed by a chapter devoted to the evaluation, documentation, and description of abnormal findings. Next, the scanning protocol chapters offer scanning protocols for the major blood vessels and organs of the abdomen (including full and limited studies), the male and female pelvic organs, and obstetrics. Scanning protocols for the scrotum, thyroid gland, breast, and neonatal brain are also included. The protocol chapters conclude with scanning protocols for vascular and cardiac studies.

Applicable protocols are patterned after the scanning guidelines of the American Institute of Ultrasound in Medicine, which, along with an abbreviation glossary, are included in the appendixes of the text. The scanning protocol chapters selectively address organ, vasculature, or fetal location, as well as anatomy, physiology, sonographic appearance, and normal variations. In addition, patient preparation, position, and breathing techniques are discussed. Steps are specified for transducer placement, surveys, and required images. Other features to assist the reader are illustrations for anatomy; patient positions; the placement of, position of, and direction to move the transducer; and illustrations of nearly all ultrasound images.

What's New

The fourth edition has been completely redesigned to enhance readability by offering more images on each page and presenting the information in an attractive, 2-color design. We added pedagogy to each chapter, including learning objectives and key words as well as updated end-of-chapter review questions, to aid the reader's understanding of the material. In addition, more than 300 new images have been included to demonstrate superior quality scans from the latest state-of-the-art ultrasound equipment. New transducer location drawings on images help the reader understand exactly where on the body to scan to produce a particular image. Also exclusive to this edition is a new chapter covering musculoskeletal protocols for those interested in this specialty.

Because the scanning methods under discussion are derived from the authors' professional experiences, most chapters highlight the techniques that we have found to work best. However, the success of scanning depends on the skill of the individual; thus finding one's personal approach to solving imaging problems is not only expected but inevitable. Therefore, in addition to our personal way of doing things, we discuss alternatives and encourage you to explore other approaches.

The text reflects the assumption that the reader has thorough knowledge of gross and sectional anatomy. An in-depth course in normal anatomy and sectional anatomy are key prerequisites for comprehending scanning techniques. As an overview, gross anatomy and reference illustrations are at the beginning of most protocol chapters.

The sonographer's role in medicine is unique among those of other allied health professionals specializing in imaging modalities because sonographic image accuracy depends on the skill of the operator, not just the technical aspects of the machine. That single reason is sufficient to support the premise that scanning skills must equal the level of importance attached to a sonographer's knowledge of physics, physiology, pathology, and anatomy. Currently, practical considerations prevent the American Registry of Diagnostic Medical Sonography from evaluating scanning ability. Therefore, feedback from sonography educators and sonologists and comparison of films with established guidelines and scanning protocols are vital to mastering the art of ultrasound scanning.

When performed at the highest level, the collective factors that define "sonographer" become an integral part of patient evaluation. It is my hope that this text provides the tools to facilitate scanning and documenting studies and, as a result, directly contributes to the achievement of excellence in the daily practice of ultrasound scanning.

Betty Bates Tempkin, BA, RT(R), RDMS

Acknowledgments

Many thanks to Developmental Editors Beth LoGiudice and John Tomedi of Spring Hollow Press, my Project Manager Mary Stueck at Elsevier, and Lois Schubert at Top Graphics. Their coordinated efforts and individual expertise make this a great new edition and they were a pleasure to work with.

I am always inspired and motivated by the feedback I receive from other sonographers, students, instructors, physicians, and peer reviews. I love hearing from you, and try to incorporate your suggestions in each new edition.

A special thank you to the American Institute of Ultrasound in Medicine (AIUM) for agreeing to include applicable AIUM guidelines in the book. This collaboration greatly benefits the reader and ultimately the ultrasound community.

Finally, to those who touch my heart—David, Max, and my closest friends—sincere thanks for your continued support and interest!

Betty Bates Tempkin, BA, RT(R), RDMS

Contents

xiii

GENERAL PRINCIPLES

CHAPTER 1

Guidelines

Betty Bates Tempkin

Key Words

Acoustic enhancement	Hyperechoic
Anechoic	Hypoechoic
Attenuate	Isosonic/isoechoic
Bull's eye	Parenchyma
Echogenic	Scanning survey
Heterogenous	Through transmission
Homogeneous	

Objectives

At the end of this chapter, you will be able to:

- Define the key words.
- Name the prerequisites to use this text.
- Outline the clinical aspects of sonography.
- Apply the sonographic terms used to describe normal body structures.
- Distinguish the various patient positions used for scanning.
- Describe the required professional and clinical standards for sonographers.
- Employ the ergonomics associated with scanning.
- Summarize basic imaging criteria.
- List common requirements for image documentation.
- Prepare a study/case to an interpreting physician.
- Name the criteria for describing sonographic findings.
- Answer the review questions at the end of the chapter.

How to Use This Text

- **Know Gross and Sectional Anatomy.** Structures are accurately identified on sonographic images by their location, *not* their sonographic appearance because it may be altered by pathology or other factors. Because sonography images the body in cross-sections (similar to CAT [computerized axial tomography] scan and MRI [magnetic resonance imaging] images), an in-depth course in gross and sectional anatomy should be a prerequisite to this text. Only as a reference, most chapters include brief sections on anatomy and physiology.
- **Know the Normal Sonographic Appearance of Body Structures and the Terms Used to Describe Them.** An understanding of the

normal sonographic appearance provides the baseline against which to recognize variations and abnormalities. Normal structural characteristics vary in sonographic appearance as discussed in Table 1-1.

- **Know the Different Patient Positions Used When Scanning.** Using different patient positions is common practice and encouraged to achieve the best sonographic images. Utilize the various patient positions as illustrated in Figure 1-1.
- **Learn Scanning Survey Steps.** A scanning survey is a detailed inclusive observation. All ultrasound examinations should begin with a comprehensive scanning survey of the area of interest and adjacent structures in at least two scanning planes. Typically, no images are taken during a survey because that would interrupt the thorough and methodical investigation of the area(s) of interest and the ability to accurately detect any normal variations or abnormalities. It is becoming common practice in many institutions to use cine clips/videos during the survey to provide more data to the interpreting physician. All scanning protocol chapters illustrate and describe how to position a patient, manipulate the transducer, and how to thoroughly evaluate an area of interest before taking representative images. It can be helpful to practice these survey steps and transducer manipulations on yourself (with the machine off to comply with safety practices) or on scanning phantoms. In this text, the enumeration of survey steps makes scanning easier and ensures thoroughness and accuracy.
- **Learn the Required Images.** Using a scanning protocol and its required images is essential for methodical and organized documentation and for comparable studies. Follow a scanning protocol as you would follow steps in a recipe. In this text, the enumeration of required images for each examination promotes the establishment of standards and improves examination quality. Applicable protocols are patterned after the scanning guidelines of the American Institute of Ultrasound in Medicine.

Professional Standards

- Dress appropriately and always wear a personal identification badge.
- Introduce yourself to patients; put them at ease and make them as comfortable as possible.
- Make sure you have the correct patient; check identification bracelets (or patient numbers) against patient charts.
- Briefly explain the examination process to the patient and then offer to answer any questions. Speak in a slow, clear, and concise manner.
- It is standard practice to obtain a brief medical history from patients. Avoid using medical terms that a patient may not understand.

Table 1-1 Sonographic Appearance of Normal Body Structures and the Terms Used to Describe Them	
Structures	**Sonographic Appearance**
ORGAN PARENCHYMA	• Organ **parenchyma** (the bulk of tissue comprising an organ) is described in terms of echo texture. • Described as having **homogeneous** (uniform composition throughout) echo texture with ranges in **echogenicity** (echoes produced by reflections of the sound beam) that are determined by a structure's density, its distance from the sound beam, and the angle at which the beam strikes the structure. • *Example:* Normal liver parenchyma may be described as homogeneous and moderately echogenic. • The echogenicity of organ textures is often compared. *Example:* The liver appears **isosonic/isoechoic** (the same echogenicity) or slightly **hyperechoic** (echoes brighter than surrounding tissues) compared to renal parenchyma and slightly **hypoechoic** (echoes not as bright as surrounding tissues) compared with the pancreas.
MUSCLES	• Described in terms of echo texture. • Muscles often have slightly echogenic linear striations when viewed longitudinally. • Generally, muscles appear hypoechoic compared to most solid body structures.
PLACENTA	• Described in terms of echo texture. • The echo texture of the placenta varies some throughout a pregnancy but it can generally be described as having homogeneous echo texture with moderate to high echogenicity by vascular components, giving the placenta a **heterogeneous** (mixed echo pattern) appearance. • Later in pregnancy, the otherwise homogeneous texture may be interrupted by vascular components. • Comparatively, the placenta is more echogenic or hyperechoic relative to the adjacent myometrium of the uterus.
TISSUE	• Described in terms of echo texture. • Described as having homogeneous echo texture with moderate echogenicity and strongly reflective borders. • The easily distinguishable abdominopelvic subcutaneous tissue layers anterior to the abdominopelvic muscles are a good example.
FLUID-FILLED STRUCTURES: Blood vessels, ducts, umbilical cord, amniotic sac, brain ventricles, ovarian follicles, renal calyces, urine-filled urinary bladder, bile-filled gallbladder	• Described as having **anechoic** (echo free) lumens (or interiors) and highly echogenic or bright walls. • They exhibit **acoustic enhancement** or **through transmission** (the area of increased echogenicity behind fluid-filled structures) of the sound beam, making them easy to distinguish sonographically.

Continued

Table 1-1	Sonographic Appearance of Normal Body Structures and the Terms Used to Describe Them—cont'd
Structures	**Sonographic Appearance**
GASTROINTESTINAL (GI) TRACT	• Bowel wall is composed of five layers. The first, third, and fifth layers appear hyperechoic compared to the darker appearance of the second and fourth layers.
	• The sonographic appearance of the GI tract lumen depends on its contents. Therefore, its appearance varies from anechoic (e.g., when fluid is present), to highly echogenic (e.g., gas, air, or collapsed lumen), to a complex or mixed appearance displaying anechoic portions (fluid) and echogenic portions (e.g., digested food, gas, air, or feces).
	• All or individual portions of the GI tract may cast a posterior shadow depending on its air or gas content. Air and gas reflect the sound beam, preventing through transmission of the beam, thus creating a shadow.
	• An empty collapsed bowel has a distinctive appearance called a "**bull's eye**" due to the contrast between the highly echogenic collapsed lumen and the darker, barely echogenic walls.
BONES, FAT, AIR, FISSURES, LIGAMENTS, DIAPHRAGM	• Described as highly **echogenic** (bright).
	• The degree of echogenicity depends on the density of the structure, its distance from the sound beam, and the angle at which the beam strikes the structure.
	• Because these structures either reflect or **attenuate** (absorb, impede, stop, decrease) the sound beam, they cast a posterior shadow and appear hyperechoic compared to adjacent structures.
	• Note that the crura of the diaphragm may appear hypoechoic to adjacent structures.

An understanding of the normal sonographic appearance of body structures provides the baseline against which to recognize variations and abnormalities.

- Practice courteous and respectful interaction with all patients and staff.
- Conversations around the area of patients and directly with patients should be proper and professional. **Never** talk about the sonographic findings or give a patient your opinion of the study results. **Only physicians can legally render a diagnosis.**

Clinical Standards

- Be familiar with your institution's universal precautions protocol.
- Be familiar with isolation policies.
- Be familiar with sterile procedures.
- Be familiar with procedures to assist physicians with special studies.
- When required, assist the patient in dressing in a hospital gown.

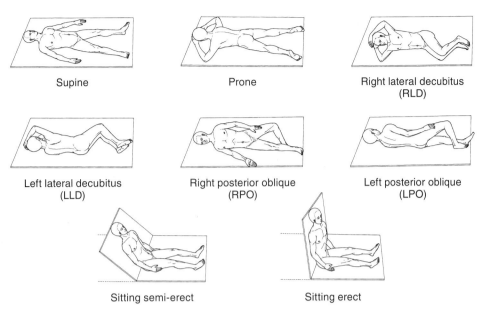

Supine   Prone   Right lateral decubitus
                                                            (RLD)

Left lateral decubitus   Right posterior oblique   Left posterior oblique
       (LLD)   (RPO)   (LPO)

Sitting semi-erect   Sitting erect

Figure 1-1 Standard Patient Positions. Different patient positions are used during an ultrasound examination depending on the area of interest being evaluated. The best patient position(s) is determined by what will produce the optimal view. It is standard practice to use different patient positions during a study to evaluate various structures. Note that any change in patient position must be noted on the images as part of standard labeling. The best patient position(s) should be established during the survey and ideally the same position should be used during image documentation. Occasionally, during image documentation of a particular structure, patient position must be changed to obtain a better image representation. If this occurs, the required images have to be retaken from the beginning of the series for that particular structure and the change in patient position must be noted on the images.

- When helping a patient into or out of a wheelchair, be certain that both brakes are locked and the leg and footrests are pushed out of the way.
- Assist the patient with any medical equipment attachments.
- Before a patient gets on or off the examination table or stretcher, make sure it is stationary with the brakes set.
- Have a handled step stool available for shorter patients or those who require more assistance.
- If the patient is already on a stretcher, avoid bumping into walls when wheeling the stretcher into the examination room. After the stretcher is situated, set the brakes.
- Drape the patient properly for the examination and make sure he or she is as comfortable as possible.
- Some transabdominal pelvic studies require the patient to have a full urinary bladder. This can cause the patient discomfort; therefore, every effort should be made to perform the study as quickly as possible.
- Invasive or endocavital studies require informing the patient about the details of the procedure and obtaining a signed informed consent before the procedure can take place. A family

member or referring physician can grant permission if the patient is incapacitated.

- It is recommended that endocavital procedures be witnessed by another health care professional; the witness's initials should be recorded on the images and on any permanent written record of the examination.

Ergonomics and Proper Use of Ultrasound Equipment

- Utilize proper body mechanics when moving patients, ultrasound equipment, stretchers, and wheelchairs.
- Use wedges and cushion blocks to assist in positioning the patient.
- Adjust equipment to user size, and have any accessories on hand before scanning.
- Scanning chairs should be ergonomically designed to maintain the sonographer's proper posture and allow for easy movement. Many manufacturers currently offer these chairs.
- Chairs should be height adjustable and include an adjustable lumbar support to encourage an upright posture.
- Chairs should swivel, allowing easy rotation from patient to machine without affecting body alignment.
- Scanning tables should be specifically designed for the comfort of the patient as well as the sonographer's use. They should have open access from all sides and be height adjustable.
- Transducers should be lightweight and balanced to reduce wrist torque.
- Transducers should be easily accessed.
- Transducer cables should be suitable in length for unrestricted use. Manufacturers now offer lightweight transducer cables and a smaller foot print for the transducer, easing strain on the sonographer's hand and wrist. Some manufacturers even offer a wireless transducer for their equipment.
- Cable support devices should be utilized to reduce wrist and forearm torque.
- The monitor and control panel should be ergonomically designed so the height and tilt can be adjusted to accommodate standing or seated users.

Imaging Criteria

- Begin with a transducer best suited to the structure(s) of interest. Use real time, transabdominal or endocavital scanners with sector or curved linear transducers.
- Use a coupling agent such as gel to remove the air between the transducer and the surface of the patient's skin.

- Patient comfort and the amount of transducer pressure exerted on the patient is an important consideration. Experiment by using different amounts of transducer pressure on your own skin surface.
- Perform comprehensive surveys. A scanning survey is a detailed inclusive observation. All ultrasound examinations should begin with a survey of the area of interest and adjacent structures in at least two scanning planes.
- No images are taken during the survey. This is the time to adjust technique, establish the best patient position(s) and breathing technique(s), thoroughly and methodically investigate the areas of interest, and rule out normal variants or abnormalities.
- Adjust the field size to best view the area of interest.
- Focus near and far gain settings to enhance visualization of the area of interest.
- Set contrast to delineate structures well from one another.
- Adjust gain settings so borders are well defined.
- Power settings should be low. Compensate with an adjusted time-gain compensation (TGC) slope.
- Avoid areas of fade-out whenever possible. Try increasing or adjusting the TGC slope or switch to a more powerful transducer.
- Each scanning protocol includes specific survey steps for the individual organ or structure. For the abdomen, when combined, these surveys comprise a complete abdominal survey. Typically, a survey of the entire abdomen begins with a survey of the aorta, followed by the inferior vena cava and liver, then the remaining abdominal organs and associated structures.
- If an abnormality is identified during the survey, it is surveyed in at least two scanning planes following completion of the general survey of the area(s) of interest.

Image Documentation Criteria

- The following information must be included on all documentation:
  - Patient's name and identification number.
  - Date and time.
  - Scanning site (name of hospital or private office).
  - Name or initials of the person performing the scanning ultrasound examination.
  - Endocavital studies should be witnessed by another health professional, and the witness's name or initials should be included on documentation.
  - Transducer megahertz.
  - Area of interest: general area and specific area. *Example:* Aorta is the general area and the proximal aorta is the specific area.

- • Patient position.
- • Scanning plane.
- Film labeling should be confined to the margins surrounding the image. Never label over the image unless you take the very same image again without any labels. Labels could cover important diagnostic information for the interpreting physician.
- Use up-to-date, calibrated, ultrasound machinery.
- Documented areas of interest must be represented in at least two scanning planes. Single plane representation of a structure is not enough confirmation.
- Documented areas of interest must be imaged in a logical sequence. Follow imaging protocol examples. Note that cine clips of your real-time imaging may benefit the interpreting physician.
- Abnormalities are documented in at least two scanning planes *following* the general protocol images for a complete study of the area(s) of interest. Note that cine clips may be very useful to aid in the delineation of various abnormalities.
- Operator-dependent, real-time scanning makes it impractical to take ultrasound images every 1 or 2 cm through a structure. Therefore, fewer representative images are given to the physician for diagnostic interpretation. **The images are a small representation of the whole, a small sample that must accurately represent the findings determined during the survey.** Note that cine clips/video may help the physician interpret your real-time scanning.

Case Presentation

- Case presentation is the method of presenting the images and related details of a study to the interpreting physician.
- State the examination and the reason for it.
- Present the patient history.
- Relate the patient's laboratory test results and any other known correlative information such as reports and films from other imaging modality studies.
- Present the documentation in the sequence it was taken.
- Be able to discuss and justify the techniques and procedures used.
- Be able to describe the ultrasound findings using appropriate sonographic terminology.

Describing Sonographic Findings

- After a study is completed, some institutions require sonographers to provide a technical observation, a written summary of the ultrasound findings that accompany the images. Written documentation of any type almost always becomes part of a patient's medical record. For this reason, the sonographer's technical impression should be documented in such a way as not to be legally compromising. In other words, sonographers should *never* provide interpretive results or diagnoses. That would not only be unjustified (according to a sonographer's level of education, training, and experience) it would be potentially legally compromising. **Only physicians are justified (according to their level of education, training, and experience) to render diagnoses.**

- Writing or describing technical observations requires restraint and the careful selection of appropriate terminology. Technical observations should be confined to descriptions of the ultrasound findings based on echo pattern and size. The origin (or location), number, composition, and any complications associated with adjacent structures are also included for descriptions of abnormal findings (see Chapter 3 for examples).

- It is important to note that if a sonographer fails to mention an abnormality in his or her technical observation but demonstrates the abnormality on the images, he or she has performed within the legal guidelines of the scope of the practice for diagnostic medical sonographers.

Review Questions

Answers on page 628.

1. Structures are accurately identified on ultrasound images by
   a) scanning plane interpretation.
   b) their sonographic appearance.
   c) two dimensional cross-sections.
   d) their location.

2. Organ parenchyma is described in terms of
   a) echo texture.
   b) sonographic characteristics.
   c) reflections.
   d) location.

3. When an organ is described as hypoechoic to another organ it means the hypoechoic organ appears
   a) brighter relative to the other.
   b) less echogenic relative to the other.
   c) visualized inferior to the other.
   d) visualized posterior to the other.

4. Degrees of echogenicity depend on
   a) a structure's shape and how far it is from the sound beam.
   b) a structure's density, attenuation factor, and shape.
   c) the angle at which the beam strikes a structure, its density, and shape.
   d) a structure's density, distance from the sound beam, and the angle at which the beam strikes it.

5. For a structure to exhibit acoustic enhancement it must
   a) have a high attenuation rate.
   b) be a blood vessel or duct.
   c) be fluid filled.
   d) have a high impedance factor.

6. Structures that cast a shadow
   a) either reflect or attenuate the sound beam.
   b) let the sound beam pass through.
   c) are always posterior to adjacent structures.
   d) exhibit acoustic posterior through enhancement.

7. The sonographic appearance of the kidneys is described as heterogeneous. Renal cortex, however, is described as
   a) hypoechoic.
   b) homogeneous.
   c) anechoic.
   d) hyperechoic.

8. The sonographic appearance of the gastrointestinal tract lumen
   a) is a distinctive "bull's eye" appearance.
   b) is dependent on its contents.
   c) is hypoechoic relative to its walls.
   d) is highly reflective.

9. Documented areas of interest
   a) must be represented in single scanning planes.
   b) must cover every 2 cm of a structure.
   c) must be represented in at least two scanning planes.
   d) must include survey images.

10. If a patient asks a sonographer questions regarding their study, the sonographer should
    a) give them their opinion then explain that the physician makes the final diagnosis.
    b) confine their remarks to either "normal" or "abnormal."
    c) explain to the patient that they will have to wait for the physician's diagnosis.
    d) provide them with a copy of their technical observation.

11. If the liver appears isosonic compared to the right kidney, it is described as
    a) heterogeneous.
    b) having different echogenicities.
    c) having the same echogenicity.
    d) appearing brighter.

12. If the spleen is described as having uniform composition throughout, it appears
    a) heterogeneous.
    b) complex.
    c) diffuse.
    d) homogeneous.

13. If the pancreas appears hyperechoic compared to the liver, it is described as
    a) heterogeneous.
    b) having different echogenicities.
    c) having the same echogenicity.
    d) appearing brighter.

14. A scanning survey is
    a) the time to take the required images.
    b) the sonographic term for measurements.
    c) a detailed inclusive observation.
    d) only performed in the abdomen.

15. Abnormal findings/pathology should be described according to
    a) size only.
    b) echo pattern, size, origin, number, composition, and any complications associated with adjacent structures.
    c) echogenicity, number, and size.
    d) echo pattern only.

CHAPTER 2

Scanning Planes and Scanning Methods

Betty Bates Tempkin

Key Words

Angle of incidence	Obliqued Orientation
Axial views	Positional orientation
Coronal planes	Pressure
Focal zone	Sagittal planes
Long axis	Short axis
Longitudinal views	Transverse planes
Measure	

Objectives

At the end of this chapter, you will be able to:
- Define the key words.
- Explain the way ultrasound uses body/scanning planes to image the body.
- Differentiate between scanning planes and views/sections.
- Interpret scanning planes.
- Apply scanning methods and manipulate the transducer.
- Produce accurate measurements.
- Identify surface landmarks.
- Answer the review questions at the end of the chapter.

Scanning Planes Defined

The scanning planes used in sonography are the same as anatomic body planes. Their interpretations depend on the location of the transducer and the sound wave approach (where the sound waves enter the body).
- Ultrasound scanning planes are:
  - **Sagittal Planes:** The mid or median sagittal plane divides the body into equal right and left sections. Parasagittal planes are to the right or left of midline and divide the body into unequal right and left sections. For this book's purpose, unless "mid" or "median" sagittal plane is specified, the term "sagittal" implies a parasagittal plane (Figure 2-1).
  - **Transverse Planes:** Divide the body into unequal superior and inferior sections (Figure 2-1).
  - **Coronal Planes:** Divide the body into unequal anterior and posterior sections (Figure 2-1).

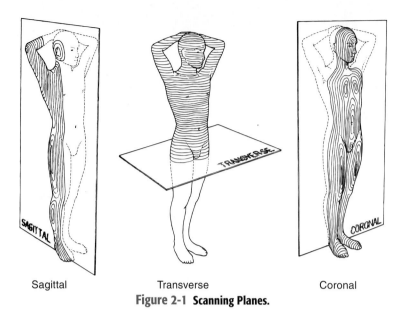

| Sagittal | Transverse | Coronal |

Figure 2-1 Scanning Planes.

- Scanning planes are used to establish the direction that the ultrasound beam enters the body and the anatomic portion of anatomy being visualized from that particular direction.
- Scanning planes are often **obliqued** (slanted; angled) by very slightly twisting/rotating the transducer. The degree of the oblique is determined by how the structure of interest lies in the body. Most body structures lie at a slight angle; they usually do not lie in a straight line up and down or straight across the body. The oblique scanning plane affords visualization of the greatest margins of a structure.
- Scanning planes provide two-dimensional ultrasound images.
- Body structures are generally viewed longitudinally and axially. **Longitudinal views** show a structure's length and depth. **Axial views** show width and depth. Do not confuse scanning planes with views. For example, "transverse" is not a view, it is a scanning plane.

Scanning Planes Interpreted

Sagittal Scanning Plane

Scanning in **sagittal planes** means that the ultrasound beam is entering the body from either an anterior or posterior direction and that the anatomic portion of body structures being visualized from that particular direction are:
- Anterior
- Posterior
- Superior
- Inferior

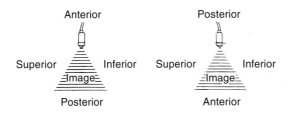

NOTE: Right and left lateral are not seen on a sagittal scan; therefore, the transducer must be moved to either the right or left of a sagittal plane to visualize adjacent anatomy.

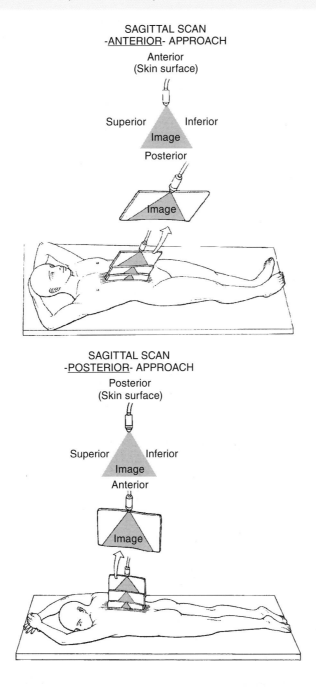

Transverse Scanning Plane

Scanning in **transverse planes** means that the ultrasound beam is entering the body from either an anterior, posterior, or lateral direction and that the anatomic portion of body structures being visualized from that particular direction are:

- Beam entering from an anterior or posterior direction:
  - Anterior
  - Posterior
  - Right lateral
  - Left lateral

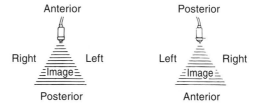

- Beam entering from a right or left lateral direction:
  - Lateral (right or left)
  - Medial
  - Anterior
  - Posterior

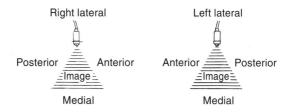

NOTE: Superior and inferior are not seen on a transverse scan; therefore, the transducer must be moved either superiorly or inferiorly from a transverse plane to visualize adjacent anatomy.

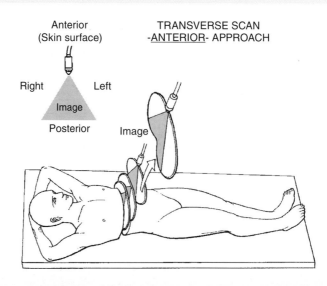

TRANSVERSE SCAN
-<u>POSTERIOR</u>- APPROACH

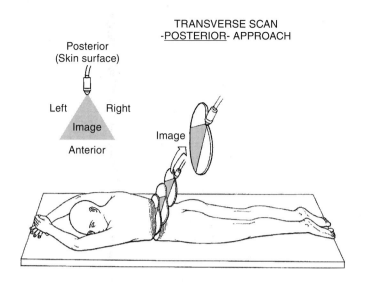

TRANSVERSE SCAN
-<u>LEFT LATERAL</u>- APPROACH

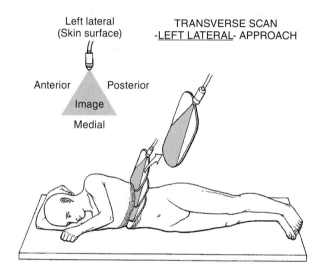

TRANSVERSE SCAN
-<u>RIGHT LATERAL</u>- APPROACH

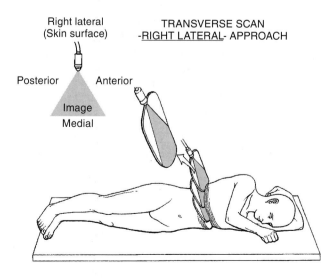

Coronal Scanning Plane

Scanning in **coronal planes** means that the ultrasound beam is entering the body from either a right or left lateral direction and that the anatomic portion of body structures being visualized from that particular direction are:

- Lateral (right or left)
- Medial
- Superior
- Inferior

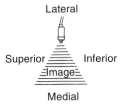

NOTE: Anterior and posterior are not seen on a coronal scan; therefore, the transducer must be moved either anteriorly or posteriorly from a coronal plane to visualize adjacent anatomy.

CORONAL SCAN
-LEFT LATERAL- APPROACH

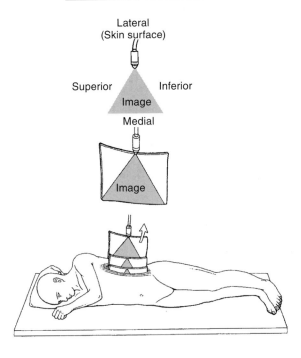

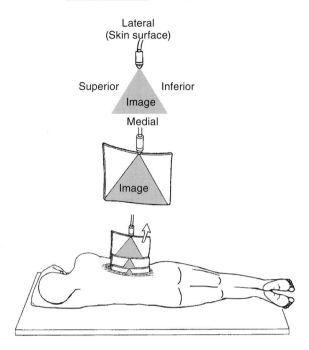

Scanning Methods

NOTE: The primary role of a sonographer is to provide interpretable images for diagnosis by a physician. This goal is totally dependent on the skill of the operator. Becoming an accomplished sonographer happens with practice and the development of good scanning methods.

Transducers
- Much has been accomplished with regard to the various types and designs of transducers used in diagnostic ultrasound. The new types and styles offer better penetration, better resolution, and better frame rates. Also, ergonomically designed transducers assist the sonographer in producing optimal images and providing enhanced patient care.
- Transducers come in a variety of shapes and sizes. The shape of the transducer determines the field of view, and the frequency (MHz) of the sound waves emitted determines how deep the sound waves penetrate and affects the clarity of the image.
- The depth of the structure being imaged ultimately determines which transducer should be used. Low frequency transducers have the most penetration whereas high frequency transducers have less penetration and are used for more superficial structures.

- Conventional diagnostic ultrasound transducers include:
  - **Curved array:** 10-4, 8-5, 5-2, 5-1 MHz. Typically used for abdominal, obstetric and gynecological imaging.
  - **Sector array:** 12-4, 5-1, 4-1 MHz. Generally used for intercostal scanning.
  - **Linear array:** 18-5, 12-5, 9-3, 8-4 MHz. Typically used for small or superficial structures and extremity Doppler.
  - **Endocavital:** 10-3, 9-5, 8-5 MHz. Used for endovaginal and endorectal imaging.
  - **TEE:** 7-3 MHz. Used for transesophageal echocardiography.
  - **Hockey stick:** 12.5 MHz. Intraoperative imaging.
  - **3D:** 7-3 MHz. Three dimensional imaging.
- All transducers have a focal zone; an area where the sound beam is narrow and imaging is at its best. A transducer's focal zone is usually indicated by a small triangle just to the right of the image. When scanning, every effort should be made to position the area(s) of interest in that focused area to obtain the best images.

How to Use the Transducer

- Scanning should be a series of fluid motions. Practice rocking and sliding the transducer to scan through body structures.
- Transducers can be easily manipulated into different positions which provide you with multiple options for thoroughly evaluating an area(s) of interest and obtaining the best images (Figure 2-2).
- The angle of incidence, or the angle at which the sound beam strikes the surface of a structure, affects the image. When the transducer/sound beam angle is perpendicular, more sound waves are reflected back, fewer are lost or scattered, and the result is a better, more accurate image.
- Applying the correct amount of pressure with the transducer can improve image quality. Typically, pressure should be applied evenly and lightly but in some cases, more pressure is applied to reach the focal zone or compress a vein. Experiment with using more or less scanning gel as it affects the pressure as well. Note that the pressure should never cause discomfort to the patient.
- Positional orientation of the transducer verifies the scanning plane. In most cases, the manufacturer of the transducer sets the positional orientation. Sagittal scanning plane orientation, for example, is usually indicated by a notch or raised portion on the top surface of the transducer. Once the transducer orientation is established, the scanning plane can be changed by rotating the transducer 90 degrees.

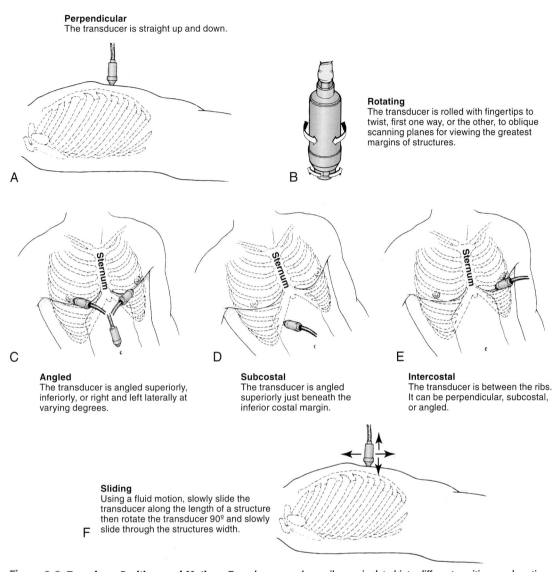

Perpendicular
The transducer is straight up and down.

A

Rotating
The transducer is rolled with fingertips to twist, first one way, or the other, to oblique scanning planes for viewing the greatest margins of structures.

B

Angled
The transducer is angled superiorly, inferiorly, or right and left laterally at varying degrees.

C

Subcostal
The transducer is angled superiorly just beneath the inferior costal margin.

D

Intercostal
The transducer is between the ribs. It can be perpendicular, subcostal, or angled.

E

Sliding
Using a fluid motion, slowly slide the transducer along the length of a structure then rotate the transducer 90° and slowly slide through the structures width.

F

Figure 2-2 Transducer Positions and Motions. Transducers can be easily manipulated into different positions and motions for optimal imaging. They include the following: **A**, Perpendicular, **B**, Rotating, **C**, Angled, **D**, Subcostal, **E**, Intercostal, **F**, Sliding.

How to Take Accurate Images and Measurements

- Scan according to how a structure is oriented or how it lies within the body. The orientation, or lie, is determined by the length or long axis (maximum length) of a structure. The long axis of a structure can be seen in any scanning plane depending on how that structure lies in the body. *For example*:
  - The pancreas lies from right to left, across the body, at a slight angle; therefore its long axis is seen in a transverse oblique scanning plane (Figure 2-3). Oblique the scanning plane by holding the transducer perpendicular and very slowly, slightly rotate it one way then the other until the required degree of oblique is achieved.

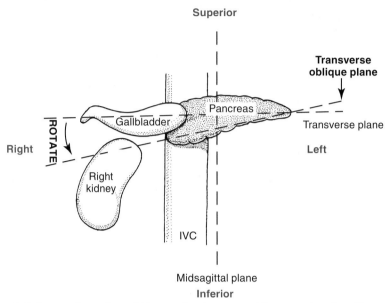

Figure 2-3 Pancreas long axis would be seen in a transverse oblique scanning plane. The sonographer can resolve the long axis by slightly rotating the transducer and scanning through the pancreas until the long axis is resolved, as demonstrated in this figure.

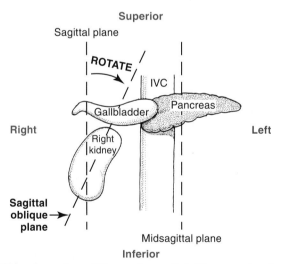

Figure 2-4 Right kidney long axis would be seen in a sagittal oblique scanning plane. Notice how the long axis is resolved by slightly rotating the transducer.

- In a true sagittal plane a kidney cannot be viewed in its entirety because the kidneys are positioned at an angle in the body. Therefore, the sagittal plane must be at an oblique to match that angle (Figure 2-4). Oblique the scanning plane by holding the transducer perpendicular and very slowly, slightly rotate it one way then the other until the required degree of oblique is achieved.

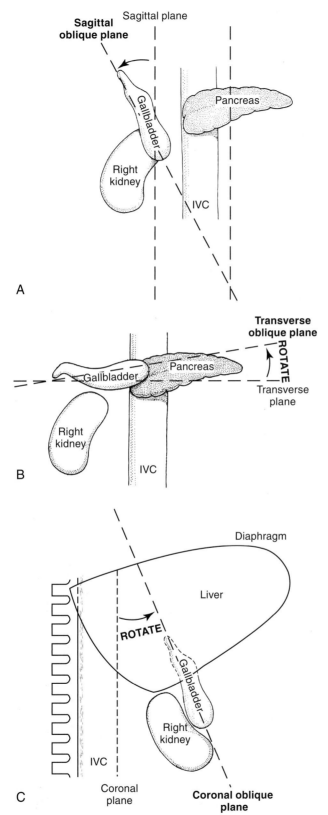

Figure 2-5 The orientation (longitudinal lie/long axis) of the gallbladder (GB) is variable because it is suspended by a long mesentery and can lie in different locations throughout the abdomen. As illustrated in the figures, once the orientation is determined, the sonographer can slightly rotate the transducer, scanning through and evaluating the GB, until the long axis is established. **A**, GB long axis will be seen in a sagittal oblique plane. **B**, GB long axis will be visualized in a transverse oblique plane. **C**, GB long axis will be seen in a coronal longitudinal plane.

- The long axis of the gallbladder can be seen in any of the three scanning planes because of its variable position in the body (Figure 2-5). Once the orientation of the gallbladder has been determined oblique the scanning plane by holding the transducer perpendicular and very slowly, slightly rotate it one way then the other until the required degree of oblique is achieved.
- From the long axis scanning plane, slowly rotate the transducer 90 degrees into the **short axis** plane for anteroposterior views and width measurements, which are taken at a structure's widest margins.
- To accurately **measure** structures, begin by scanning as perpendicular to the structure as possible for the truest representation of its size. As previously discussed, if the sound beam is not perpendicular to the structure, the size of the structure is distorted on the image. The degree of distortion depends on the degree of the angle of the sound beam (or the angle of incidence).
- Typical measurements are calculated in volumes *based on*:

$$L \times W \times AP = \text{Volume}$$

L represents length, **W** is width, and **AP** is the anteroposterior dimension.

Surface Landmarks

- The following surface landmarks are used as references when scanning:

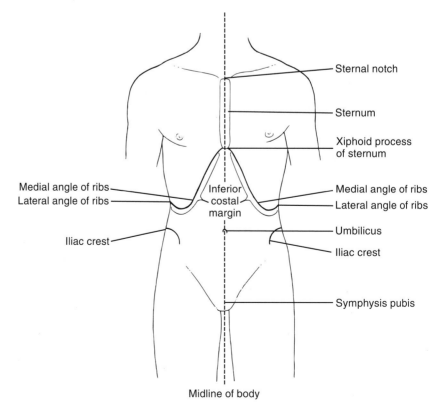

Sternal notch

Sternum

Xiphoid process of sternum

Medial angle of ribs
Lateral angle of ribs

Inferior costal margin

Medial angle of ribs
Lateral angle of ribs

Iliac crest

Umbilicus

Iliac crest

Symphysis pubis

Midline of body

Review Questions

Answers on page 628.

1. Coronal planes divide the body into unequal _____ and _____ sections.

2. When scanning in a coronal plane, the ultrasound beam enters the body from
   a) either an anterior or posterior direction.
   b) a posterior direction.
   c) a medial direction.
   d) either a right or left lateral direction.

3. Transverse planes divide the body into unequal _____and _____ sections.

4. When scanning in a transverse plane, the ultrasound beam enters the body from
   a) either an anterior, posterior, right lateral, or left lateral direction.
   b) either an anterior or posterior direction.
   c) a right or left lateral direction.
   d) either an anterior, posterior, or medial direction.

5. Sagittal planes divide the body into unequal _____ and _____ sections.

6. When scanning in a sagittal plane, the ultrasound beam enters the body from
   a) either an anterior or posterior direction.
   b) either an anterior, posterior, right lateral, or left lateral direction.
   c) either an anterior, posterior, or medial direction.
   d) either a right or left lateral direction.

7. Scanning planes are _____ dimensional.

8. The anatomic area(s) *not* seen in a coronal plane
   a) are lateral and medial.
   b) is superior.
   c) are anterior and posterior.
   d) is inferior.

9. The anatomic area(s) *not* seen in a transverse plane
   a) are lateral and medial.
   b) is medial.
   c) are superior and inferior.
   d) are anterior and posterior.

10. The anatomic area(s) *not* seen in a sagittal plane
    a) is posterior.
    b) is lateral.
    c) are superior and inferior.
    d) are anterior and posterior.

11. Scanning planes are often obliqued (by very slightly twisting the transducer). The degree of the oblique is determined by _____ _____.

12. The oblique scanning plane affords visualization of the
    _____.

13. The _____ of the structure being imaged ultimately deter-
    mines which transducer should be used.

14. When scanning, every effort should be made to position the area(s)
    of interest in the transducer's _____ to obtain
    the best images.

PART II

PATHOLOGY

CHAPTER 3

Scanning Protocol for Abnormal Findings/Pathology

Betty Bates Tempkin

Key Words

Ascites	Infiltrative diffuse disease
Calculi	Intraorgan features
Complex (mass)	Localized disease
Cystic (mass)	Mass
Diffuse disease	Necrosis
Extraorgan features	Origin
Focal diffuse disease	Septations
Heterogeneous	Solid (mass)
Homogeneous	True cyst

Objectives

At the end of this chapter, you will be able to:

- Define the key words.
- Recognize the classic sonographic appearances of abnormal findings and pathology and the sonographic terms used to describe them.
- Relate pathologic sonographic findings to interpreting physicians in an accurate and professional manner.
- Explain the universal scanning protocol for documenting abnormal sonographic findings/pathology regardless of the type.
- Answer the review questions at the end of the chapter.

Criteria for Evaluating Abnormal Findings/Pathology

Once a sonographer becomes practiced at recognizing the echo patterns of normal anatomy, it stands to reason that any change in that normal appearance would suggest an abnormality is present. Even if a sonographer does not know what the change or deviation in the normal echo pattern is caused by, *recognizing it as a deviation is what is most important.*

- During an ultrasound scan:
  - *Differentiate* abnormal echo patterns from normal echo patterns.
  - *Document* any differences in echo pattern appearance.

NOTE: While you are scanning, experiment using different amounts of transducer pressure (keeping patient comfort in mind) to improve imaging.

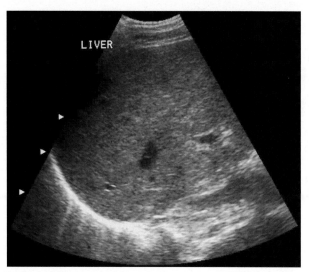

Figure 3-1 Infiltrative Diffuse Disease. When diffuse disease is infiltrative it spreads throughout an entire organ. Depending on the progression of the disease, changes in the appearance of the organ's parenchyma range from subtle to severe. In this case, the liver was obviously enlarged and there were subtle changes in the appearance of the parenchyma.

- After the scan:
  - *Describe* any difference in echo pattern appearance using sonographic terminology to provide the interpreting physician with the comprehensive details of the study.
- All pathology visualized by ultrasound in some way disrupts the normal *echo pattern* of the organ or structure involved and may also alter its *shape, size, contour, position,* or *textural appearance.*
- Key findings can be used to help detect *parenchymal changes of an organ.* When the normal **homogeneous** (uniform) texture of organ parenchyma is interrupted by disease, the parenchyma assumes an irregular or **heterogeneous** pattern. The changes may be **diffuse disease**—either *infiltrative* throughout the organ or *focal* in a specific area; or the changes may be **localized disease**, consisting of single or multiple masses.
  - **Infiltrative diffuse disease:**
    - *Spreads* throughout an entire organ.
    - May appear subtle to very obvious depending on the severity and progression of the disease. Look for characteristic changes in *overall* organ echo texture, size, shape, and position, and any associated complications with adjacent structures (Figure 3-1). With advanced diffuse disease, the appearance of the parenchyma may also be interrupted with multiple necrotic or blood filled spaces. Each diffuse disease has its own distinctive criteria that may include all or only some of these characteristics.
  - **Focal diffuse disease:**
    - Look for *isolated areas* with a change in organ echo texture, size, and possible displacement of adjacent structures (Figure 3-2).

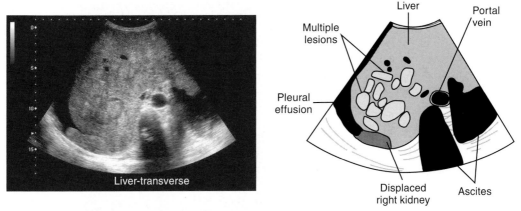

Figure 3-2 Focal Diffuse Disease. This image shows how focal diffuse disease *disrupts* the normal appearance of organ paren-chyma. Observe the multiple lesions. Notice how the *size* of the liver appears enlarged, *displacing* the right kidney posteriorly.

- **Localized disease (masses):**
  - Look for a mass or multiple masses, which are circumscribed to a specific area. A mass may be classified according to its composition as **solid** (all tissue), *cystic* (fluid filled), or *complex* (tissue and fluid) (Figure 3-3).
- Certain disease processes are accompanied by the formation of *calculi*, which interrupt the normal appearance of an organ. Typically, calculi or "stones" are distinguished by the fact that they impede (reflect, absorb, stop, decrease) sound waves, creating an echogenic or bright anterior surface and dark to anechoic posterior shadow (Figure 3-4). These acoustic shadows usually have sharp, well-defined edges.
- Some abnormalities are a result of *obstruction* due to calculi, disease, or compromise from an adjacent enlarged organ or mass. All of these present sonographically as deviations from the normal appearance and size of the structure(s) they are associated with (Figure 3-5).
- Abnormalities such as vascular aneurysms are due to a *break down* or weakening of structure, which present sonographically as deviations from the normal appearance and size (Figure 3-6).
- There are certain body structures such as *lymph nodes* that are generally not appreciated sonographically unless they are abnormal (Figure 3-7).

Criteria for Documenting Abnormal Findings/Pathology

- Pathology must be surveyed in at least *two* scanning planes *following* the survey of the primary area(s) of interest. This is not to say that the abnormality is not evaluated as the area of interest is evaluated, but it ensures that a total evaluation is made of a structure, not just its abnormal part.

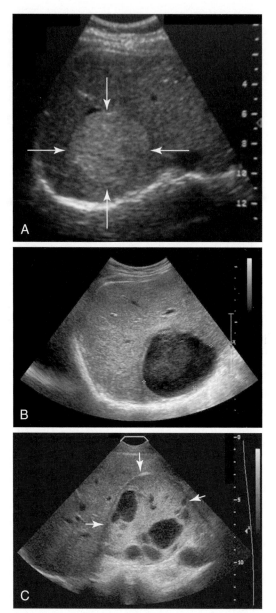

Figure 3-3 Types of Masses. A mass is classified according to its composition; solid, cystic, complex. **A,** This is a *solid*, echogenic mass in the liver (noted by *arrows*). It appears hyperechoic relative to the surrounding liver. Notice how the mass is circumscribed to a specific area. **B,** This is *cystic* mass (noted by the measurement calipers). It appears specific to one area and is primarily anechoic with echogenic internal debris. Note the increased posterior through transmission indicating fluid. **C,** This is a *complex* mass (noted by *arrows*). It appears confined to one area and heterogeneous; composed of echogenic, solid portions and anechoic, cystic portions (indicated by increased posterior through transmission).

- Image documentation must be in at least *two* scanning planes. Single-plane representation of an abnormality is not enough confirmation.
- Image documentation must include a volume measurement of an abnormality. Volume measurements: $L \times W \times AP = V$ (length × width × the anteroposterior dimension).
  - Careful placement of measurement calipers at the leading margins of an abnormality provides accurate dimensions.

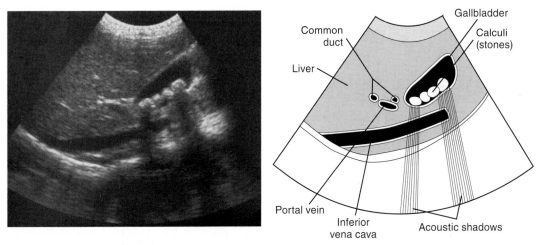

Figure 3-4   Calculi. Typically, calculi or "stones" are distinguished by the fact that they impede (reflect, absorb, stop, decrease) sound waves This creates a bright anterior surface and dark to anechoic posterior shadow. Note the well-defined, sharp edges of the shadows.

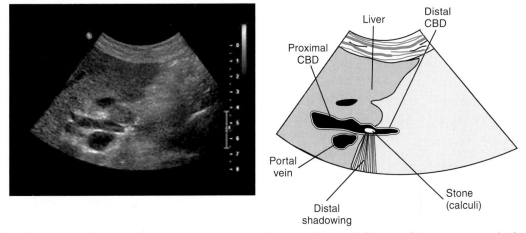

Figure 3-5   Obstruction. Some abnormalities are a result of obstruction due to calculi (stone), disease, or compromise from an adjacent enlarged organ or mass. In this case, a stone within the common bile duct (CBD) is obstructing the flow of bile; consequently, the proximal portion of the CBD is dilated. (Courtesy Adrian Goudie, MD, Ultrasoundvillage.com.)

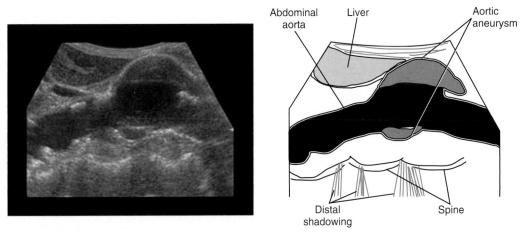

Figure 3-6   Breakdown. Some abnormalities, such as the aortic aneurysm seen in this image, are due to a break down or weakening of structure. (Courtesy Dr. T.S.A. Geertsma, Ziekenhuis Gelderse Vallei, Ede, The Netherlands.)

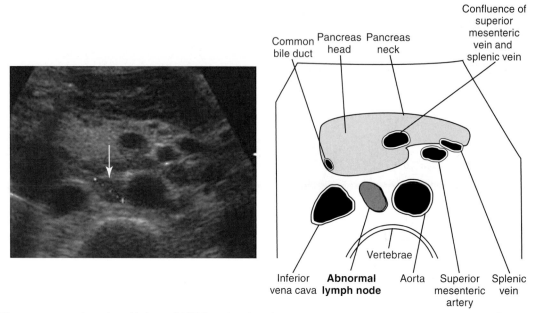

Figure 3-7 Lymph Nodes. This image highlights a lymph node *(arrow);* typically, they are not appreciated sonographically unless they are abnormal.

- When multiple masses are present and can be differentiated from each other, they should be measured individually.
- Image documentation must include views of the abnormality with high- and low-gain settings in at least two scanning planes to resolve the composition.
- Remember, you can document an abnormality without knowing what it is. It is not necessary to be familiar with specific diseases and abnormalities to document them sonographically. A sonographer benefits, however, from having a broader knowledge of specific abnormalities and pathologic processes. The goal is to provide the physician with interpretable images.
- **The required images are a small representation of what a sonographer visualizes during a study. Therefore, the images should provide the interpreting physician with the most telling and technically accurate information available.**

Criteria for Describing the Sonographic Appearance of Abnormal Findings/Pathology

- The purpose of learning how to accurately and appropriately describe the sonographic appearance of pathology is essential to staying within the scope of a sonographer's legal parameters. This need arises with the understanding that physicians exclusively render diagnoses.
- You can document and describe an abnormality without knowing what it is. From the examples in this section, you will see that it is not necessary to be familiar with specific diseases and abnormalities

to describe them sonographically. A sonographer benefits, however, from having a broader knowledge of specific abnormalities and pathologic processes.

- While the findings in the next image are typical of diffuse liver disease/cirrhosis, an example of how a sonographer should describe the findings is:

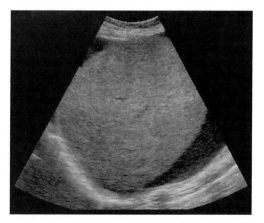

"Enlarged right lobe of the liver, visualization of intrahepatic vessels is markedly decreased. Ascites noted anteriorly and inferiorly."

- One example of *focal disease* is pancreatitis which causes focal enlargement of the head of the pancreas. Pressure from the enlarged head can obstruct, constrict, or dilate the common bile duct. In some cases, the duodenum becomes obstructed as well. While the findings in the following image are consistent with pancreatitis, an example of how a sonographer should describe the findings is:

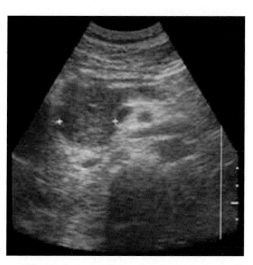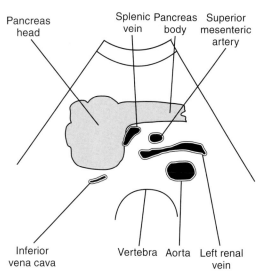

"Pancreas appears heterogeneous. Head appears focally enlarged. Irregular contour of the head is noted. The inferior vena cava and

left renal vein appear compressed posteriorly by the head. The distal portion of the left renal vein appears dilated. The common bile duct, gastroduodenal artery, and duodenum are not visualized."

- Masses should be described according to *origin, size, composition, number,* and any *associated complications with adjacent structures or body system.*
  - Masses are generally distinctive in appearance and unless very small, they are readily identified. In some cases, the organ or structure that a mass arises from is obvious; in others, it can be challenging to resolve depending on the size and because of the close proximity of body structures. When determining the origin (location of origination) it may be helpful to classify a mass as intraorgan or extraorgan:
    - Intraorgan features to look for are:
      - *Disruption* of the normal internal architecture
      - External *bulging* of organ capsules
      - *Displacement* or shift of adjacent structures
    - Extraorgan features include:
      - *Displacement* of other organs and structures
      - *Obstruction* of other organs or structures from view
      - Internal *invagination* of organ capsules
      - *Discontinuity* of organ capsules
    - Large masses usually present the greatest challenge when you're trying to determine their origin especially if their size obstructs the organ or structure they arise from and also if adjacent organs or structures are involved (Figure 3-8).
    - In some cases the exact origin of an abnormality cannot be sonographically distinguished so the location or

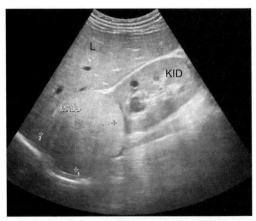

Figure 3-8 Determining the Origin of a Large Mass. In some cases, determining the origin of a mass can be challenging especially if the mass is large. In this image the liver (L) appears to be being pushed anteriorly by a large extrahepatic, right upper quadrant mass. The kidney (KID) appears to be compromised by the mass and the adrenal gland is not visualized. A conclusive determination cannot be made from this single view, therefore the mass could be either renal or adrenal in origin.

site is described by structures immediately adjacent to the abnormality.

- The *size* of a mass must be documented with a volume measurement. As previously discussed, volume measurements are **L × W × AP = V** (length × width × the anteroposterior dimension).

- Sonography cannot definitively distinguish between malignant and benign masses. However, providing the interpreting physician with ultrasound images of the correct composition of an abnormality can help to increase the percentage of correct diagnoses made before biopsies or surgery. *Composition* is determined by evaluating a mass or masses at high- and low-gain technical settings. This technical range should demonstrate any variations in echodensities.

  ▪ **Solid masses:** are described in terms of echo texture. The level of echogenicity and appearance of tissue texture depend on what type of localized disease is present, the degree of its echodensity, and its effect on internal architecture. The sonographic appearance of solid masses is variable. They can appear isosonic/isoechoic to the organ parenchyma they are part of, distinguishable only by its walls or they can appear anechoic, homogeneous, or heterogeneous with low, moderate, or highly reflective echo textures. Vascular, interstitial, and collagen components, and the presence of any necrosis (breakdown) can influence the appearance of solid or soft tissue masses. In some cases, the walls may be poorly defined and the contour can appear irregular.

  ▪ Although a conclusive determination cannot be made from a single image, it is highly probable that the solid mass (SOL) in this image is adrenal in origin and obstructing the view of the small adrenal gland. LIV, liver; R KID, right kidney; SOL, space occupying lesion; DIAPH, diaphragm. A sonographer should describe this image as:

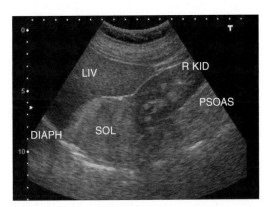

"Extrahepatic right upper quadrant mass pushing the liver superiorly and the kidney inferiorly. Mass appears solid, heterogeneous, and

hyperechoic compared to the liver and kidney. Contour is primarily smooth. There are no visible calcifications. The kidney appears separate from the mass. The adrenal gland is not visualized."

- **Cystic masses:** are described as being either a true cyst or cystic in nature. To be considered a **true cyst** the mass in question must meet 3 sonographic criteria:
  1. It must not contain internal echoes; it must appear anechoic. In some cases, it is normal to visualize "cystic noise" or low level echoes near the anterior wall of the mass, however, echoes *never* occur in the posterior portion of a true cyst.
  2. The walls of the cyst must be well-defined, thin, and smooth.
  3. The mass must exhibit posterior through transmission.
- A sonographer should describe the following image of a true cyst as:

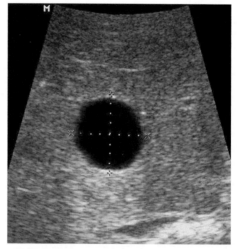

"Anechoic liver mass with well-defined, thin, smooth walls. Increased posterior through transmission present. 2.5 cm anteroposteriorly, 2.5 cm wide."

- If one of the three criteria is not met, the mass is not a true cyst. A mass that meets one or more of these criteria is said to be **cystic** in nature as seen in the next image showing an abnormal fluid collection (ascites) in the pancreas. A sonographer should describe these findings as:

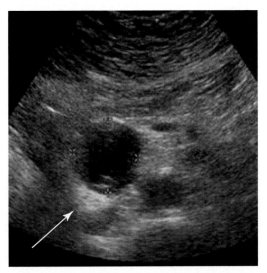

"Anechoic mass in the head of the pancreas (between measurement calipers). Echogenic debris noted in the posterior portion of the mass. Walls appear thick and irregular. Increased posterior through transmission present (arrow). 2 cm anteroposteriorly, 1.8 cm wide." (Courtesy Koenraad Mortelé, MD, Beth Israel Deaconess Medical Center, Boston, Mass.)

- Some cystic masses contain single or multiple septations: thin, bright, membranous inclusions as demonstrated in the following image. A sonographer should describe the findings as:

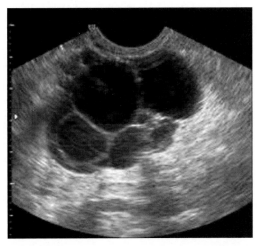

"Primarily cystic ovarian mass with smooth borders and increased posterior through transmission. Contains bright, thin inclusions and low level echoes posteriorly."

- **Complex masses:** a mass containing fluid and solid components is described as complex. Complex masses may be *primarily cystic* or *primarily solid.* Wall appearance of a complex mass is variable, from well-defined and smooth to poorly defined and irregular. Note that the internal composition of a mass may change with time. An example is a solid mass, which degenerates (**necrosis**). This process usually means that the solid mass begins to liquefy and thereby assume a complex appearance.
- This image of a complex mass should be described by a sonographer as:

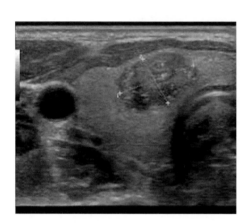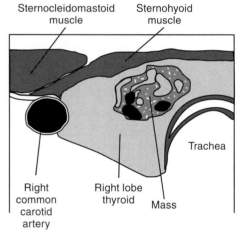

"Primarily solid, heterogeneous, complex mass in the right lobe of the thyroid gland. Anechoic areas noted in the posterior portion of the mass. Very small bright areas noted throughout. No shadowing is present. Walls appear smooth but uneven.

Required Images for Abnormal Findings/Pathology

NOTE: The required images of pathology should always follow the standard protocol images for the specified study.

1. Longitudinal image of the pathology *with measurement from the most superior to most inferior margin.*

   Labeled: **"ORGAN"** or **"SITE LOCATION"** and **"SCANNING PLANE"**

NOTE: In cases where the origin of an abnormality cannot be determined, adjacent structures must be noted for a site location. Look for bright, echogenic interfaces where fat separates adjacent structures.

2. Same image and labeling as number 1, *without calipers.*

> **NOTE:** Use the same "frozen" image as used for Number 1, just remove the measurement calipers because they could possibly cover significant diagnostic information for the interpreting physician.

3. Axial image *with measurements from the most anterior to most posterior margin and from the most lateral to lateral or lateral to medial margin.*

   Labeled: **"ORGAN"** or **"SITE LOCATION"** and **"SCANNING PLANE"**

4. Same image and labeling as number 3, *without calipers.*
5. Longitudinal image with high gain technique.

   Labeled: **"ORGAN"** or **"SITE LOCATION," "SCANNING PLANE,"**
   "HIGH GAIN"

6. Axial image *with high gain technique.*

   Labeled: **"ORGAN"** or **"SITE LOCATION," "SCANNING PLANE,"**
   "HIGH GAIN"

7. Longitudinal image *with low gain technique.*

   Labeled: **"ORGAN"** or **"SITE LOCATION," "SCANNING PLANE,"**
   "LOW GAIN"

8. Axial image *with low gain technique.*

   Labeled: **"ORGAN"** or **"SITE LOCATION," "SCANNING PLANE,"**
   "LOW GAIN"

> **NOTE:** Depending on the size and complexity, additional images may be necessary to document the full extent of the abnormality. These additional views must be documented in at least two scanning planes.

Review Questions

Answers on page 628.

1. The required images for abnormal sonographic findings are
   a) organ specific.
   b) the same for all abnormalities, no matter the type.
   c) taken in place of standard protocol images of the area of interest.
   d) single plane representations.

2. Diffuse changes in the appearance of organ parenchyma can be classified as
   a) hyperechoic and hypoechoic.
   b) infiltrative and focal.
   c) diffuse and localized.
   d) single or multiple masses.

3. A mass should always be described as
   a) diffuse disease.
   b) either solid or complex.
   c) either solid, cystic, or complex.
   d) heterogeneous.

4. Focal disease is
   a) in a specific area.
   b) spreads throughout an entire organ.
   c) anechoic.
   d) localized.

5. Localized disease represents
   a) diffuse disease.
   b) single or multiple masses.
   c) infiltrative disease.
   d) organ displacement.

6. To be classified a true cyst, a mass must
   a) appear anechoic, exhibit increased posterior acoustic enhancement, and have well-defined thick walls.
   b) appear echo free with well-defined, smooth, thin walls and exhibit internal "cystic noise."
   c) appear anechoic, exhibit posterior "cystic noise", and have well-defined, smooth walls.
   d) appear echo free with well-defined, smooth, thin walls, and exhibit increased posterior acoustic enhancement.

7. A complex mass
   a) is primarily cystic in nature.
   b) appears uniform and well-defined.
   c) has a high echodensity.
   d) is solid and liquid.

8. Intraorgan features of a mass include
   a) shift of adjacent structures, disruption of normal internal architecture, internal invagination of vasculature.
   b) obstruction of other organs or structures from view, disruption of normal internal architecture, discontinuity of organ capsules.
   c) shift of adjacent structures, disruption of normal internal architecture, external bulging of organ capsules.
   d) displacement of other organs and structures, obstruction of other organs or structures from view, internal invagination of organ capsules.

9. Composition of an abnormality is resolved
   a) by determining wall thickness, and echodensity.
   b) at high gain technical settings.
   c) by the amount of high-and low-gain technique required to visualize wall thickness.
   d) through a range of high- and low-gain technical settings.

10. Masses should be described according to
    1) _____, 2) _____, 3)_____, 4) _____,
       and 5) _____.

11. Describe the following:

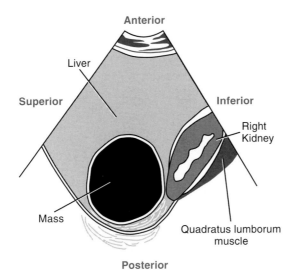

_____
_____
_____
_____

12. Describe the findings in this image:

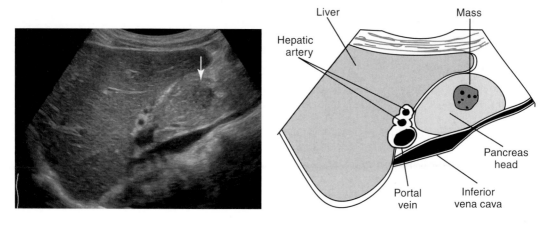

_____
_____
_____

13. Describe the findings in this image:

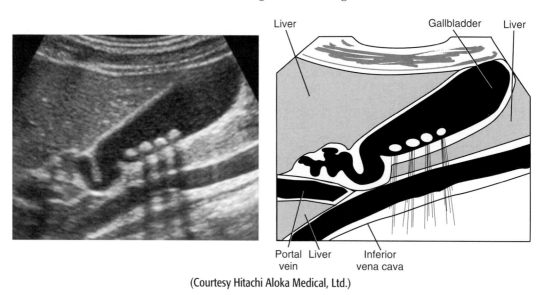

(Courtesy Hitachi Aloka Medical, Ltd.)

_____
_____
_____

14. Describe the findings in this image:

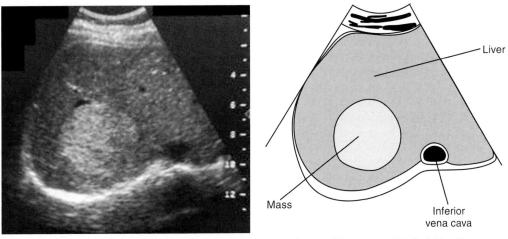

(Courtesy J Anthony Parker, MD, PhD, Joint Program in Nuclear Medicine, Harvard Medical School.)

_____

_____

_____

15. Describe the following:

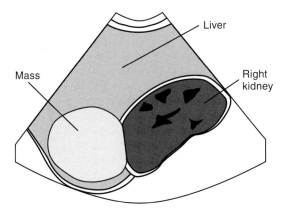

_____

_____

_____

PART III

ABDOMINAL SCANNING PROTOCOLS

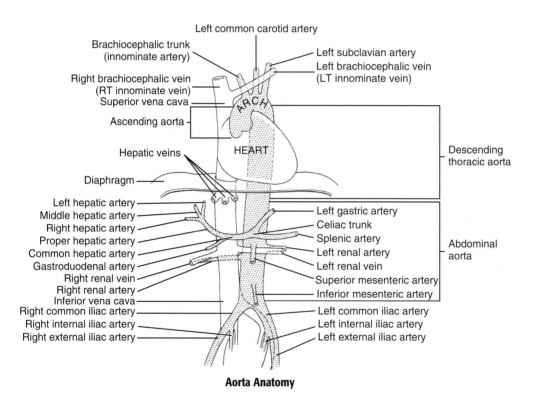

Left common carotid artery

Brachiocephalic trunk
(innominate artery)

Right brachiocephalic vein
(RT innominate vein)

Superior vena cava

Ascending aorta

Hepatic veins

Diaphragm

Left hepatic artery
Middle hepatic artery
Right hepatic artery
Proper hepatic artery
Common hepatic artery
Gastroduodenal artery
Right renal vein
Right renal artery
Inferior vena cava
Right common iliac artery
Right internal iliac artery
Right external iliac artery

Left subclavian artery
Left brachiocephalic vein
(LT innominate vein)

ARCH

HEART

Descending
thoracic aorta

Left gastric artery
Celiac trunk
Splenic artery
Left renal artery
Left renal vein
Superior mesenteric artery
Inferior mesenteric artery

Abdominal
aorta

Left common iliac artery
Left internal iliac artery
Left external iliac artery

Aorta Anatomy

CHAPTER 4

Abdominal Aorta Scanning Protocol

Betty Bates Tempkin

Key Words

Abdominal aorta	Media
Adventitia	Proximal
Celiac artery (CA)	Retroperitoneum
Common hepatic artery	Right renal artery (RRA)
Common iliac arteries	Splenic artery
Gastric artery	Superior mesenteric artery (SMA)
Inferior mesenteric artery (IMA)	Thoracic aorta
Intima	Tortuous
Left renal artery (LRA)	

Objectives

At the end of this chapter, you will be able to:

- Define the key words.
- Identify the sonographic appearance of the aorta, its branches, and the terms used to describe them.
- List the transducer options for scanning the aorta.
- Name the various suggested breathing techniques for patients when scanning the aorta.
- Identify suggested patient position (and options) when scanning the aorta.
- Describe patient prep for an abdominal aorta study.
- Describe the survey steps and how to evaluate the entire length, width, and depth of the aorta and its branches.
- Identify the order and exact locations to take representative images of the aorta.
- Describe normal variations of the abdominal aorta.
- Answer the review questions at the end of the chapter.

Overview

Location

- The **aorta** originates at the left ventricle of the heart then ascends posterior to the pulmonary artery; it arches to the left then descends (**thoracic aorta**) *posterior to the diaphragm* into the **retroperitoneum** (portion of abdominopelvic cavity posterior to the peritoneal sac) of the abdominal cavity (**abdominal aorta**).

- The abdominal aorta is *vertically orientated* in the body. It descends, anterior to the spine, just to the left of the midline then *bifurcates* into the common iliac arteries anterior to the body of the fourth lumbar vertebra.

Anatomy
- The largest artery in the body
- Consists of three muscle layers:
  1. Intima (innermost)
  2. Media (middle)
  3. Adventitia (outer)
- 3 anterior branches:
  1. Celiac artery (CA) **trunk:** also known as "celiac axis," branches into the left gastric artery, common hepatic artery, and splenic artery
  2. Superior mesenteric artery (SMA): just inferior to the CA, divides into several small arteries that supply the ascending portion of the colon and largest portion of the small intestine
  3. Inferior mesenteric artery (IMA): inferior to the SMA and renal arteries, divides into several small arteries that supply the transverse and descending portions of the colon and the rectum
- 2 lateral branches:
  1. Right renal artery (RRA): located a few centimeters within the origin of the SMA, it courses anterior to the spine and posterior to the inferior vena cava in route to the right kidney
  2. Left renal artery (LRA): located a few centimeters within the origin of the SMA, it courses left lateral to the spine and posterior to the tail of the pancreas in route to the left kidney
- Size is normal up to 3 cm in diameter, gradually tapering toward the bifurcation
- Can be very **tortuous** (marked by twists, turns, or bends)

Physiology
- Supplies the organs, bones, and connective structures of the body with oxygen and nutrient-rich blood.

Sonographic Appearance
- Anechoic lumen surrounded by bright, echogenic walls.
- Because the aorta is vertically orientated in the body, longitudinal and long axis views are seen in coronal scanning planes and sagittal scanning planes as demonstrated in the following image. The aorta appears like a large long tube, anechoic with bright walls, immediately anterior to the spine, and immediately posterior to

the esophageal gastric junction, crus of the diaphragm, SMA, and splenic artery.

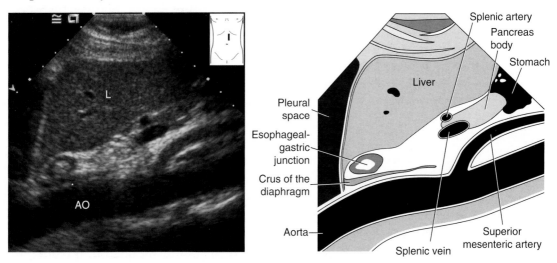

- Short axis (or axial) sections of the aorta are seen in transverse scanning planes. The following transverse scanning plane image shows how easy it is to recognize the short axis section of the aorta in the posterior portion of the image, immediately anterior and just to the left of the spine. It appears large, round, and anechoic with bright walls.

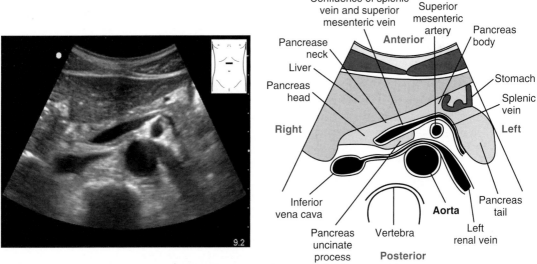

(Courtesy Geoffrey E. Hayden, MD, Charleston, S.C.)

Note the axial section of the SMA branch. It appears "separate" from the aorta because following the rise of its trunk from the aorta's anterior wall, it runs in front of, or anterior to, and parallel to the aorta. The space left between the aorta and SMA affords passage of the left renal vein (LRV) seen here in longitudinal section, on its way to the inferior vena cava (IVC).

- The proximal (closest to origin) portion of the abdominal aorta is described as the area seen *inferior to the diaphragm* and *superior to the CA trunk*; it lies anterior to the spine and posterior to the esophageal gastric junction and liver.
- The **mid** portion of the abdominal aorta is seen *from the CA trunk running along the length of the SMA*; it lies anterior to the spine and posterior to the CA, SMA, splenic artery, splenic vein, body of the pancreas, a portion of the stomach, and the liver.
- The **distal** (farthest from origin) portion of the abdominal aorta is described *as inferior to the SMA and superior to the bifurcation*; it lies anterior to the spine and posterior to the bowel.

Normal Variants
- Normal variations of the abdominal aorta are rare but include:
  - Markedly tortuous
  - May lie on the right side of the inferior vena cava
  - May include an anterior pulmonary branch close to the CA trunk

Preparation

Patient Prep
- The patient should fast for at least 6 to 8 hours before the ultrasound study.
- If the patient has eaten, still attempt the examination.

Transducer
- **3.0 MHz or 3.5 MHz.**
- 5.0 MHz for thin patients.

Breathing Technique
- Normal respiration.
- Deep, held respiration.

NOTE: Different breathing techniques should be used whenever the suggested technique does not give the desired results.

Patient Position
- Supine.
- Right lateral decubitus, left lateral decubitus, left posterior oblique, right posterior oblique, or sitting semierect to erect as needed.

NOTE: Different patient positions should be used whenever the suggested position does not give the desired results.

Abdominal Aorta Survey Steps

Abdominal Aorta • Longitudinal Survey

NOTE: While you are scanning, experiment using different amounts of transducer pressure (keeping patient comfort in mind) to improve imaging.

Sagittal Plane • Transabdominal Anterior Approach

1. Begin scanning with the transducer perpendicular, at the midline of the body, just inferior to the xiphoid process of the sternum.

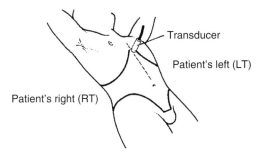

2. Slightly move or angle the transducer to the patient's right and identify the longitudinal, anechoic section of the distal inferior vena cava (IVC), just posterior to the liver.

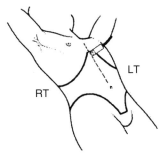

NOTE: Use the diaphragm to differentiate the IVC from the aorta. The IVC passes through the highly reflective diaphragm that can be visualized in the superior portion of the image; the aorta lies posterior to the diaphragm.

3. Return to the midline and slightly move or angle the transducer to the patient's left and identify the longitudinal, anechoic section of the proximal aorta just posterior to the liver.

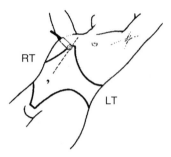

4. While viewing the proximal aorta, it may be necessary to slightly twist/rotate the transducer, first one way, then the other, to resolve the longest sections and long axis of the aorta. Additional slight twists can help reveal the proximal aorta's anterior branches, the CA, and the SMA, if they are not already visualized. Now, very slightly rock or move the transducer from right to left, scanning completely through each side of the aorta. Continue this as you slowly slide the transducer inferiorly following along the length of the aorta. Keep your eyes on the screen; use the image as a guide, evaluating the appearance of the aorta until you scan completely through the middle and distal portions to the bifurcation (usually seen at the level of the umbilicus) and right and left common iliac arteries.

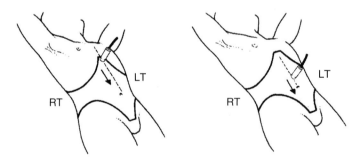

5. In some cases, the bifurcation site and common iliac arteries can be better visualized with the transducer angled from a lateral position. At the level of the most distal portion of the aorta, move the transducer slightly toward the patient's left, then angle the transducer at varying degrees aiming the sound beam back toward the aorta until you relocate the distal portion. Keeping this angle, very slowly slide the transducer inferiorly until the bifurcation site and common iliac arteries come into view.

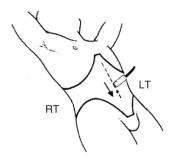

NOTE: The longitudinal sections of the distal aorta and bifurcation (into the right and left common iliac arteries) can be difficult to resolve from a sagittal plane. In most cases, visualization is easier from a coronal plane, left lateral approach as described below. While middle and proximal portions of the aorta tend to be better visualized from a transabdominal sagittal plane, alternatively, they may also be evaluated from the coronal plane, left lateral approach.

Distal Aorta and Bifurcation • Coronal Plane • Left Lateral Approach

Patient Position: Right Lateral Decubitus (or Supine, Sitting Semierect to Erect)
1. Begin with the transducer perpendicular, midcoronal plane, just superior to the iliac crest.
2. Use the inferior pole of the left kidney as a landmark; it is usually easy to visualize at this level or by sliding the transducer slightly superiorly.
3. When the inferior pole is located, the distal aorta, bifurcation site, and common iliac arteries should be seen in the medial and inferior portions of the image. It may be necessary to slightly twist/rotate the transducer at varying degrees to oblique the coronal plane and resolve the long axis of the distal aorta, bifurcation site, and common iliac arteries.
4. To evaluate the middle and proximal aorta, move the transducer superiorly from the level of the bifurcation or scan intercostally, looking for the aorta medially.
5. To avoid moving the patient, the survey of the bifurcation in the decubitus position can be done following the axial survey of the aorta.

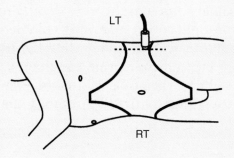

Abdominal Aorta • Axial Survey
Transverse Plane • Transabdominal Anterior Approach

1. Begin scanning with the transducer perpendicular, at the midline of the body, just inferior to the xiphoid process of the sternum.

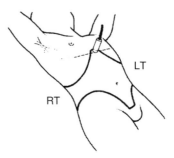

2. Angle the transducer superiorly until the heart is identified by its pulsations. Keeping your eyes on the screen, very slowly return the transducer to a perpendicular position while looking for the round, anechoic axial section of the aorta to come into sight just to the left of midline, anterior to the spine.

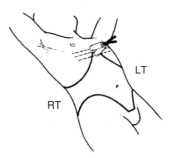

> **NOTE:** An alternative method for locating the axial section of the proximal aorta begins by viewing a longitudinal section of the proximal aorta from a sagittal plane. From that position, slowly rotate the transducer 90 degrees into the transverse plane. The axial view of the aorta should come directly into sight.

3. With the proximal aorta in sight, very slightly rock or move the transducer from right to left, scanning completely through the aorta. Continue this as you slowly slide the transducer inferiorly. Keep your eyes on the screen; use the image as a guide to avoid losing sight of the aorta. Note and evaluate the aorta's anterior branches. Slightly twisting/rotating the transducer can

help to distinguish the CA (and its branches—the left gastric, common hepatic, and splenic arteries) and just inferior to that, the SMA.

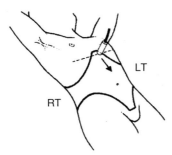

4. Continue rocking and sliding the transducer inferiorly through the middle and distal aorta to the bifurcation. Note and evaluate the mid aorta's lateral branches, the renal arteries. At the level of the bifurcation, the view will change from one large, round, echo-free structure (the aorta) to two small, round, echo-free structures (the iliac arteries), one seen on each side of midline. Evaluate the common iliac arteries by scanning through them inferiorly until you lose sight of them.

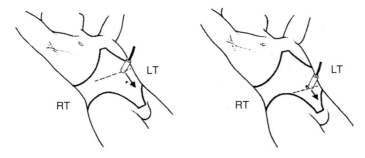

Abdominal Aorta Required Images

Abdominal Aorta • Longitudinal Images
Sagittal Plane • Transabdominal Anterior Approach

NOTE: The required images are a small representation of what a sonographer visualizes during a study. Therefore, the images should provide the interpreting physician with the most telling and technically accurate information available.

1. Longitudinal image of the **PROXIMAL AORTA** (inferior to the diaphragm and superior to the celiac trunk).

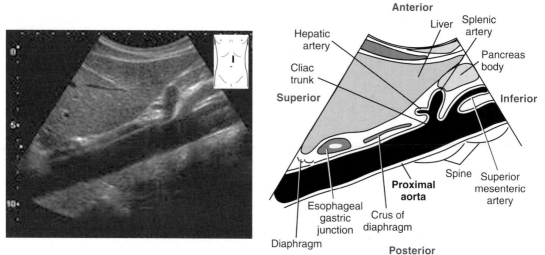

Labeled: **AORTA SAG PROX** (Courtesy Toshiba Medical Systems Corp.)

2. Longitudinal image of the **MID AORTA** (inferior to the celiac trunk and along the length of the SMA).

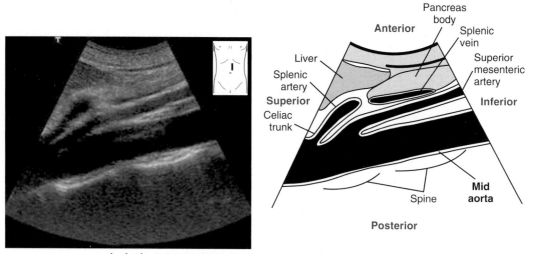

Labeled: **AORTA SAG MID** (Courtesy Ultrasoundpaedia.com.)

3. Longitudinal image of the **DISTAL AORTA** (inferior to the SMA and superior to the bifurcation).

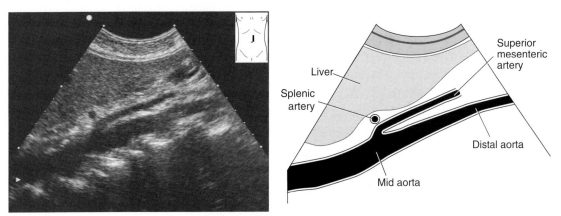

Labeled: **AORTA SAG DISTAL**

4. Longitudinal image of the **AORTA BIFURCATION** (common iliac arteries).

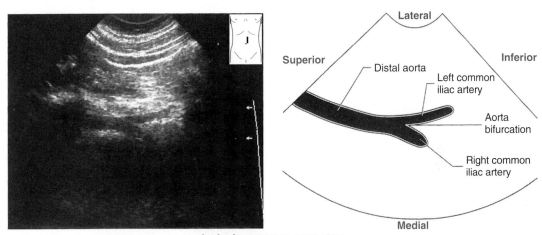

Labeled: **AORTA SAG BIF** or
AORTA SAG BIF LT OBL or
AORTA LT COR BIF

NOTE: To avoid moving the patient, longitudinal images of the bifurcation in the decubitus position can be taken following the axial images. Although the coronal plane approach can be used with the patient supine, the decubitus position is generally easier and can be helpful if the patient has obscuring bowel gas anteriorly.

Abdominal Aorta • Axial Images
Transverse Plane • Transabdominal Anterior Approach

> **NOTE:** The anteroposterior size of the abdominal aorta is routinely measured and documented because most ultrasound studies of the aorta are done to rule out an aneurysm—abnormal dilatation of the weakened vessel's wall. The biggest risk factor for rupture of an aneurysm is size. Note that the most common location of abdominal aortic aneurysms is infrarenal.

5. Axial image of the **PROXIMAL AORTA** (inferior to the diaphragm and superior to the celiac trunk) with anterior to posterior measurement *(calipers outside wall to outside wall)*.

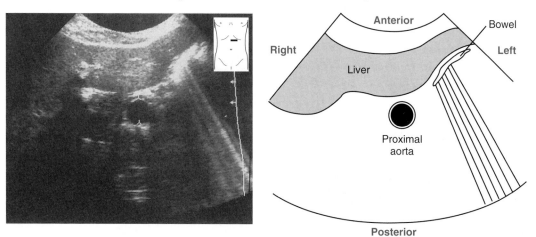

Labeled: **AORTA TRV PROX**

6. Same image as 5 *without measurement calipers.*

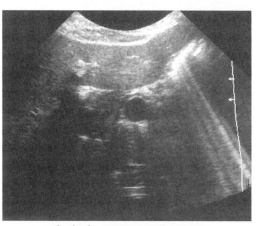

Labeled: **AORTA TRV PROX**

7. Axial image of the **MID AORTA** (inferior to the celiac trunk, at the level of the renal arteries, and along the length of the SMA) with anterior to posterior measurement *(calipers outside wall to outside wall).*

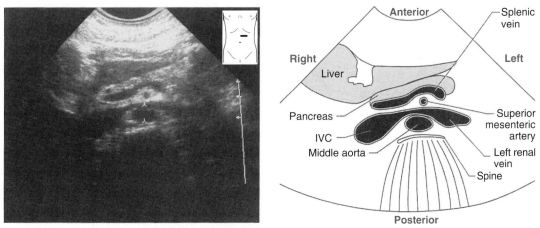

Labeled: **AORTA TRV MID**

8. Same image as 7 *without measurement calipers.*

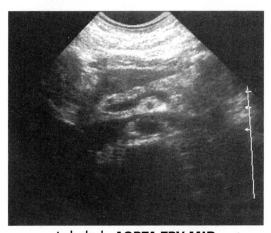

Labeled: **AORTA TRV MID**

NOTE: If the renal arteries are not represented on the previous images, an additional image(s) of the renal arteries should be taken here and labeled accordingly:

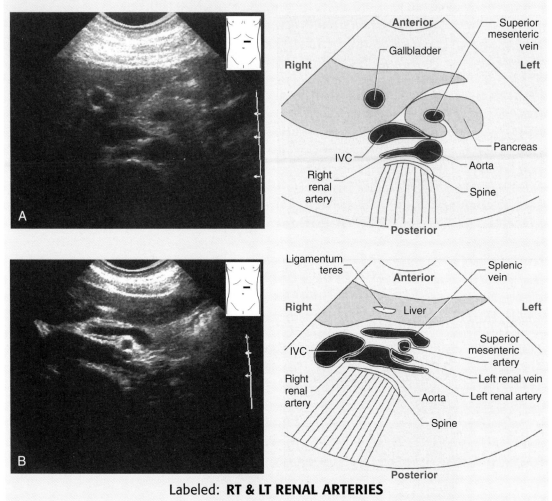

Labeled: **RT & LT RENAL ARTERIES**

9. Axial image of the **DISTAL AORTA** (inferior to the SMA and superior to the bifurcation) with anterior to posterior measurement *(calipers outside wall to outside wall).*

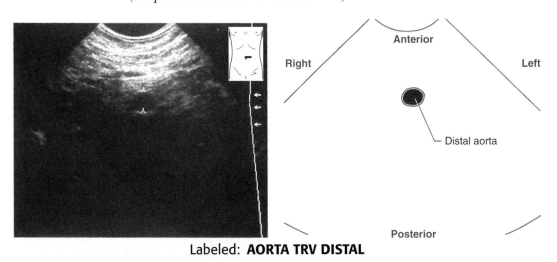

Labeled: **AORTA TRV DISTAL**

10. Same image as 9 *without measurement calipers.*

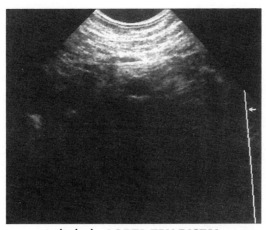

Labeled: **AORTA TRV DISTAL**

11. Axial image of the **AORTA BIFURCATION** (common iliac arteries).

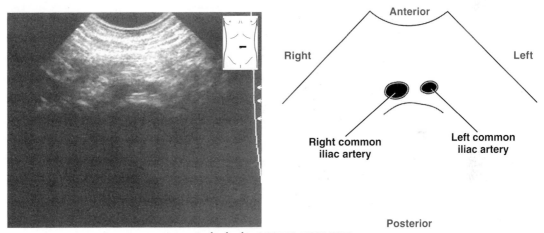

Labeled: **AORTA TRV BIF**

Required Images When the Abdominal Aorta is Part of Another Study

1. Longitudinal image of the **PROXIMAL** and **MID AORTA.**

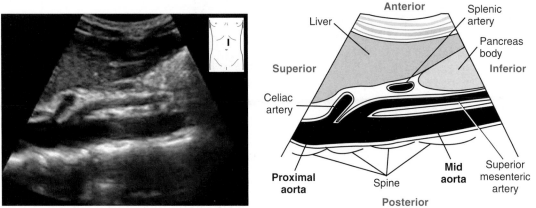

Labeled: **AORTA SAG MID**

2. Axial image of the **MID AORTA** at the level of the renal arteries.

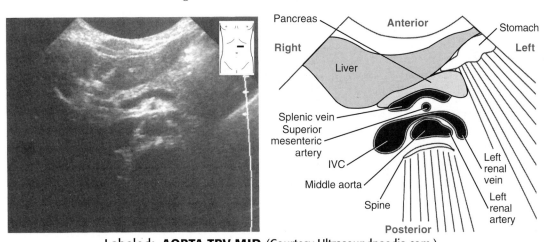

Labeled: **AORTA TRV MID** (Courtesy Ultrasoundpaedia.com.)

Review Questions

Answers on page 628.

1. The lie of the aorta within the body is
   a) mid sagittal.
   b) superior to inferior.
   c) transverse oblique.
   d) transverse.

2. The long axis of the aorta is visualized best in a
   a) sagittal or coronal scanning plane.
   b) transverse scanning plane.
   c) axial section.
   d) right lateral decubitus position.

3. Longitudinal views of the splenic artery and common hepatic artery are seen in a
   a) sagittal or coronal scanning plane.
   b) transverse scanning plane.
   c) sagittal scanning plane.
   d) coronal section.

4. Axial views of the SMA are seen in a
   a) sagittal or coronal scanning plane.
   b) transverse scanning plane.
   c) sagittal scanning plane.
   d) longitudinal section.

5. Longitudinal views of the renal arteries are seen in a
   a) sagittal or coronal scanning plane.
   b) transverse scanning plane.
   c) sagittal scanning plane.
   d) sagittal section.

6. The size of the aorta is normal up to
   a) 3 cm.
   b) 1.5 cm.
   c) 2 cm.
   d) 3.5 cm.

7. The proximal abdominal aorta is the portion
   a) between the diaphragm and CA trunk.
   b) between the diaphragm and caudate lobe of the liver.
   c) just inferior to the CA trunk.
   d) that ascends from the heart.

8. The mid portion of the abdominal aorta is
   a) between the diaphragm and CA trunk.
   b) inferior to the celiac trunk and along the length of the SMA.
   c) between the CA trunk and IMA.
   d) between the CA trunk and SMA trunk.

9. Beginning posteriorly, and in correct order by the location in the body, the abdominal aorta is
   a) to the left of the spine, posterior to the splenic and common hepatic arteries, the SMA, splenic vein, tail of the pancreas, left lobe of the liver.
   b) anterior and just to the left of the spine, posterior to the gastro-esophageal junction, CA, SMA, splenic vein, body of the pancreas, portion of the stomach, left lobe of the liver.
   c) anterior to the spine, posterior to the gastroesophageal junction, splenic vein, body of the pancreas, portion of the stomach, left lobe of the liver.
   d) anterior to the spine and kidneys, posterior to the gastroesophageal junction, splenic vein, body of the pancreas, portion of the stomach, left lobe of the liver.

10. The distal abdominal aorta is the portion
    a) that lies between the renal arteries and IMA.
    b) inferior to the SMA trunk and superior to the bifurcation.
    c) posterior to the head of the pancreas.
    d) the bifurcation.

11. The aorta is posterior to all of the following except the
    a) left renal vein.
    b) SMA.
    c) esophageal gastric junction.
    d) pancreas head.

12. A(n) _____ section of the RRA is seen _____.
    a) axial, in a transverse scanning plane between axial sections of the superior mesenteric vein and inferior vena cava.
    b) longitudinal, in a transverse scanning plane posterior to an axial section of the inferior vena cava and longitudinal section of the right renal vein.
    c) axial, in a sagittal scanning plane between axial sections of the SMA and aorta.
    d) longitudinal, in a transverse scanning plane posterior to the SMA.

13. Which of the following is *not* a direct branch of the abdominal aorta?
    a) celiac trunk.
    b) renal artery.
    c) mesenteric artery.
    d) external iliac artery.

14. What is the most common location of an abdominal aortic aneurysm?
    a) suprarenal.
    b) aortic arch.
    c) infrarenal.
    d) thoracic.

15. The biggest risk factor for rupture of an abdominal aortic aneurysm is
    a) location.
    b) size.
    c) velocity of flow through the vessel.
    d) age of the patient.

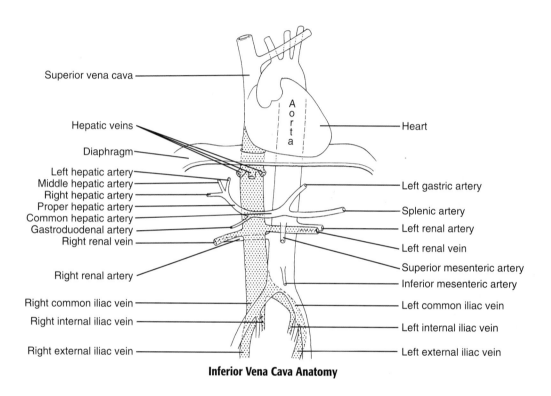

Superior vena cava

Hepatic veins

Diaphragm

Left hepatic artery
Middle hepatic artery
Right hepatic artery
Proper hepatic artery
Common hepatic artery
Gastroduodenal artery
Right renal vein

Right renal artery

Right common iliac vein

Right internal iliac vein

Right external iliac vein

Aorta

Heart

Left gastric artery

Splenic artery

Left renal artery

Left renal vein

Superior mesenteric artery
Inferior mesenteric artery

Left common iliac vein

Left internal iliac vein

Left external iliac vein

Inferior Vena Cava Anatomy

CHAPTER 5

Inferior Vena Cava Scanning Protocol

Betty Bates Tempkin

Key Words

Adventitia	Medial sacral vein
Common iliac veins	Mid IVC
Distal IVC	Proximal IVC
Hepatic veins	Renal veins
Iliac veins	Retroperitoneum
Inferior phrenic vein	Right adrenal vein
Inferior vena cava (IVC)	Right ovarian or testicular vein
Intima	Tortuous
Lumbar veins	Valsalva maneuver
Media	

Objectives

At the end of this chapter, you will be able to:

- Define the key words.
- Distinguish the sonographic appearance of the inferior vena cava (IVC), its tributaries, and the terms used to describe them.
- Describe the transducer options for scanning the IVC.
- List the various suggested breathing techniques for patients when scanning the IVC.
- List the suggested patient position (and options) when scanning the IVC.
- Describe the patient prep for an IVC study.
- Name the survey steps and explain how to evaluate the entire length, width, and depth of the IVC and its tributaries.
- Explain the order and exact locations to take representative images of the IVC.
- Answer the review questions at the end of the chapter.

Overview

Location

- The inferior vena cava (IVC) originates at the junction of the two common iliac veins anterior to the body of the fifth lumbar vertebra. The IVC is *vertically oriented* in the body; it ascends through the retroperitoneum (portion of abdominopelvic cavity posterior to the peritoneal sac) anterior and just to the right of the spine and then passes *through the diaphragm* to enter the right atrium of the heart.

- As the IVC ascends through the retroperitoneum on its way to the heart it passes through a deep fossa on the posterior surface of the liver between the caudate lobe and bare area.

Anatomy

- The inferior portion of the body's largest vein.
- Consists of 3 muscle layers:
  1. **Intima** (innermost)
  2. **Media** (middle layer)
  3. **Adventitia** (outer)
- Tributaries:
  1. 3 hepatic veins
  2. 2 renal veins
  3. 2 common iliac veins
  4. **Right adrenal vein**
  5. **Right ovarian vein** or **testicular vein**
  6. **Inferior phrenic vein**
  7. **4 lumbar veins**
  8. **Medial sacral vein**
- Size is variable and normal up to 4 cm
- Can be very **tortuous** (marked by twists, turns, or bends)

Physiology

- The IVC returns deoxygenated blood from the tissues to the heart for oxygenation and recirculation.

Sonographic Appearance

- Anechoic lumen surrounded by bright, echogenic walls.
- During real-time examination it is not uncommon to visualize multiple, small, moving echoes within the lumen of the IVC, which are thought to be related to the flow of blood.
- During real-time evaluation the IVC demonstrates significant variation in diameter relative to arterial vessels. The IVC is seen to increase in size with deep inspiration or the **Valsalva maneuver** (exhaling with airways closed–mouth shut, nose pinched shut) and decrease in size during expiration. Note that a momentary collapse of the IVC can be observed by having a patient "sniff."
- Since the IVC is vertically orientated in the body, longitudinal and long axis views are seen in coronal scanning planes and sagittal scanning planes as demonstrated in the following image. The IVC appears like a large long tube, anechoic with thin, bright walls, immediately anterior to the spine and right renal artery and immediately posterior to the head of the pancreas, portion of the distal common bile duct,

portion of the portal vein, and the right lobe of the liver. Note that the space between the IVC and the spine affords passage of the right renal artery, seen here in an axial section, on its way to the right kidney.

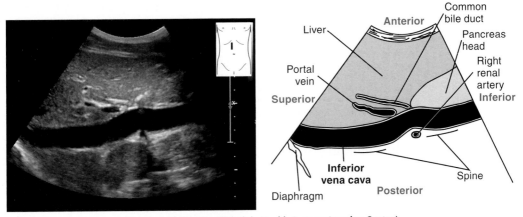

(Courtesy University of Virginia Health Systems Imaging Center.)

- Short axis (or axial) sections of the IVC are seen in transverse scanning planes. The following transverse scanning plane image shows how easy it is to recognize the short axis section of the mid portion of the IVC in the posterior portion of the image, immediately anterior to the right renal artery and anterior and just to the right of the spine, and immediately posterior to the head of the pancreas and the gallbladder. It appears large, round, anechoic with bright, thin walls, and at this level the right and left renal vein tributaries are easily identified. Notice how the space between the IVC and the spine affords passage of the right renal artery, seen here in a longitudinal section, on its way to the right kidney.

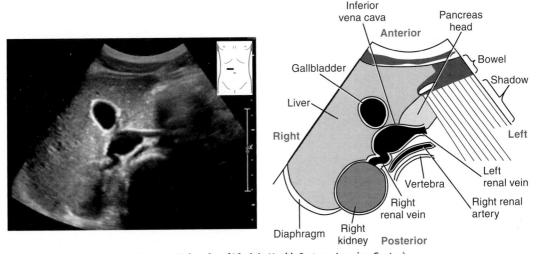

(Courtesy University of Virginia Health Systems Imaging Center.)

- The proximal (closest to origin) portion of the IVC is described as the area seen extending from its origin at *the common iliac veins to the area just inferior to the renal vein tributaries.*
- The mid portion of the IVC is seen at the *level of the renal vein tributaries, posterior to the head of the pancreas.*
- The distal (farthest from origin) portion of the IVC is seen extending from the area *just superior to the renal vein tributaries to the right atrium of the heart;* it includes the hepatic vein tributaries located just inferior to the diaphragm.
- The 3 hepatic veins, 2 renal veins, and 2 common iliac veins are the IVC tributaries that are routinely visualized with ultrasound. The remaining tributaries are usually too small to distinguish.

Normal Variants
- Duplication.
- Total or partial absence.
- May be particularly short.
- Visceral transposition lying to the left of the aorta.
- Crosses to lie to the left of the aorta.
- Joins with the azygos vein; enters the superior vena cava.

Preparation

Patient Prep
- The patient should fast for at least 6 to 8 hours before the ultrasound examination.
- If the patient has eaten, still attempt the examination.

Transducer
- **3.0 MHz or 3.5 MHz.**
- 5.0 MHz for thin patients.

Breathing Technique
- **Normal respiration** or deep, held respiration.

> **NOTE:** Different breathing techniques should be used whenever the suggested breathing technique does not produce the desired results. The diameter of the IVC will vary depending on the level of respiration. Normal veins increase with held respiration or the Valsalva maneuver.

Patient Position
- **Supine.**
- Left lateral decubitus, right lateral decubitus, left posterior oblique, right posterior oblique, or sitting semierect to erect as needed.

NOTE: Different patient positions should be used whenever the suggested position does not produce the desired results.

Inferior Vena Cava Survey Steps

Inferior Vena Cava • Longitudinal Survey
Sagittal Plane • Transabdominal Anterior Approach

NOTE: While you are scanning, experiment using different amounts of transducer pressure (keeping patient comfort in mind) to improve imaging.

1. Begin scanning with the transducer perpendicular, at the midline of the body, just inferior to the xiphoid process of the sternum.

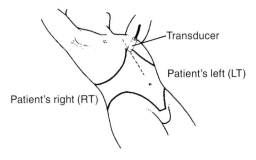

2. Slightly move or angle the transducer to the patient's left and identify the longitudinal, anechoic, section of the proximal aorta just posterior to the liver.

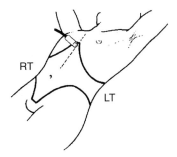

NOTE: Use held respiration or locate the diaphragm to differentiate the IVC from the abdominal aorta. As mentioned, varying respiration changes the size of the IVC. The IVC passes through the highly reflective diaphragm that can be visualized in the superior portion of the image; the aorta lies posterior to the diaphragm.

3. Return to the midline and slightly move or angle the transducer to the patient's right; identify the longitudinal, anechoic, section of the distal IVC just posterior to the liver.

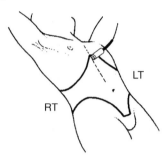

4. While viewing the distal IVC, it may be necessary to slightly twist/ rotate the transducer, first one way, then the other, to resolve the longest sections and long axis of the IVC. When the long axis is located, barely twisting/rotating the transducer can help resolve the hepatic vein tributaries, which are seen within the liver, emptying into the IVC anteriorly (Figure 5-1, *A*). Now, very slightly rock or move the transducer from right to left, scanning completely through each side of the IVC. Continue this and slowly slide the transducer inferiorly following along the length of the IVC. Keep your eyes on the screen; use the image as a guide, evaluating the appearance of the mid and proximal IVC until you reach the right and left common iliac veins (usually at or just beyond the level of the umbilicus).

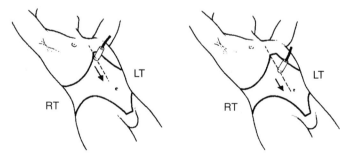

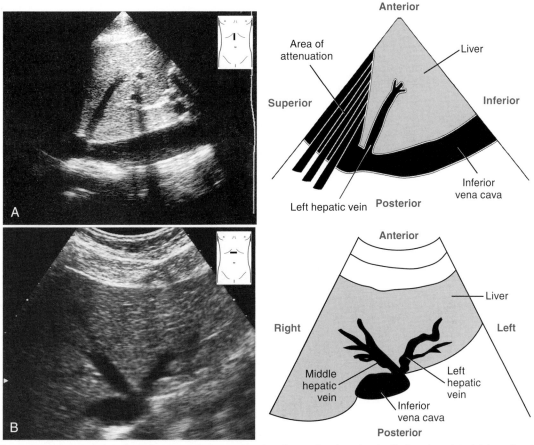

Figure 5-1 Hepatic Vein Tributaries. A, Sagittal scanning plane image showing a longitudinal section of the left hepatic vein emptying into the long section of the inferior vena cava (IVC). **B,** Axial section of the IVC from a transverse scanning plane, showing sections of the middle and left hepatic veins emptying into the anterior portion of the IVC.

5. In some cases, the convergence of the common iliac veins can be better visualized with the transducer angled from a lateral position. At the level of the most proximal portion of the IVC, move the transducer slightly toward the patient's right then angle the transducer at varying degrees aiming the sound beam back toward the IVC until you relocate the proximal portion. Keeping this angle, very slowly slide the transducer inferiorly until the convergence site and right and left common iliac veins come into view.

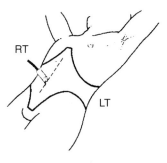

NOTE: The longitudinal sections of the convergence of the right and left common iliac veins into the proximal IVC can be difficult to resolve from a sagittal plane. In most cases, visualization is easier from a coronal plane, right lateral approach as described below. While distal and middle portions of the IVC tend to be better visualized from a transabdominal sagittal plane, alternatively, they may also be evaluated from the coronal plane, right lateral approach.

Proximal IVC and Common Iliac Veins • Coronal Plane • Right Lateral Approach

Patient Position: Left Lateral Decubitus (or Supine, Sitting Semierect to Erect)

1. Begin with the transducer perpendicular, midcoronal plane, just super to the iliac crest.
2. Use the inferior pole of the right kidney as a landmark; it is usually easy to visualize at this level or by sliding the transducer slightly superiorly.
3. When the inferior pole is located, the proximal IVC, convergence site, and common iliac veins should be seen in the medial and inferior portions of the image. It may be necessary to slightly twist/rotate the transducer at varying degrees to oblique the coronal plane and resolve the long axis of the proximal IVC, convergence site, and right and left common iliac veins.
4. To evaluate the middle and distal portions of the IVC, move the transducer superiorly from the level of the convergence site or scan intercostally, looking for the IVC medially.
5. To avoid moving the patient, the survey of the proximal IVC, convergence site, and common iliac veins in the decubitus position can be done following the axial survey of the IVC.

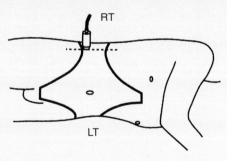

Inferior Vena Cava • Axial Survey
Transverse Plane • Transabdominal Anterior Approach

1. Begin scanning with the transducer perpendicular, at the midline of the body, just inferior to the xiphoid process of the sternum.

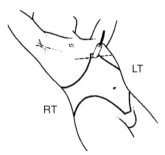

2. Angle the transducer superiorly until the heart is identified by its pulsations. Keeping your eyes on the screen, very slowly return the transducer to a perpendicular position while looking for the oval or round, anechoic IVC to come into sight just to the right of the midline; anterior to the spine.

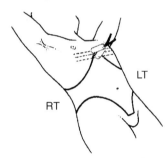

3. With the distal IVC in sight, very slightly rock or move the transducer from right to left, scanning completely through the IVC. Continue this as you slowly slide the transducer inferiorly. Keep your eyes on the screen; use the image as a guide to avoid losing sight of the IVC. Note and evaluate the anterior hepatic vein tributaries as they empty into the IVC (Figure 5-1, *B*).

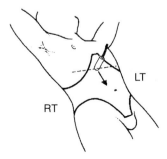

4. Continue rocking and sliding the transducer inferiorly through the middle and proximal IVC to the convergence of the common iliac veins. Note and evaluate the IVC's lateral tributaries, the renal veins. At the level of the common iliac veins, the view will change from one large, round, echo-free structure (the IVC) to two small, round, echo-free structures (the iliac veins), one seen on each side of the midline. Evaluate the common iliac veins by scanning through them inferiorly until you lose sight of them.

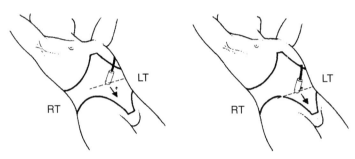

NOTE: An alternative method for locating the axial section of the distal IVC begins by viewing a longitudinal section of the distal IVC from a sagittal plane. From that position, slowly rotate the transducer 90 degrees into the transverse scanning plane. The axial view of the IVC should come directly into sight.

Inferior Vena Cava Required Images

Inferior Vena Cava • Longitudinal Images
Sagittal Plane • Transabdominal Anterior Approach

NOTE: The required images are a small representation of what a sonographer visualizes during a study. Therefore, the images should provide the interpreting physician with the most telling and technically accurate information available.

NOTE: Measurements of the IVC are not required unless indicated by pathology.

1. Longitudinal image of the **DISTAL IVC** to include the diaphragm and hepatic vein(s).

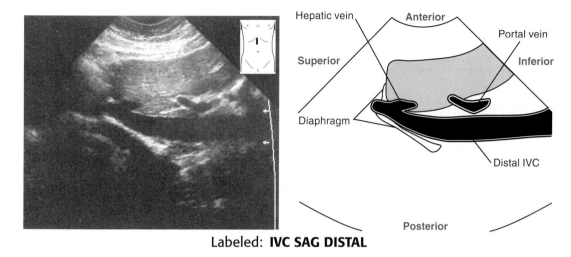

Labeled: **IVC SAG DISTAL**

2. Longitudinal image of the **MID IVC** at the level of the head of the pancreas.

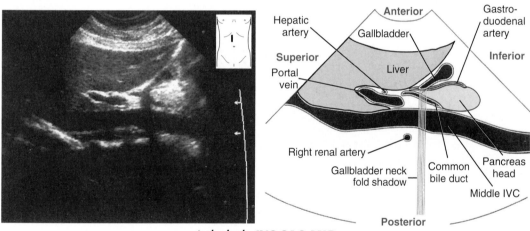

Labeled: **IVC SAG MID**

3. Longitudinal image of the **PROXIMAL IVC.**

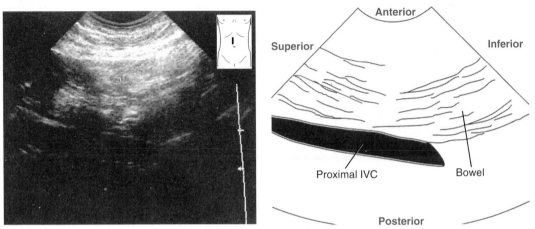

Labeled: **IVC SAG PROX**

4. Longitudinal image of the **COMMON ILIAC VEINS.**

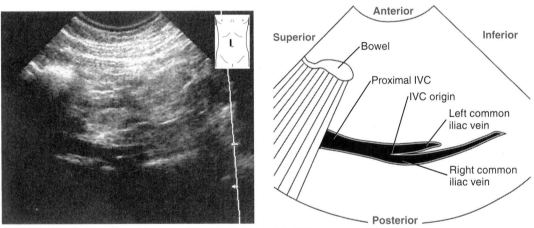

Labeled: **SAG CIV** or
SAG CIV RT OBL or
RT COR CIV

NOTE: To avoid moving the patient, longitudinal images of the common iliac veins in the decubitus position can be taken following the axial images. Although the coronal plane approach can be used with the patient supine, the decubitus position is generally easier and can be helpful if the patient has obscuring bowel gas anteriorly.

Inferior Vena Cava • Axial Images
Transverse Plane • Transabdominal Anterior Approach
5. Axial image of the **DISTAL IVC** to include the hepatic veins.

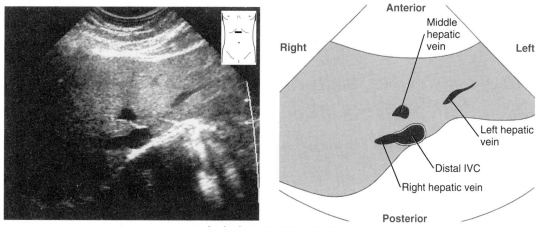

Labeled: **IVC TRV DISTAL**

6. Axial image of the **MID IVC** at the level of the renal veins.

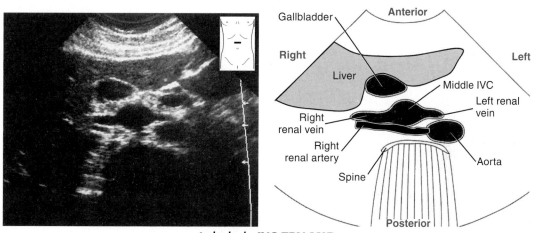

Labeled: **IVC TRV MID**

7. Axial image of the **PROXIMAL IVC.**

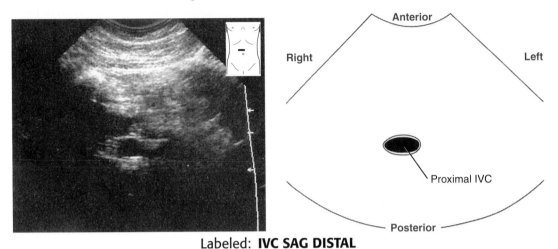

Labeled: **IVC SAG DISTAL**

8. Axial image of the **COMMON ILIAC VEINS.**

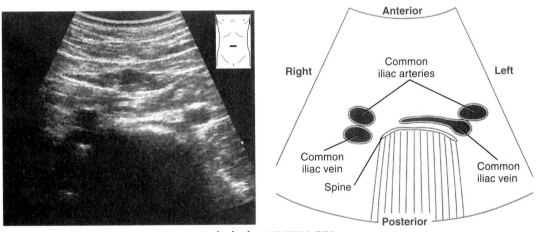

Labeled: **IVC TRV CIV**

Required Images When the Inferior Vena Cava is Part of Another Study

1. Longitudinal image of the **DISTAL** and **MID IVC.**

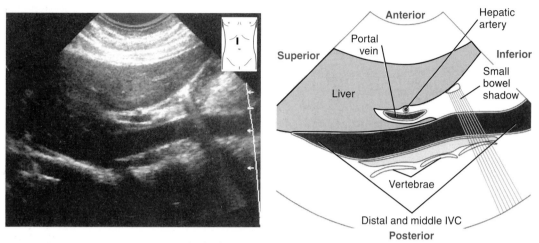

Labeled: **IVC SAG DISTAL/MID**

2. Axial image of the **DISTAL IVC** to include the hepatic veins.

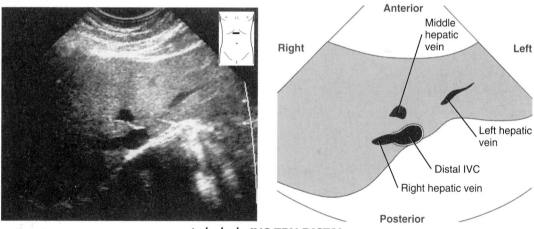

Labeled: **IVC TRV DISTAL**

Review Questions

Answers on page 628.

1. The lie of the IVC within the body is
   a) midsagittal.
   b) superior to inferior.
   c) oblique.
   d) transverse.

2. The long axis of the IVC is seen from a(n)
   a) sagittal or coronal scanning plane.
   b) transverse scanning plane.
   c) axial section.
   d) left lateral decubitus position.

3. Longitudinal views of the renal vein tributaries are seen in a
   a) sagittal or coronal scanning plane.
   b) transverse scanning plane.
   c) midsagittal plane.
   d) longitudinal section.

4. Axial views of the renal vein tributaries are seen in a
   a) sagittal or coronal scanning plane.
   b) transverse scanning plane.
   c) midsagittal plane.
   d) longitudinal section.

5. The IVC
   a) tributaries include the splenic vein.
   b) tributaries include the splenic vein and superior mesenteric vein.
   c) passes through a deep fossa on the inferior surface of the liver at the level where it is anterior to the left renal artery.
   d) passes through a deep fossa on the posterior surface of the liver between the caudate lobe and bare area.

6. The size of the IVC is normal up to
   a) 4 cm
   b) 1.5 cm
   c) 2 cm
   d) 3.5 cm

7. The proximal IVC is the portion
   a) that extends superiorly from the common iliac veins to just below the level of the renal veins.
   b) adjacent to the diaphragm and posterior to the body of the liver.
   c) posterior to the head of the pancreas at the level of the renal veins.
   d) that enters the heart.

8. The mid portion of the IVC is
   a) the portion that extends superiorly from the common iliac veins to just below the level of the renal veins.
   b) adjacent to the diaphragm and posterior to the body of the liver.
   c) posterior to the head of the pancreas at the level of the renal veins.
   d) the portion that enters the heart.

9. The distal IVC is the portion
   a) that extends superiorly from the common iliac veins to just below the level of the renal veins.
   b) that extends superior to the renal veins to the right atrium of the heart.
   c) posterior to the head of the pancreas at the level of the renal veins.
   d) just superior to the common iliac veins.

10. Beginning posteriorly, and in correct order by the location in the body, the IVC is
    a) just to the right of and at the same level as the spine, posterior to the splenic and common hepatic arteries, body of the pancreas, right lobe of the liver.
    b) anterior and just to the right of the spine, anterior to the right renal artery, posterior to the head of the pancreas, gastroduodenal artery, portal splenic confluence, and the liver.
    c) anterior to the spine, posterior to the gastroesophageal junction, splenic vein, head of the pancreas, portion of the duodenum, right lobe of the liver.
    d) anterior to the spine and kidneys, posterior to the gastroesophageal junction, splenic vein, head of the pancreas, portion of the duodenum, right lobe of the liver.

11. The left renal vein has a(n) _____ course compared with the right renal vein.
    a) identical
    b) shorter
    c) wider
    d) longer

12. All of the following are IVC tributaries except the
    a) hepatic veins.
    b) right renal vein.
    c) superior mesenteric vein.
    d) left renal vein.

13. The *primary* function of the IVC is to
    a) carry deoxygenated blood from the heart.
    b) serve as a lymph drainage channel.
    c) carry deoxygenated blood to the heart.
    d) regulate metabolism.

14. The right and left common iliac veins are _____ the right and left common iliac arteries.
    a) posterior to
    b) anterior to
    c) wider than
    d) longer than

15. The IVC is medial to all of the following except the
    a) right adrenal gland.
    b) caudate lobe.
    c) right kidney.
    d) right ureter.

16. The IVC is anterior to all of the following except the
    a) transverse duodenum.
    b) right crus of the diaphragm.
    c) right adrenal gland.
    d) psoas major muscle.

17. The IVC is right lateral to all of the following except the
    a) aorta.
    b) caudate lobe.
    c) left renal vein.
    d) portal splenic confluence.

18. The IVC is posterior to all of the following except the
    a) uncinate process.
    b) spine.
    c) hepatic veins.
    d) common bile duct.

19. The IVC passes through a deep fossa on the posterior surface of the
    liver between the _____ and _____.
    a) caudate lobe and gallbladder fossa
    b) spine and right lateral lobe
    c) caudate lobe and bare area
    d) bare area and diaphragm

20. Normally, the diameter of the IVC will _____ during the
    Valsalva maneuver or inspiration.
    a) decrease
    b) increase
    c) collapse
    d) stay the same

21. The orientation of the IVC within the body is
    a) vertical oblique.
    b) vertical.
    c) oblique.
    d) horizontal.

22. Which of the following vessels runs posterior to the IVC?
    a) left renal vein
    b) right hepatic artery
    c) right renal artery
    d) left renal artery

23. The IVC lies along the posterior surface of what lobe of the liver?
    a) left
    b) caudate
    c) quadrate
    d) anterior segment of the right

24. In the following transverse scanning plane image, a(n) _____ section of the IVC is visualized.

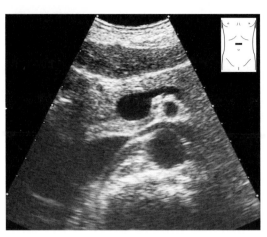
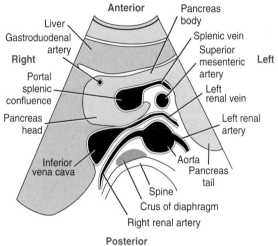

a) transverse
b) longitudinal
c) sagittal
d) axial

25. In the transverse scanning plane image above, a(n) _____ section of the left renal vein is visualized.
a) transverse
b) longitudinal
c) sagittal
d) axial

26. In the following sagittal scanning plane image, a(n) _____ section of the IVC is visualized.

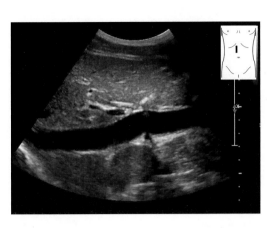 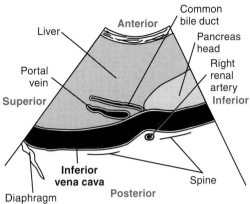

   a) transverse
   b) longitudinal
   c) sagittal
   d) axial

27. In the sagittal scanning plane image above, a(n) _____ section of the right renal artery is visualized.
   a) transverse
   b) longitudinal
   c) sagittal
   d) axial

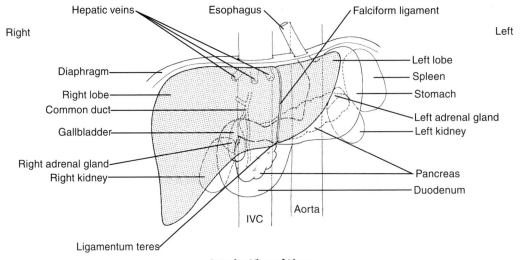

Hepatic veins

Esophagus

Falciform ligament

Right

Left

Diaphragm

Left lobe

Spleen

Right lobe

Stomach

Common duct

Left adrenal gland

Gallbladder

Left kidney

Right adrenal gland

Right kidney

Pancreas

Duodenum

Aorta

IVC

Ligamentum teres

Anterior View of Liver

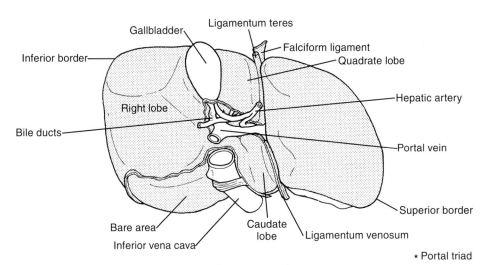

Gallbladder

Ligamentum teres

Inferior border

Falciform ligament

Quadrate lobe

Right lobe

Hepatic artery

Bile ducts

Portal vein

Superior border

Bare area

Caudate lobe

Inferior vena cava

Ligamentum venosum

∗ Portal triad

View of Liver From Below

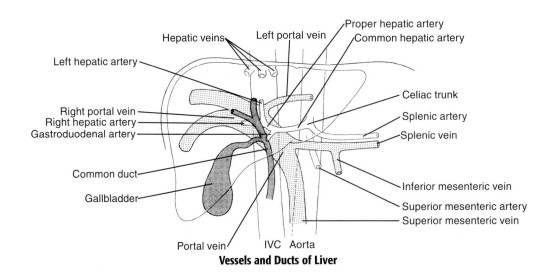

Hepatic veins

Left portal vein

Proper hepatic artery

Common hepatic artery

Left hepatic artery

Right portal vein

Celiac trunk

Right hepatic artery

Splenic artery

Gastroduodenal artery

Splenic vein

Common duct

Inferior mesenteric vein

Gallbladder

Superior mesenteric artery

Superior mesenteric vein

Portal vein

IVC   Aorta

Vessels and Ducts of Liver

CHAPTER 6

Liver Scanning Protocol

Betty Bates Tempkin

Key Words

Anterior surface	Left triangular ligament
Biliary tract	Ligamentum teres
Caudate lobe	Ligamentum teres fissure
Common hepatic artery	Ligamentum venosum fissure
Coronary ligament	Main lobar fissure
Cystic artery	Middle hepatic artery
Falciform ligament	Porta hepatis
Gastroduodenal artery	Portal triad
Gastrohepatic ligament	Portal vein
Glisson's capsule	Portal venous system
Hepatic ducts	Posterior surface
Hepatic veins	Proper hepatic artery
Hepatoduodenal ligament	Quadrate lobe
Inferior surface	Right functional lobe
Intraperitoneal	Right hepatic artery
Left functional lobe	Right lobe
Left hepatic artery	Right triangular ligament
Left intersegmental fissure	Superior surface
Left lobe	

Objectives

At the end of this chapter, you will be able to:

- Define the key words.
- Distinguish the sonographic appearance of the liver and the terms used to describe it.
- Describe the transducer options for scanning the liver.
- List the various suggested breathing techniques for patients when scanning the liver.
- List the suggested patient position (and options) when scanning the liver.
- Describe the patient prep for a liver study.
- Distinguish normal variants of the liver.
- Name the survey steps and explain how to evaluate the entire length, width, and depth of the liver.
- Explain the order and exact locations to take representative images of the liver.
- Answer the review questions at the end of the chapter.

Overview

Location

- The liver occupies the right side of the upper abdomen and often extends beyond the midline of the body to the left side. Generally, it lies between the level of the nipples to the level of the eighth or ninth rib.
- Except for a bare area that encompasses most of the liver's posterior surface, it is **intraperitoneal** (enclosed in the sac formed by the parietal peritoneum). Additional interruptions of the peritoneum at the liver include the gallbladder fossa, **porta hepatis** (the area of the hilus/opening where the portal vein and hepatic artery enter the liver and the common duct exits), falciform ligament attachment, and portions around the inferior vena cava (IVC).
- The liver is the most anterior visceral organ of the peritoneal cavity. The left lobe and majority of the right lobe are surrounded by the rib cage. The remaining portion of the right lobe is usually in contact with the abdominal wall.
- Superior, posterior, and anterior liver surfaces abut the diaphragm.
- The **left lobe** of the liver lies in the left hypochondriac and epigastric regions. It is bounded in front by the rib cage and abdominal wall and posteriorly it rests on the stomach.
- The **right lobe** occupies the right hypochondrium. It is bounded in front by the rib cage and abdominal wall and posteriorly it rests on the gallbladder, head of the pancreas, right adrenal gland, and right kidney (primarily the superior pole).
- The **caudate lobe** is located on the posterior surface of the liver and lies posterior to the porta hepatis between the fissure for the ligamentum venosum and the IVC.

Anatomy

- The liver is considered the largest internal organ of the body. Its mass displaces the gas-filled components of the digestive system, providing an acoustic window for viewing upper abdominal and retroperitoneal structures.
- Size and shape are variable. Anteroposterior size is normal up to 15 cm. Viewed anteriorly, it has a basic wedge shape, tapering toward the left side. The right lobe is significantly larger than the left lobe.
- The entire liver is encased by **Glisson's capsule**, a thick, fibrous, connective tissue layer that contains nerves, blood vessels, and lymphatic vessels. In turn, the encased liver is largely covered by the peritoneum.
- The liver is divided into *lobes* according to anatomy and into *segments* according to function:

Liver Lobes

Using the traditional anatomic system, the liver is divided based on the sonographic identification of specific anatomic landmarks.

(a) Left lobe: Anatomically separated from the right lobe by the falciform ligament on its superior surface. Divided from the caudate lobe by the fissure for the ligamentum venosum and on its inferior (visceral) surface from the quadrate lobe by the fissure for the ligamentum teres.

(b) Right lobe: Anatomically separated from the left lobe by the falciform ligament on its superior (diaphragmatic) surface and by the left intersegmental fissure on its inferior surface. Riedel's lobe, a normal anatomic variant, is a projection of the right lobe that can extend as far as the iliac crest.

(c) Caudate lobe: Anatomically separated from the left lobe by the fissure for the ligamentum venosum. Boundaries are the IVC on the right, its margin on the left, which forms the hepatic boundary of the superior recess of the lesser sac, and the porta hepatis anteriorly.

(d) Quadrate lobe: Distinguished sonographically and physiologically as the medial portion of the left lobe. The porta hepatis borders posteriorly, the margin of the liver anteriorly, the gallbladder fossa right laterally, and on the left, the fissure for the ligamentum teres.

Liver Segments

Liver segments are based on hepatic function. Segments are determined according to blood supply and biliary drainage. Segmental liver anatomy is clinically significant for localizing potentially resectable liver lesions.

(a) **Two main functional divisions:** right and left. Middle hepatic veins located in the main lobar fissure delineate the liver into intrahepatic (functional), right and left lobes:

- The **right functional lobe** is everything to the right of the plane through the gallbladder fossa and IVC (analogous to the anatomic right lobe).
  - *Two divisions: anterior segment and posterior segment:* The right hepatic vein, located in the right intersegmental fissure, delineates the anterior and posterior segments. These segments are also separated by the right portal vein that passes centrally within them.
- The **left functional lobe** is everything to the left of the plane through the gallbladder fossa and IVC (analogous to the anatomic left lobe, caudate lobe, and quadrate lobe).
  - *Two divisions: medial segment and lateral segment:* The medial segment is analogous to the traditional quadrate lobe. The

lateral segment is analogous to the anatomic left lobe. The ascending portion of the left portal vein (in the left intersegmental fissure) delineates the medial and lateral segments. These segments are also separated by the left hepatic vein (in the left intersegmental fissure) superiorly and the ligamentum teres inferiorly.

(b) **Caudate lobe:** the portion of the liver lying posterior to the porta hepatis, between the fissure for the ligamentum venosum and the IVC.

• *No divisions:* It distinctly receives hepatic arterial and portal venous blood from both the right and left systems, which otherwise individually supply respective right and left lobes. The left portal vein separates the caudate lobe from the medial segment of the left lobe. The left portal vein runs anterior to the caudate and posterior to the medial segment. The fissure for the ligamentum venosum runs along the left anterior margin of the caudate separating it from medial and lateral segments of the functional left lobe.

Liver Surfaces

The different *surfaces* of the liver include distinctions among the *posterior, anterior, superior,* and *inferior* surfaces.

(a) Posterior surface:
• Caudate lobe.
• Bare area.
• Deeply indented area centrally where it lies on the spine.
• Fossae for the IVC and ligamentum venosum.
• Attachment to the diaphragm by loose connective tissue.
• Most of this surface is not covered by peritoneum.

(b) Anterior surface:
• Lies inside the peritoneum immediately posterior to the xiphoid process of the sternum.
• Is part of the diaphragmatic surface until it loses contact on the left at the seventh or eighth costal cartilage and on the right anywhere from the 6th to the 10th costal cartilage.
• Is accentuated by a deep notch. The ligamentum teres ascends from the umbilicus to the umbilical notch of the anterior surface.

(c) Superior surface:
• Is intraperitoneal.
• Is a convex diaphragmatic, smooth surface, separated from the pleura, lungs, pericardium, and heart by the dome of the diaphragm.

(d) Inferior surface:
• Is covered by peritoneum except at the porta hepatis and site of the gallbladder attachment.

- Is a concave visceral surface accentuated by fossae and indentations from organs that rest against its surface.
- Of the left lobe is deeply indented by the anterior surface of the stomach.
- Of the right lobe is accentuated by the hepatic flexure of the colon, right kidney and adrenal gland, and the duodenum, where it lies adjacent to the gallbladder neck.
- Anterior mid portion is the **quadrate lobe** (medial left lobe) bound by the falciform ligament on the left.
- Posterior mid portion of the inferior surface is the caudate lobe. The posterior portion of the caudate forms a part of the anterior boundary of the lesser sac.

Liver Ligaments

Liver ligaments attach the liver to the diaphragm, stomach, anterior abdominal wall, and retroperitoneum. Liver ligaments are viewable with ultrasound because of the fat and collagen within and around these structures. This makes them quite hyperechoic relative to hepatic parenchyma. The different types of liver ligaments include the *falciform ligament, ligamentum teres, coronary ligament, right* and *left triangular ligaments, gastrohepatic ligament*, and *hepatoduodenal ligament*.

(a) **Falciform ligament:** Parietal peritoneal, anteroposterior fold that attaches the bare area of the liver to the right rectus muscle of the anterior abdominal wall. It extends from the diaphragm to the umbilicus, running along the liver's anterior surface. It is continuous with the ligamentum teres, which is contained within its layers. On the liver's superior (diaphragmatic) surface, it is described as the anatomical divider of the right and left lobes and along with the ligamentum teres, functionally designates the boundary of the left lobe's medial and lateral segments.

(b) **Ligamentum teres:** Fibrous, round ligament formed by the obliterated left umbilical vein. Arises from the umbilicus and courses within the falciform ligament to the umbilical notch on the anterior surface of the liver. Coursing along the inferior (visceral) surface, it continues as the ligamentum venosum (obliterated ductus venosus) running posteriorly to the IVC.

(c) **Coronary ligament:** Parietal peritoneal, bifold layer that attaches the liver's posterior surface to the diaphragm. Anterior and posterior layers are continuous anteriorly with the falciform ligament and laterally with the triangular ligaments.

(d) **Right and left triangular ligaments:** Formed by continuations of the coronary ligament. Triangular extensions on the right from the far right border of the bare area to the diaphragm and on the left from the superior surface of the left lobe to just anterior of the esophageal opening in the diaphragm.

(e) **Gastrohepatic ligament**: Visceral peritoneal, bifold layer also known as the lesser omentum. From the undersurface of the liver, it is continuous with the ligamentum venosum. Ascending, it attaches the undersurface with the lesser curvature of the stomach and the first portion of the duodenum.

(f) **Hepatoduodenal ligament**: Portion of the lesser omentum that is located on the right free edge of the gastrohepatic ligament. Extends to the duodenum and right hepatic flexure and forms the ventral portion of the foramen of Winslow or the epiploic foramen. Surrounds the portal triad immediately adjacent to the porta hepatis.

Liver Fissures

Liver *fissures* are the normal grooves or folds throughout the liver that typically form the spaces that contain various blood vessels or ligaments. Ultrasound can identify the fissures associated with the liver due to the fat and collagen within and around them, which makes them highly reflective relative to liver parenchyma. Types of liver fissures include *main lobar fissure, left intersegmental fissure, fissure for the ligamentum venosum*, and *fissure for the ligamentum teres*.

(a) **Main lobar fissure**: Runs obliquely between the neck of the gallbladder and right portal vein. Contains the middle hepatic vein and separates the right and left hepatic lobes. Its course is short and variable.

(b) **Left intersegmental fissure**: Subdivides the right lobe into anterior and posterior portions.

(c) **Ligamentum venosum fissure**: Contains the gastrohepatic ligament and separates the left lobe and caudate lobe.

(d) **Ligamentum teres fissure**: Forms the left boundary of the quadrate or medial portion of the left lobe.

Liver Vessels and Ducts

The liver receives nutrient rich blood from the hepatic artery and the portal vein, which is highly saturated with oxygen. The hepatic veins drain the liver of deoxygenated blood. The hepatic ducts transport bile, a fluid made in the liver, to the bile ducts. The bile ducts convey the bile to the gallbladder for storage. When bile is needed to aid digestion of fat, the bile ducts carry it into the duodenum. Structures that make up the liver vessels and ducts include the *hepatic arteries, hepatic veins, portal vein, portal venous system, hepatic ducts*, and *portal triad*.

(a) **Hepatic arteries**: Supply the liver with oxygenated blood from the aorta. The celiac axis branch of the aorta divides into the splenic, left gastric, and common hepatic arteries.

• The **common hepatic artery** runs directly toward the right side of the body, anterior to the portal vein and left of the common bile duct. Here, it divides into the **gastroduodenal artery** and the proper hepatic artery.

- The **proper hepatic artery** divides into two main branches, the **right and left hepatic arteries** which supply the right and left segmental lobes, respectively.
- The **middle hepatic artery** generally arises from the left hepatic artery.
- The **cystic artery** arises from the right hepatic artery.

(b) **Hepatic veins:** The right, *middle*, and *left* hepatic veins drain the blood from the liver and empty it into the IVC.

(c) **Portal vein:** The *main* portal vein enters the liver at the porta hepatis, posterior to the hepatic artery and common bile duct. It then divides into the *right* and *left* branches. These branches become intersegmental veins that branch into medial and lateral portions of the left lobe and anterior and posterior portions of the right lobe.

(d) **Portal venous system:** Supplies the greatest percentage of total blood flow to the liver. Formed by the confluence of three tributaries:

(1) *Splenic vein*

(2) *Superior mesenteric vein*

(3) *Inferior mesenteric vein*

Commonly referred to as the *portal splenic confluence*. This system carries blood from the spleen and bowel to the liver.

(e) **Hepatic ducts:** Enzymatic bile is manufactured in the liver then transferred via the *right* and *left* hepatic ducts from the liver to the extrahepatic bile ducts at the porta hepatis. As the right and left hepatic ducts emerge from liver parenchyma at the porta hepatis, they unite to form the *common hepatic duct*, which courses inferomedially where it is joined by the *cystic duct* to form the *common bile duct*. The common bile duct descends to cross behind the first portion of the duodenum to enter into or run along the posterior portion of the parenchyma of the head of the pancreas. From there it courses slightly toward the right and enters the second portion of the duodenum, where it ends at the ampulla of Vater. The extrahepatic bile ducts (common hepatic, cystic, common bile) maintain communication between the liver and gastrointestinal tract.

(f) **Portal triad:** Refers to the *proper hepatic artery*, *common duct*, and *portal vein* at the level of the porta hepatis. When there is a question of dilated bile ducts, a distinction between these structures is important. The following oblique, transverse scanning plane image shows that at the level of the porta hepatis, the portal vein (1) lies posterior to the proper hepatic artery (2), which is on the left and the common duct (3), located on the right. The appearance of the axial sections of the portal triad is often referred to as "Mickey's sign" as they resemble a face and two ears.

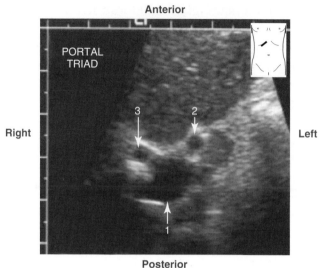

(From Brant WE: *The Core Curriculum: Ultrasound.*
Lippincott Williams & Wilkins, 2001.)

Physiology

- **Vascular Functions:** The vascular functions of the liver include
  the storage and filtration of blood. The liver expands to act as a
  blood reservoir in times of excess blood volume and supplies extra
  blood in times of diminished blood volume. Kupffer cells that line
  hepatic sinuses cleanse the blood of up to all but approximately
  1% of bacteria found in portal blood from the intestine. It detoxi-
  fies drugs such as alcohol and barbiturates.
- **Metabolic Functions:** The liver is a primary center of metabolism, supporting multiple body systems and activities. It assists
  the digestive and excretory systems by metabolizing fats, carbohydrates, and proteins to form bile and urea and in the process syn-
  thesizes many substances that are sent to other areas of the body
  to perform a vast number of body functions. The liver uptakes
  and stores glycogen, vitamins, and iron. It also forms most of the
  substances utilized in blood coagulation and excretes drugs, hormones, and other substances into bile and ultimately the feces.
- **Secretory and Excretory Bile Functions:** Produces and
  secretes bile through the **biliary tract** (ductal path) into the small
  bowel where it is used for the digestion of fat.

Sonographic Appearance

- As seen in the following image, the normal liver is described as homogeneous, with midgray to moderately echogenic *parenchyma*. Portions of blood vessels that appear anechoic may be seen scattered throughout liver parenchyma. Normal liver parenchyma is generally described as hyperechoic compared to normal renal cortex, as seen in this image, and hypoechoic compared to the normal pancreas.

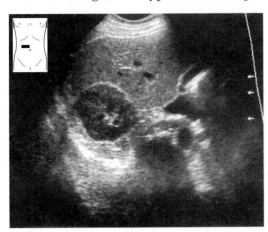
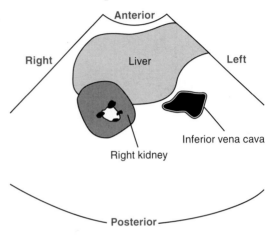

- Hepatic *vessels* and *ducts* display anechoic lumens surrounded by variations of bright, echogenic walls. The next image shows how portal veins and hepatic veins appear as anechoic, tubular structures branching throughout the liver. It is important to be able to distinguish portal veins from hepatic veins. Some sonographers use the difference often noted in the sonographic appearance of their walls. Typically, as demonstrated in the image, portal vein walls appear highly echogenic due to the reflective collagen that encases them, while the walls of hepatic veins appear as if they have no distinguishable margins because their walls contain minimal collagen. Note that this, however, is not a reliable way to make the distinction between these two vessels, because smaller portal vein branches may lack these surrounding echoes and in some cases, bright, reflective walls have been visualized surrounding the larger hepatic vein tributaries. These vessels have different branching patterns as well. Therefore, to correctly differentiate between portal veins and hepatic veins, follow their branches back toward the porta hepatis or IVC, respectively.

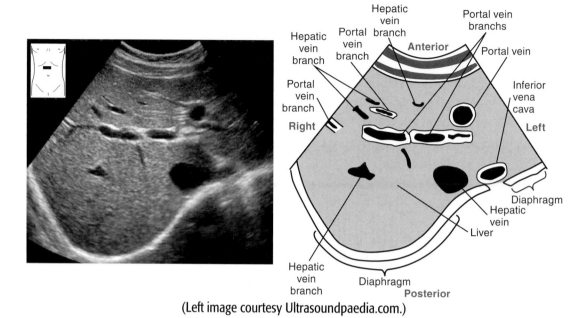

(Left image courtesy Ultrasoundpaedia.com.)

- The *ligaments* and *fissures* of the liver appear highly reflective due to the fat and collagen within and around them. In the images below, *A*, shows the bright, reflective ligamentum venosum and *B*, demonstrates the thin, bright main lobar fissure.

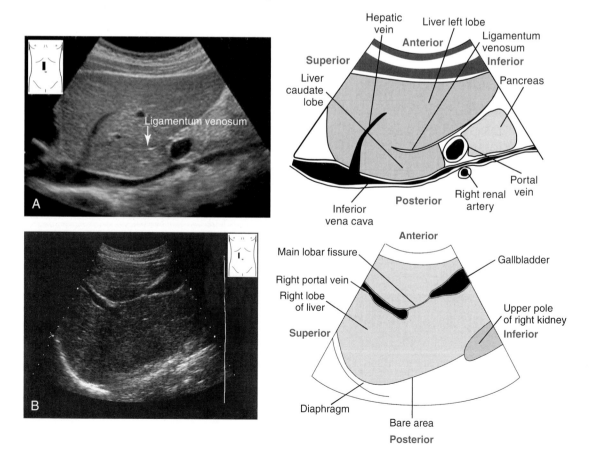

Normal Variants

- **Reidel's lobe:** Inferior extension of the right lobe.
- **Absence of left lobe:** Very rare. Results from occlusion of the left hepatic vein due to abnormal extension of neonatal spasm of the ligamentum venosum.
- **Multiple size and shape variations.**

Preparation

Patient Prep

- The patient should fast for 8 to 12 hours before the study. This ensures normal gallbladder and biliary tract dilatation and reduces the stomach and bowel gas anterior to the pancreas. This is significant because the liver, biliary tract, gallbladder, and pancreas are interdependent systems.
- If the patient has eaten, still perform the examination.

Transducer

- **3.0 MHz** or **3.5 MHz.**
- 5.0 MHz for very thin patients. It may be necessary to use 5.0 MHz for a patient's left lobe and 3.0 or 3.5 MHz for the right lobe.

Breathing Technique

- **Deep, held inspiration.**

NOTE: Different breathing techniques should be used whenever the suggested breathing technique does not produce the desired results.

Patient Position

- **Supine.**
- Left lateral decubitus, left posterior oblique, sitting semierect to erect or prone as needed.

NOTE: Different patient positions should be used whenever the suggested position does not produce the desired results.

Liver Survey Steps

Liver • Longitudinal Survey
Sagittal Plane • Transabdominal Anterior Approach

> **NOTE:** While you are scanning, experiment using different amounts of transducer pressure (keeping patient comfort in mind) to improve imaging.

1. Begin to scan the liver with the transducer perpendicular, at the midline of the body, just inferior to the xiphoid process of the sternum. Have the patient take in a deep breath and hold it. The general area of the left lobe should come into view as the most anterior structure in the image. Identify the ligamentum venosum, caudate lobe, and IVC or aorta.

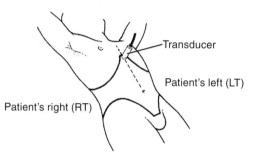

> **NOTE:** Depending on liver shape and patient respiration, varying degrees of subcostal and inferior angles may have to be used when scanning the liver longitudinally to completely survey the liver margins. In some cases intercostal scanning will be necessary.

2. While viewing the left lobe, use subcostal angles and very slowly move the transducer to the patient's left, lateral and inferior along the costal margin until you have evaluated the entire left lobe. Note the aorta posteriorly.

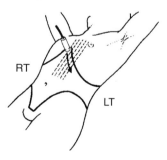

3. Return to midline just inferior to the xiphoid process to begin evaluating the right lobe. Use subcostal angles and slowly move the transducer to the patient's right, lateral and inferior along the costal margin until you are beyond the right lateral, inferior lobe. You should be able to identify the IVC, hepatic veins, portal vein, portal triad, porta hepatis, main lobar fissure, bile ducts, gallbladder (dilated or collapsed), right kidney, and perinephric space.

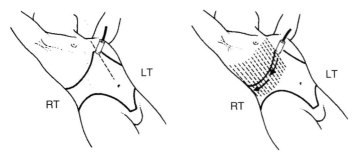

4. Move the transducer back onto the right lateral inferior lobe. Place the transducer at the most lateral edge of the right costal margin and use a *very* sharp subcostal angle to view the right lateral superior lobe. Move or angle the transducer right lateral and sweep through and beyond the right lateral superior lobe. Identify the dome of the right lobe and adjacent pleural space.

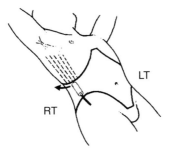

NOTE: Even with sharp subcostal transducer angles the longitudinal views of the right lateral superior lobe in a sagittal plane can be difficult to visualize. As an alternative, try sagittal plane intercostal scanning or scanning in the coronal plane from the patient's right side.

Alternative 1: Right Lateral Superior Lobe of Liver • Sagittal Plane • Intercostal Approach

Patient position: Supine, left posterior oblique or sitting semi-erect to erect

1. Begin scanning with the transducer perpendicular in an inter-costal space anterior to the area of the right lateral superior lobe. Suspended respiration may make the area easier to view.
2. Move the transducer to adjacent intercostal spaces to evaluate the entire right lateral superior lobe.
3. Angling the transducer within the intercostal spaces and using different breathing techniques can aid evaluation.
4. Note the dome of the right lobe and the adjacent pleural space.

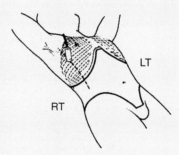

Alternative 2: Right Lateral Superior Lobe of Liver • Coronal Plane • Right Lateral Subcostal Approach

Patient position: Supine, left posterior oblique, left lateral decubitus, sitting semierect to erect

1. Begin scanning at the mid coronal plane with the transducer angled subcostal from the inferior costal margin.
2. With the patient holding their breath, vary the degree of the transducer angle until all of the margins of the right lateral superior lobe have been evaluated.
3. Note the dome of the right lobe and the adjacent pleural space.

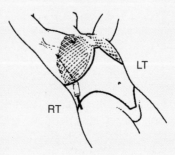

Alternative 3: Right Lateral Superior Lobe of Liver • Coronal Plane • Right Lateral Intercostal Approach

Patient position: Supine, left posterior oblique, left lateral decubitus, sitting semierect to erect

1. Begin scanning with the transducer perpendicular, midcoronal plane, just inferior to the costal margin. Move superiorly into the first intercostal space.
2. Have the patient use suspended or deep, held respiration, as you move the transducer superiorly through the adjacent intercostal spaces until you scan through and beyond the right lateral superior lobe.
3. Angling the transducer within the intercostal spaces and using different breathing techniques can aid evaluation.
4. Note the dome of the right lobe and the adjacent pleural space.

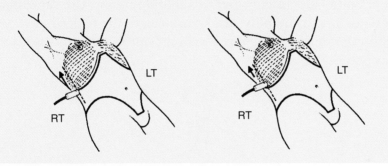

Liver • Axial Survey

Transverse Plane • Transabdominal Anterior Approach

1. Begin the axial evaluation of the liver with the transducer perpendicular, at the midline of the body, just inferior to the xiphoid process of the sternum. Have the patient take in a deep breath and hold it. The general area of the left lobe can be identified as the largest and most anterior structure in the image. Identify the ligamentum venosum, caudate lobe, hepatic vein(s), IVC, and aorta.

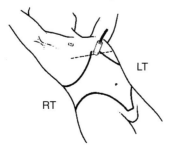

NOTE: Depending on liver shape and patient respiration, varying degrees of subcostal and inferior transducer angles may have to be used when scanning the liver from the axial plane to completely evaluate the superior and inferior liver margins. In some cases intercostal scanning may be necessary.

2. While viewing the left lobe, slowly move the transducer inferior until you scan through and beyond the left lobe. Note the portal vein and ligamentum teres.

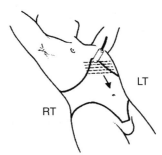

3. Depending on liver shape and size, all of the left lateral aspect of the left lobe may be seen in its entirety from midline. If not, return to midline, just inferior to the xiphoid process. Use subcostal and inferior angles and move the transducer to the patient's left, lateral and inferior along the costal margin until you scan through and beyond the left lobe.

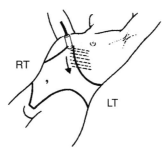

4. Return to midline, just inferior to the xiphoid process. To evaluate the right lobe, use subcostal and inferior transducer angles and very slowly move the transducer to the patient's right, lateral and inferior along the costal margin until you scan through and beyond the right lateral inferior lobe. Identify the IVC, hepatic veins, portal vein, portal triad, right and left portal branches, porta hepatis, main lobar fissure, bile ducts, gallbladder, right kidney, and perinephric space.

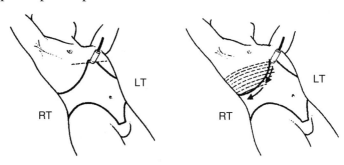

5. Move the transducer back onto the right lateral inferior lobe. Place the transducer at the most lateral edge of the right costal margin and use a very sharp subcostal angle to view the right lateral superior lobe. Move or angle the transducer right lateral and sweep through and beyond the right lateral superior lobe. Note the dome of the right lobe and adjacent pleural space.

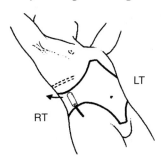

NOTE: Even with sharp subcostal transducer angles the axial views of the right lateral superior lobe in a transverse plane can be difficult to visualize. As an alternative, try transverse plane intercostal scanning or scanning in the transverse plane from the patient's right side.

Alternative 1: Right Lateral Superior Lobe of Liver • Transverse Plane • Anterior Intercostal Approach

Follow the same recommended scanning method as the one for the sagittal plane, longitudinal survey, intercostal approach of the right lateral superior lobe.

Alternative 2: Right Lateral Superior Lobe of Liver • Transverse Plane • Right Lateral Subcostal Approach

Follow the same recommended scanning method as the one for the coronal plane, longitudinal survey, subcostal approach of the right lateral superior lobe.

Alternative 3: Right Lateral Superior Lobe of Liver • Transverse Plane • Right Lateral Intercostal Approach

Follow the same recommended scanning method as the one for the coronal plane, longitudinal survey, intercostal approach of the right lateral superior lobe.

Liver Required Images

Liver • Longitudinal Images
Sagittal Plane • Transabdominal Anterior Approach

> **NOTE:** The required images are a small representation of what a sonographer visualizes during a study. Therefore, the images should provide the interpreting physician with the most telling and technically accurate information available.
>
> **NOTE:** Measurements of the liver are not required unless indicated by pathology.

1. Longitudinal image of the **LEFT LOBE** to include its inferior margin and the abdominal aorta.

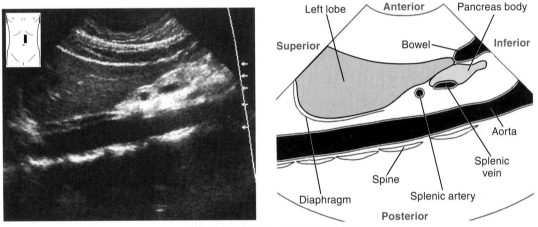

Labeled: **LIVER SAG LT LOBE**

2. Longitudinal image of the **LEFT LOBE** to include the diaphragm and caudate lobe.

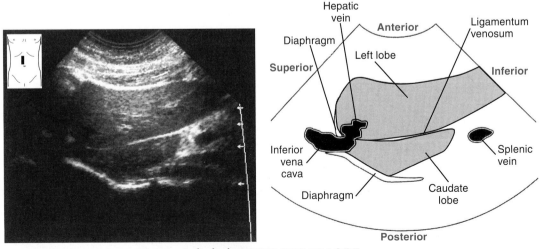

Labeled: **LIVER SAG LT LOBE**

3. Longitudinal image of the **RIGHT LOBE** to include the IVC where it passes through the liver.

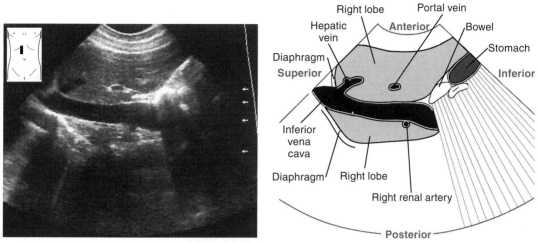

Labeled: **LIVER SAG RT LOBE**

4. Longitudinal image of the **RIGHT LOBE** to include the main lobar fissure, gallbladder, and portal vein.

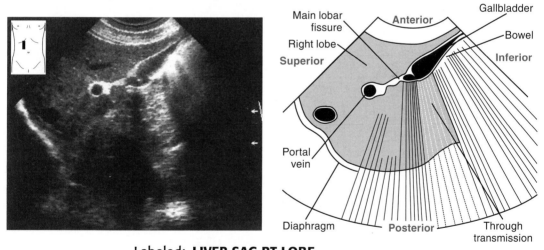

Labeled: **LIVER SAG RT LOBE**

5. Longitudinal image of the **RIGHT LOBE** to include part of the right kidney for parenchyma comparison.

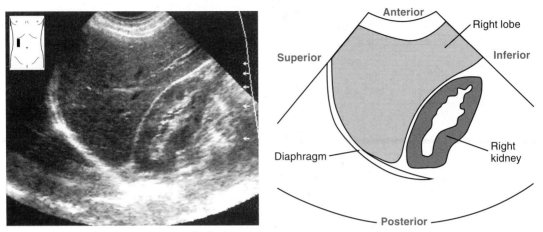

Labeled: **LIVER SAG RT LOBE**

6. Longitudinal image of the **RIGHT LOBE** to include the dome and the adjacent pleural space.

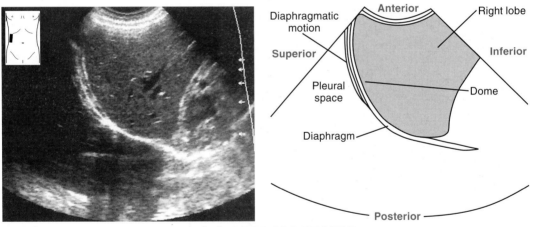

Labeled: **LIVER SAG RT LOBE**

Liver • Axial Images
Transverse Plane • Transabdominal Anterior Approach
7. Axial image of the **LEFT LOBE** to include its lateral margin.

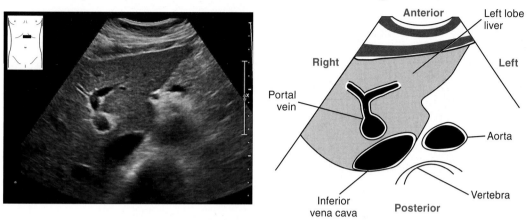

Labeled: **LIVER TRV LT LOBE**

8. Axial image of the **LEFT LOBE** to include the ligamentum teres.

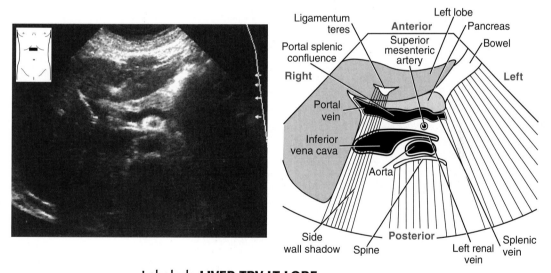

Labeled: **LIVER TRV LT LOBE**

NOTE: Depending on liver size and shape, it may be possible to take one axial image that includes the left lobe's lateral margin and the ligamentum teres. If so, label: **LIVER TRV LT LOBE**

9. Axial image of the **RIGHT LOBE** to include the hepatic veins.

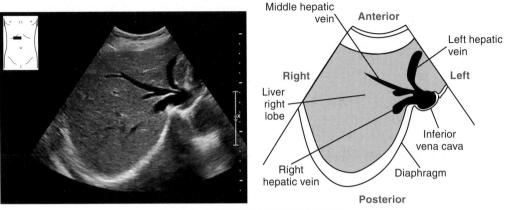

Labeled: **LIVER TRV RT LOBE**

10. Axial image of the **RIGHT LOBE** to include the right and left branches of the portal vein.

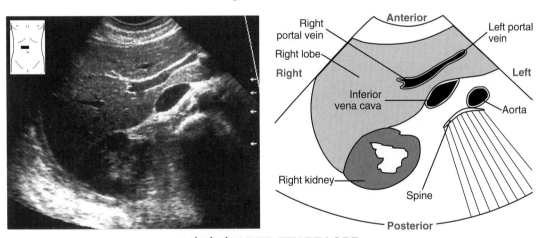

Labeled: **LIVER TRV RT LOBE**

11. Axial image of the **RIGHT LOBE** to include the main portal vein entering the porta hepatis.

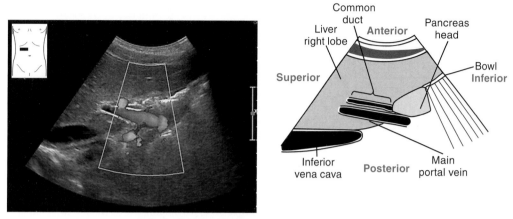

Labeled: **LIVER TRV RT LOBE**

12. Axial image of the **RIGHT LATERAL INFERIOR LOBE.**

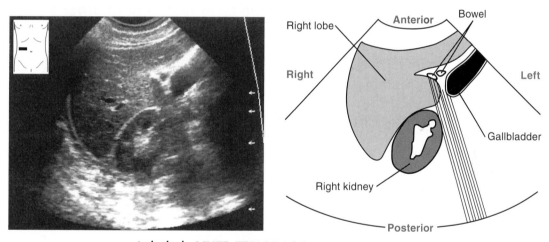

Labeled: **LIVER TRV RT LOBE**

13. Axial image of the **RIGHT LATERAL LOBE** to include the dome and the adjacent pleural space.

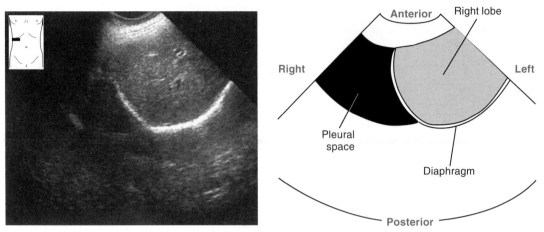

Labeled: **LIVER TRV RT LOBE**

Required Images When the Liver is Part of Another Study

- Required images of the liver are always the *same*, whether it is the primary area of interest or part of another study.

Review Questions

Answers on page 629.

1. The sonographic appearance of normal liver parenchyma may be described as
   a) hypoechoic relative to normal renal cortex.
   b) heterogeneous with low-level echoes.
   c) homogeneous with medium-level echoes.
   d) hyperechoic relative to the pancreas.

2. The vascular branches seen scattered throughout the liver parenchyma are
   a) pulmonary and hepatic veins.
   b) portal veins.
   c) hepatic veins.
   d) portal and hepatic veins.

3. The portal vein is formed by the confluence of the
   a) splenic vein, and superior and inferior mesenteric veins.
   b) superior and inferior mesenteric veins.
   c) splenic vein, pancreatic duct, and common bile duct.
   d) splenic and superior mesenteric veins.

4. The portal triad is found at the level of the _____, and consists of the _____.
   a) porta hepatis; hepatic artery, bile duct, and portal vein
   b) confluence of the portal vein; gastroduodenal artery, bile duct, and portal vein
   c) porta hepatis; hepatic artery, gastroduodenal artery, and IVC
   d) porta hepatis; cystic duct, bile duct, and portal vein

5. The liver is intraperitoneal except for interruptions at the gallbladder fossa, porta hepatis, and falciform ligament, portions around the IVC, and _____
   a) the superior surface.
   b) the anterior surface.
   c) the bare area.
   d) Glisson's capsule.

6. The liver is divided into lobes according to _____ and into segments according to _____.
   a) function; anatomy
   b) function; biliary drainage
   c) anatomy; function
   d) blood supply; biliary drainage

7. The main lobar fissure of the liver
   a) subdivides the right lobe into anterior and posterior portions.
   b) runs between the right branch of the portal vein and the neck of the gallbladder.
   c) forms the left boundary of the medial portion of the left lobe.
   d) runs between the left branch of the portal vein and the neck of the gallbladder.

8. The caudate lobe is located on which surface of the liver?
   a) Inferior
   b) Posterior
   c) Anterior
   d) Superior

9. The right, left, and middle hepatic veins
   a) converge at the porta hepatis.
   b) drain the blood from the right lobe of the liver.
   c) empty into the IVC.
   d) empty into the main portal vein.

10. A longitudinal section of the right and left branches of the portal vein is seen in a
    a) sagittal scanning plane.
    b) longitudinal view of the right lobe of the liver.
    c) transverse scanning plane.
    d) axial section of the left lobe of the liver.

11. Anteroposterior measurement of the adult liver should not be larger than
    a) 12 cm.
    b) 15 cm.
    c) 20 cm.
    d) 25 cm.

12. Which ligament separates the left lobe from the caudate lobe?
    a) Coronary
    b) Venosum
    c) Falciform
    d) Hepatoduodenal

13. Segmental lobar anatomy divides the liver into ____ lobes.
    a) Three
    b) Four
    c) Six
    d) Eight

14. The right lobe of the liver is divided into anterior and posterior segments by the _____
    a) middle hepatic vein.
    b) right hepatic vein.
    c) right portal vein.
    d) main portal vein.

15. The normal liver should have a/an _____ sonographic appearance.
    a) homogeneous
    b) heterogeneous
    c) low-level echogenicity
    d) anechoic

16. Hepatic veins _____ in size as they drain toward the IVC.
    a) remain the same
    b) increase
    c) decrease

17. What percentage of the total blood flow to the liver does the portal system supply?
    a) 30
    b) 50
    c) 75
    d) 90

18. The common bile duct and the hepatic artery follow a/an _____ course to the portal vein within the liver.
    a) medial
    b) anterior
    c) posterior
    d) superior

19. Just anterior to the portal vein within the liver lies the common bile duct and the hepatic artery.
    a) True
    b) False

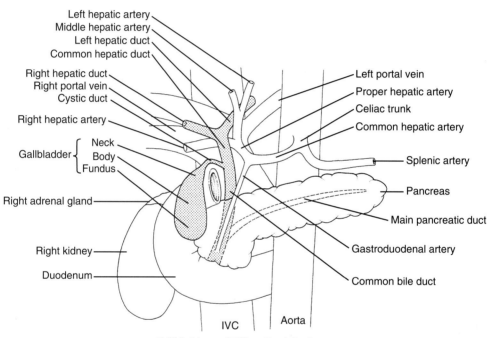

Left hepatic artery
Middle hepatic artery
Left hepatic duct
Common hepatic duct

Right hepatic duct
Right portal vein
Cystic duct

Right hepatic artery

Gallbladder { Neck
Body
Fundus

Right adrenal gland

Right kidney

Duodenum

Left portal vein
Proper hepatic artery
Celiac trunk
Common hepatic artery

Splenic artery

Pancreas

Main pancreatic duct

Gastroduodenal artery

Common bile duct

IVC   Aorta

Gallbladder and Biliary Tract Anatomy

CHAPTER 7

Gallbladder and Biliary Tract Scanning Protocol

Betty Bates Tempkin

Key Words

Ampulla of Vater	Left intrahepatic duct
Common bile duct (CBD)	Main lobar fissure (MLF)
Common duct	Main pancreatic duct
Common hepatic duct (CHD)	Porta hepatis
Cystic duct	Portal triad
Hepatic artery	Retroduodenal CBD
Intraperitoneal	Right intrahepatic duct

Objectives

At the end of this chapter, you will be able to:

- Define the key words.
- Distinguish the sonographic appearance of the gallbladder and biliary tract and the terms used to describe it.
- Describe the transducer options for scanning the gallbladder and biliary tract.
- List the various suggested breathing techniques for patients when scanning the gallbladder and biliary tract.
- List the suggested patient positions (and options) when scanning the gallbladder and biliary tract.
- Describe the patient preparation for a gallbladder and biliary tract study.
- Distinguish the gallbladder and biliary tract normal variants.
- Name the survey steps and explain how to evaluate the entire length, width, and depth of the gallbladder and biliary tract.
- Explain the order and exact locations to take representative images of the gallbladder and biliary tract.
- Answer the review questions at the end of the chapter.

Overview

Location

- The gallbladder (GB) and biliary tract are intraperitoneal structures (enclosed in the sac formed by the parietal peritoneum).
- The gallbladder is located in the fossa on the posteroinferior portion of the right lobe of the liver. The gallbladder fossa is closely

related to the **main lobar fissure (MLF)** of the liver, one of the normal folds throughout the liver that typically form the spaces that contain various blood vessels or ligaments. The MLF runs obliquely between the neck of the gallbladder and right portal vein. It contains the middle hepatic vein and separates the right and left hepatic lobes. Its course is short and variable.

- The gallbladder is extremely variable in position and location as a portion of it is attached by long mesentery, allowing for movement. The neck or narrow portion of the gallbladder, however, is fixed in its position at the main lobar fissure.
- The biliary tract or "tree" runs between the liver and the duodenum.

Anatomy

- The **right** and **left intrahepatic ducts** exit the liver at the **porta hepatis** (area of the hilus/opening where the portal vein and hepatic artery enter the liver and the common duct exits) and meet to form the **common duct**. The superior or *proximal portion* of the common duct is referred to as the **common hepatic duct (CHD)**. The CHD runs slightly inferomedially where it is joined by the **cystic duct** (directs bile from the CHD into the neck of the gallbladder) to form the *distal portion* of the common duct, the **common bile duct (CBD)**. The CBD courses inferior and medial, all the way to the duodenum.
- As the CBD courses inferomedially, it is referred to as the **retroduodenal CBD**, as it passes behind the first part of the duodenum en route to the head of the pancreas. At the head of the pancreas the CBD either *passes through* the pancreatic head or *runs along a groove* on the posterior surface of the head to meet with the **main pancreatic duct** (or duct of Wirsung, which transports and discharges pancreatic enzymes into the duodenum). Joined together or separately, the CBD and duct of Wirsung course slightly to the right to enter the second portion of the duodenum at the **ampulla of Vater**, a dilatation of the duodenum, where they empty bile and pancreatic juices to aid the digestive process.

- Normal *common duct size* is variable according to the amount of bile it contains and patient age. The common duct is known to enlarge with age. CHD is considered normal in size up to 4 mm; the CBD up to 6 mm. Following loss of GB function (as a result of cholecystectomy or gallbladder disease), the common duct assumes bile storage function and is considered normal in size up to 10 mm.
- The gallbladder is a muscular, membranous sac that has been described as pear-shaped, conical, or like a partially filled water balloon. Its narrow end is called the **neck,** a tube-like structure that joins the cystic duct. Its rounded "bottom" is called the **fundus.** The portion between the neck and fundus is called the **body.**
- The gallbladder serves as a storage site for bile; it is not essential to life. Without the gallbladder, the biliary tract (ducts) continues to transport bile from the liver to the duodenum.
- The *size of the gallbladder* is variable according to the amount of bile it is storing. It is considered normal up to 3 cm wide and 7 cm to 10 cm long. In a fasting patient, the gallbladder wall measurement is considered normal up to 3 mm.

Physiology
- The gallbladder and biliary tract are considered accessories to the digestive system because they store and transport the bile that is manufactured in the liver to the duodenum to help digest fat.
- The hepatic and biliary ducts passively transport bile directly to the second portion of the duodenum or by way of the gallbladder where bile is stored and concentrated.

Sonographic Appearance

- Since the position of the gallbladder is variable depending on the amount of bile it contains and/or the length of its mesenteric attachment its orientation in the body is also variable. Therefore, the gallbladder long axis can be visualized in any scanning plane.
- As demonstrated in the images below, *A*, the normal bile-filled gallbladder appears longitudinally as an anechoic, oblong structure with bright, thin walls and *B*, axial sections appear as anechoic, round or oval structures with bright, thin walls.

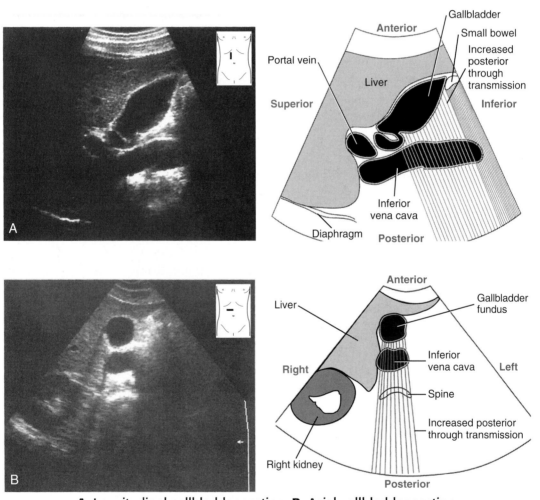

A, Longitudinal gallbladder section. **B,** Axial gallbladder section.

- The following images show how *A*, the bile-filled common duct appears longitudinally as an anechoic tubular structure with bright, thin walls and *B*, axial sections of the duct appear as small, anechoic, round structures with bright, thin walls.

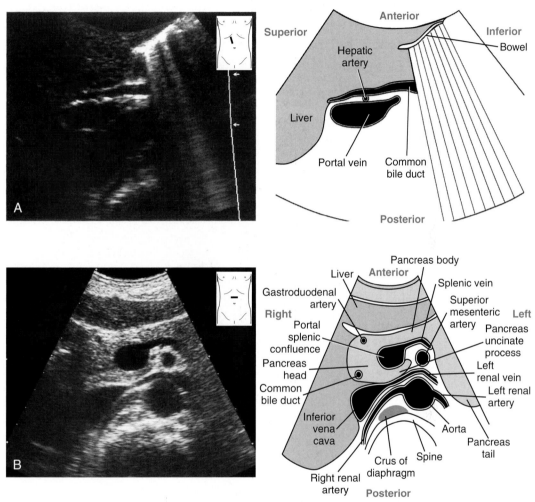

A, Longitudinal common duct section in a sagittal scanning plane.
B, Axial CBD section in a transverse scanning plane.

- When there is a question of dilated bile ducts, it is important to make a distinction between the structures that comprise the portal triad: the *proper hepatic artery, common duct*, and *portal vein* at the level of the porta hepatis. The following oblique, transverse scanning plane image shows that at the level of the porta hepatis, the portal vein (1) lies posterior to the proper hepatic artery (2), which is on the left and the CBD (3), located on the right. The appearance of the axial sections of the portal triad is often referred to as "Mickey's sign" as they resemble a face and two ears.

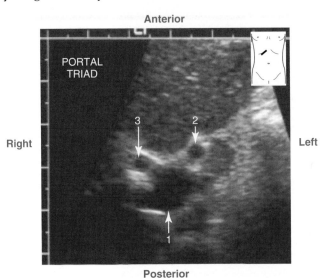

(From Brant WE: The Core Curriculum: Ultrasound. Lippincott Williams & Wilkins, 2001.)

Normal Variants
Gallbladder
- Shape variations:
  - **Segmental contractions:** These "segments" disappear when the patient changes position or fasts.
  - **Phrygian cap:** The fundus is folded over giving the gallbladder a "capped" appearance.
- Position variations:
  - The position and location of the gallbladder is variable because it is suspended by long mesentery.
  - Very rare, deep fossa, intrahepatic gallbladder.
- Septations:
  - May partially or totally divide the gallbladder.

Biliary Tract
- Duplications:
  - Although very rare, the common duct may be partially or completely duplicated.

- Level variations:
  - The level of the junction of the cystic duct and common hepatic ducts is variable.
- Septations:
  - May partially or totally divide the cystic duct, producing various degrees of double gallbladder.

Preparation

Patient Prep
- The patient should fast for 8 to 12 hours before the study. This ensures normal gallbladder and biliary tract dilatation and reduces the amount of bowel gas.
- If the patient has eaten within 4 to 6 hours, still attempt the examination.

> **NOTE:** A nonvisualized gallbladder is indicative of either gallbladder disease or the patient recently eating. Therefore, it is essential to determine when a patient last ate.

Transducer
- **3.0 MHz** or **3.5 MHz.**
- 5.0 MHz for thin patients.

Breathing Technique
- **Deep, held inspiration.**

> **NOTE:** Different breathing techniques should be used whenever the suggested breathing technique does not produce the desired results.

Patient Position
- The gallbladder and biliary tract study is performed with the patient in two different positions.
- **Supine and left lateral decubitus.**
- Left posterior oblique, sitting semierect to erect or prone as needed.

> **NOTE:** Different patient positions are required when examining the gallbladder to help differentiate certain abnormalities from each other. For example, gallstones and sludge will move and change their position within the gallbladder when the patient position is changed. Gallbladder polyps and carcinoma remain stationary.
> **NOTE:** Different patient positions should be used whenever the suggested positions do not produce the desired results.

Gallbladder and Biliary Tract Survey Steps

> **NOTE:** The gallbladder and biliary tract **must** be surveyed in **two different patient positions**.

Gallbladder • Longitudinal Survey
Sagittal Plane • Transabdominal Anterior Approach • First Patient Position

> **NOTE:** Generally, the gallbladder tends to lie in the area between the right medial angle of the ribs and the superior pole of the right kidney.

First Patient Position: Supine

1. Begin scanning with the transducer perpendicular, just inferior to the costal margin at the right medial angle of the ribs. Have the patient take in a deep breath and hold it. In most cases, the portal vein and gallbladder neck should come into view. If the gallbladder is not visualized here, locate the bright main lobar fissure of the liver that extends from the right branch of the portal vein to the gallbladder neck.

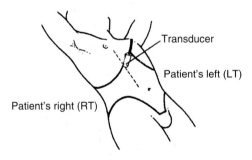

> **NOTE:** If the gallbladder is still not visualized, try moving the transducer slightly inferior and right lateral. Subcostal transducer angles can also help locate the gallbladder. In some cases, intercostal scanning may be necessary to view the gallbladder.

2. Once the gallbladder is identified, find its long axis. This can be accomplished by slightly twisting/rotating the transducer first one way, then the other, to oblique the scanning plane according to the lie of the gallbladder. Occasionally, no oblique is necessary.

> **NOTE:** If the long axis of the gallbladder cannot be resolved in the sagittal plane, rotate the transducer 90 degrees into the transverse scanning plane. Remember that gallbladder lie is variable and the scanning plane must be adjusted accordingly.

3. Assuming the long axis is identified in the sagittal plane, begin the survey by *very* slightly rocking the transducer from right to left, sweeping through both side margins of the gallbladder while at the same time *very* slowly sliding inferiorly through and beyond the fundus.

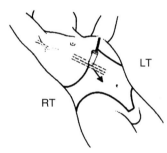

4. Continue rocking and sliding and move the transducer back onto the fundus, then *very* slowly rock and slide superiorly, surveying through and beyond the gallbladder body and neck.

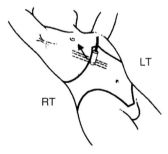

Gallbladder • Axial Survey

Transverse Plane • Transabdominal Anterior Approach • First Patient Position

1. Relocate the gallbladder long axis in the sagittal plane. Move inferiorly to view the fundus then *very* slowly rotate the transducer 90 degrees into the transverse plane. A round or oval axial section of the fundus will come into view.

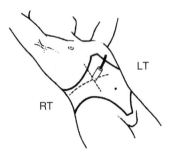

2. *Very* slightly rock the transducer superior to inferior and at the same time slowly slide inferiorly, through and beyond the fundus.

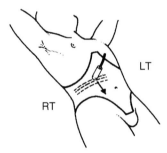

3. Continue rocking and slide the transducer superiorly back onto the fundus and continue scanning up through the body and neck until you are beyond the gallbladder.

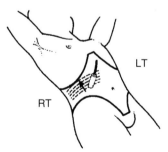

Biliary Tract • Longitudinal Survey
Sagittal Plane • Transabdominal Anterior Approach • First Patient Position

1. Begin scanning by relocating the long axis of the gallbladder. Identify the neck, main lobar fissure, and portal vein. Look for a small, anechoic, longitudinal section of the common duct just anterior to the portal vein. It may be necessary to *very* slightly twist/rotate the transducer, first one way, then the other to oblique the scanning plane according to the lie of the duct and to resolve its long axis.

   NOTE: The common duct usually lies at a right angle to the costal margin.

   NOTE: In a sagittal oblique plane, at the level of the porta hepatis, the portal vein will be traversed, seen as round or oval, in a short axis/axial section. Just inferior to this level, the portal vein appears longitudinal as it runs posterior and parallel to the common duct.

2. Barely rock the transducer right to left, sweeping through both sides of the common duct and at the same time *very slowly* slide the transducer *slightly* superior and right lateral to survey through and beyond the margin of the proximal portion of the duct. The distance moved is *very* small.

   NOTE: Notice the appearance of the small, anechoic, axial section of the hepatic artery running between the long sections of the duct and the portal vein.

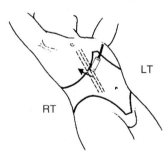

3. Move the transducer just inferior, back onto the duct then return to the level of the gallbladder neck and main lobar fissure.

4. Continue the survey by barely rocking the transducer right to left and at the same time *very slowly* slide the transducer *slightly* inferior and medial to scan through and beyond the distal portion of the duct at the level of the head of the pancreas. The distance moved is *very* small.

Remain at this level to begin the axial survey of the duct.

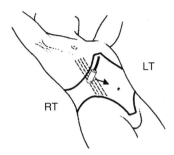

> **NOTE:** The distal portion of the duct or CBD can be difficult to visualize for the short distance that it runs behind the duodenum due to overlying bowel gas. When this occurs, continue to scan through the duodenum and pick up the duct again just on the other side of the duodenum or at the head of the pancreas. To visualize this retroduodenal portion of the duct, some institutions have patients drink enough water to fill the duodenum. The water displaces the bowel gas and serves as an acoustic "window" to view the duct.

Biliary Tract • Axial Survey
Transverse Plane • Transabdominal Anterior Approach • First Patient Position

> **NOTE:** Because of the small diameter of the common duct, a complete axial survey can be difficult. Therefore, when measurements are within normal limits it is acceptable to evaluate the axial sections of the proximal portion of the duct (the CHD) at the level of the GB neck and the distal portion of the duct (the CBD) at the level of the head of the pancreas.

1. While still in the sagittal plane relocate the long axis of the common bile duct (CBD) at the level of the head of the pancreas. *Very slowly* rotate the transducer 90 degrees into the transverse plane. Look for the small, round, anechoic section of the CBD within the posterolateral portion of the pancreas head. In most cases, the small axial section of the gastroduodenal artery can also be identified anterior to the CBD in the anterolateral portion of the pancreas head.

2. Return to the sagittal plane and relocate the long axis view of the gallbladder neck. Move the transducer *slightly* superior to the neck and a longitudinal section of the common hepatic duct (CHD) anterior to the portal vein should come into view. Resolve the long axis of the duct then *very* slowly rotate the transducer 90 degrees into the transverse plane. Look for the small, round, anechoic section of the CHD anterior to the portal vein.

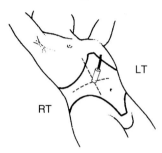

Gallbladder • Longitudinal Survey
Sagittal Plane • Transabdominal Anterior Approach •
Second Patient Position
Second Patient Position: Left Lateral Decubitus
Follow the same survey steps used for the *first patient position* for longitudinal and axial gallbladder surveys and longitudinal and axial surveys of the common duct.

Gallbladder and Biliary Tract Required Images

NOTE: The required images are a small representation of what a sonographer visualizes during a study. Therefore, the images should provide the interpreting physician with the most telling and technically accurate information available.

Gallbladder • Longitudinal Images
Sagittal Plane • Transabdominal Anterior Approach •
First Patient Position/Supine

NOTE: The gallbladder **must** be documented in **two different patient positions.**

1. **LONG AXIS** image of the gallbladder.

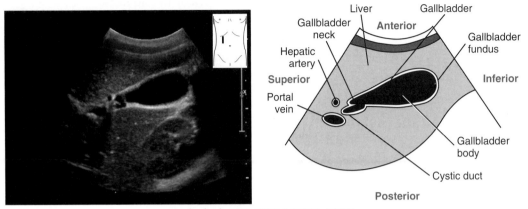

Labeled: **GB SAG LONG AXIS**

> **NOTE:** In many cases gallbladder definition is sacrificed to achieve the long axis. Therefore, additional longitudinal images of the gallbladder fundus, body, and neck should be documented.

2. Longitudinal image of the **GALLBLADDER FUNDUS** and **BODY.**

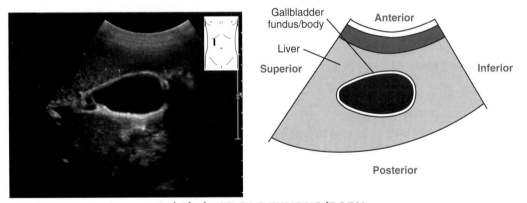

Labeled: **GB SAG FUNDUS/BODY**

3. Longitudinal image of the **GALLBLADDER NECK.**

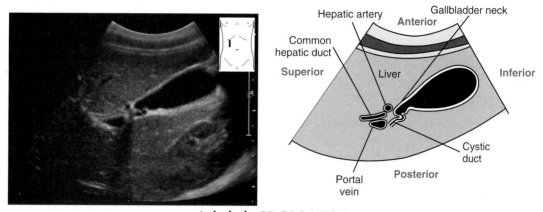

Labeled: **GB SAG NECK**

NOTE: The area where the neck of the gallbladder joins the cystic duct is described as the spiral valve due to its tortuous appearance. This reference is to appearance only because there is no valvular action.

Gallbladder • Axial Images

Transverse Plane • Transabdominal Anterior Approach • First Patient Position/Supine

4. Axial image of the **GALLBLADDER FUNDUS.**

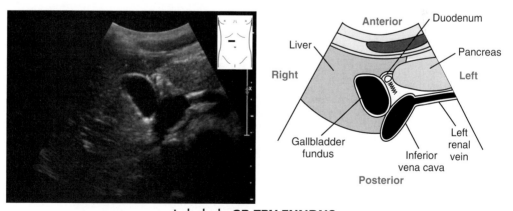

Labeled: **GB TRV FUNDUS**

5. Axial image of the **GALLBLADDER BODY.**

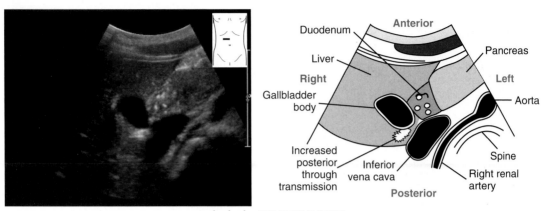

Labeled: **GB TRV BODY**

6. Axial image of the **GALLBLADDER NECK.**

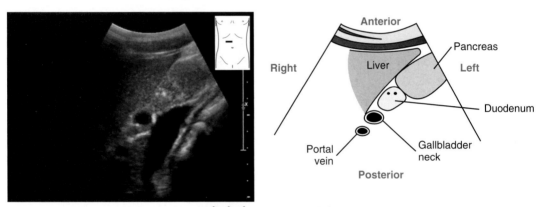

Labeled: **GB TRV NECK**

7. Axial image of the **GALLBLADDER** *with anterior wall measurement.*

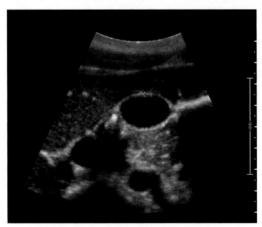

Labeled: **GB ANT WALL MS**

NOTE: Gallbladder wall thickness is typically evaluated from the short-axis. Measure the anterior wall at its most narrow point. Remember to keep the transducer perpendicular to the gallbladder wall for an accurate measurement.

Biliary Tract • Longitudinal Images
Sagittal Plane • Transabdominal Anterior Approach • First Patient Position

NOTE: Images of the common duct may be taken in the second patient position if the duct was better visualized in that position during the survey. Also, common duct images can be magnified to aide physician interpretation.
NOTE: As a general rule, CHD measurements are only required when the CBD measurement is abnormal.
NOTE: The longitudinal image of the CHD can be omitted if the duct was well visualized on the longitudinal image of the gallbladder neck or long axis gallbladder images.

8. Longitudinal image of the **COMMON HEPATIC DUCT (CHD).**

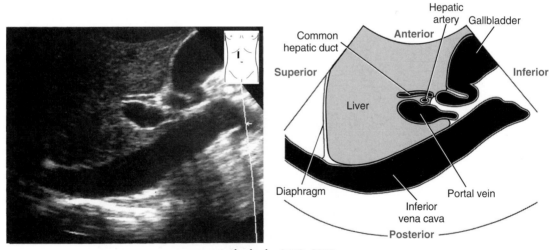

Labeled: **SAG CHD**

9. Longitudinal image of the **COMMON BILE DUCT (CBD)** *with anterior to posterior measurement (from interior margin of anterior wall to interior margin of posterior wall).*

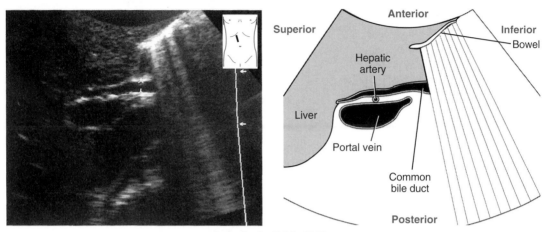

Labeled: **SAG CHD**

NOTE: Notice how the measurement of the CBD is at the widest margins of the lumen. Sometimes Doppler is helpful to differentiate the CBD and hepatic artery. Axial images and measurements are not required for the CHD and CBD unless the longitudinal CBD measurement exceeds the normal limit.

10. Same image as 9 *without calipers.*

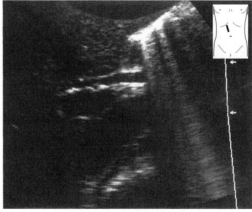

Labeled: **SAG CHD**

Gallbladder • Longitudinal Image
Sagittal Plane • Transabdominal Anterior Approach • Second Patient Position/Left Lateral Decubitus
11. **LONG AXIS** image of the gallbladder.

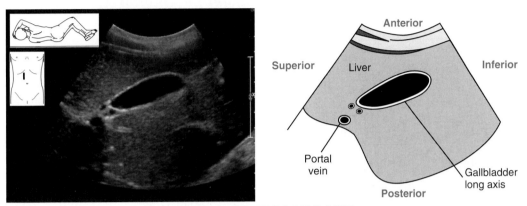

Labeled: **GB SAG LONG AXIS**

Gallbladder • Axial Image
Transverse Plane • Transabdominal Anterior Approach • Second Patient Position/Left Lateral Decubitus
12. Axial image of the **GALLBLADDER FUNDUS.**

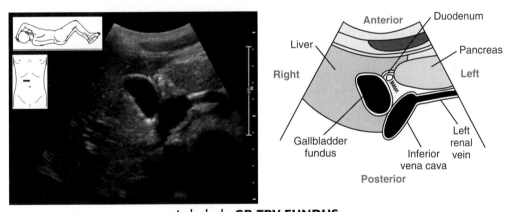

Labeled: **GB TRV FUNDUS**

Required Images When the Gallbladder and Biliary Tract are Part of Another Study

Gallbladder • Longitudinal Image
Sagittal Plane • Transabdominal Anterior Approach
1. **LONG AXIS** image of the gallbladder.

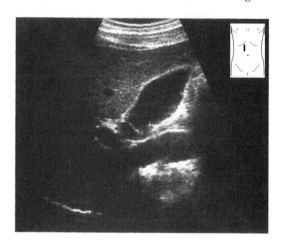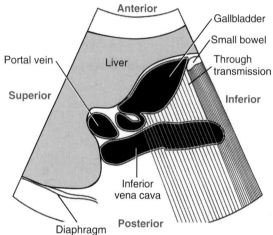

Labeled: **GB SAG LONG AXIS**

Gallbladder • Axial Image
Transverse Plane • Transabdominal Anterior Approach
2. Axial image of the **GALLBLADDER FUNDUS.**

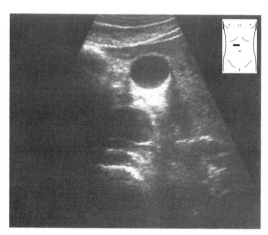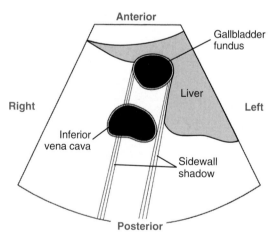

Labeled: **GB TRV FUNDUS**

Biliary Tract • Longitudinal Images
Sagittal Plane • Transabdominal Anterior Approach

NOTE: Common duct images can be magnified to aide physician interpretation.
NOTE: The longitudinal image of the CHD can be omitted if the duct was well visualized on the longitudinal image of the gallbladder neck or long axis gallbladder images.

3. Longitudinal image of the **COMMON HEPATIC DUCT (CHD).**

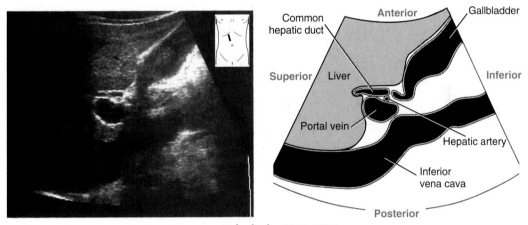

Labeled: **SAG CHD**

4. Longitudinal image of the **COMMON BILE DUCT (CBD)** *with anterior to posterior measurement (from interior margin of anterior wall to interior margin of posterior wall).*

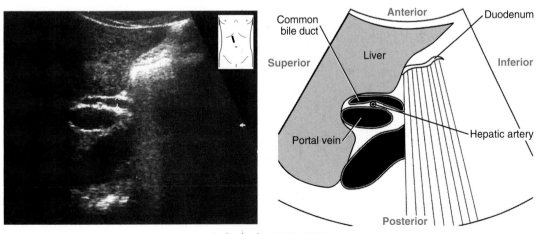

Labeled: **SAG CBD**

NOTE: Notice how the measurement of the CBD is at the widest margins of the lumen. Sometimes Doppler is helpful to differentiate the CBD and hepatic artery. Axial images and measurements are not required for the CHD and CBD unless the longitudinal CBD measurement exceeds the normal limit.

5. Same image as 4 *without calipers*.

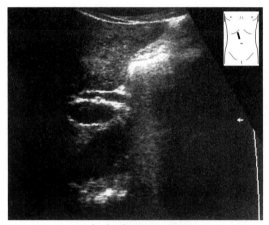

Labeled: **SAG CBD**

Review Questions

Answers on page 629.

1. The long axis of the gallbladder is visualized in
    a) a transverse scanning plane.
    b) either transverse, sagittal, or coronal scanning planes depending on its position.
    c) a sagittal scanning plane.
    d) longitudinal scanning planes.

2. What can help in the evaluation of the retroduodenal portion of the CBD?
    a) use water to displace the bowel gas.
    b) glucagon.
    c) intercostal, left lateral decubitus approach.
    d) use a sharp transducer angle right laterally from the midline.

3. In a sagittal scanning plane at the level of the porta hepatis the portal vein will be
    a) seen in long axis.
    b) seen in short axis.
    c) anterior to the common duct.
    d) anterior to the hepatic artery.

4. Different patient positions are used when evaluating the gallbladder because
    a) it distinguishes certain abnormalities from each other.
    b) single position evaluation is not enough confirmation.
    c) of the variability of the position of the gallbladder.
    d) it unfolds the gallbladder.

5. _____describes a folded gallbladder fundus.
    a) segmental contraction.
    b) Santorini's fold.
    c) biliary bend.
    d) Phrygian cap.

6. The long axis view of the common duct is seen
    a) in an oblique sagittal scanning plane.
    b) in an oblique transverse scanning plane.
    c) posterior to the long axis of the hepatic artery.
    d) posterior to the axial sections of the portal vein.

7. The gallbladder tends to lie in the
    a) retroperitoneum.
    b) midepigastrium.
    c) area between the right medial angle of the ribs and the superior pole of the right kidney.
    d) area just inferior to the level of the costal margin.

8. The CBD is located to the hepatic artery.
    a) left lateral.
    b) right lateral.
    c) inferomedially.
    d) posterior.

9. The cystic duct connects the
   a) common hepatic and CBDs.
   b) common duct and pancreatic duct.
   c) common duct and gallbladder neck.
   d) gallbladder neck and body.

10. The spiral valve
    a) closes when the gallbladder is full of bile.
    b) regulates the flow of bile from the gallbladder.
    c) is the tortuous connection of the gallbladder and cystic duct.
    d) is the tortuous connection of the gallbladder and common duct.

11. The proximal portion of the common duct is
    a) called the CBD.
    b) appears traversed when viewed at the level of the porta hepatis in a sagittal plane.
    c) called the CHD.
    d) appears traversed when viewed at the level of the pancreas head in a sagittal scanning plane.

12. The distal portion of the common duct is
    a) called the CBD.
    b) appears traversed when viewed at the level of the porta hepatis in a sagittal plane.
    c) called the CHD.
    d) appears traversed when viewed at the level of the pancreas head in a sagittal scanning plane.

13. The common duct usually lies at a right angle to the costal margin.
    a) true.
    b) false.

14. The gallbladder serves as a storage site for bile and is variable in size according to the amount of bile it is storing.
    a) true.
    b) false.

15. The CHD is considered normal in size up to
    a) 2 mm.
    b) 4 mm.
    c) 6 mm.
    d) 8 mm.

16. What is the normal diameter of the gallbladder wall?
    a) < 0.5 mm
    b) > 1.0 cm
    c) < 3 mm
    d) > 5 mm

17. The gallbladder is described in three major sections:
    a) head, neck, body.
    b) head, neck, fundus.
    c) left, middle, right.
    d) superior, medial, lateral.

18. The biliary system has three main functions. Which of the following is *not* a function?
    a) transports bile to the gallbladder.
    b) stores bile.
    c) transports bile to aid in digestion of fat.
    d) stores enzymes.

19. The biliary ducts are subdivided into intrahepatic and extrahepatic ducts.
    a) true.
    b) false.

20. A fold in the gallbladder fundus is called the Phrygian cap.
    a) true.
    b) false.

21. Intrahepatic bile ducts are not routinely visualized on ultrasound.
    a) true.
    b) false.

22. The gallbladder is an intraperitoneal organ.
    a) true.
    b) false.

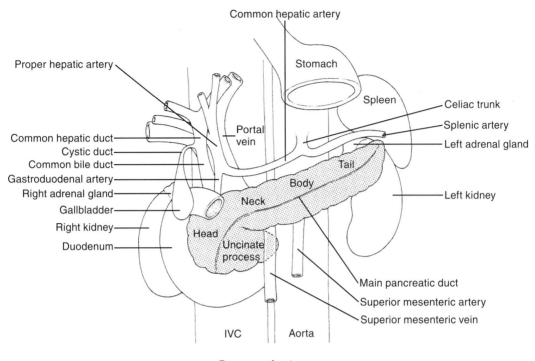

Pancreas Anatomy

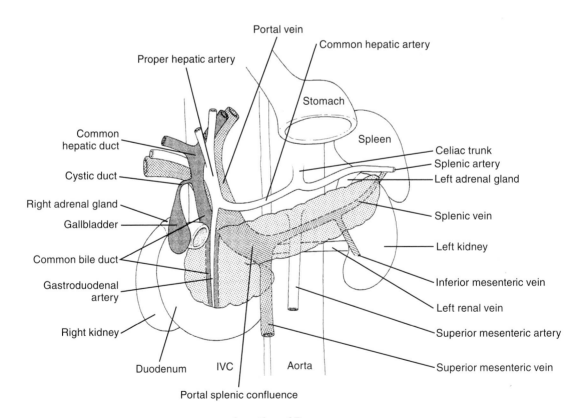

Location of Pancreas

CHAPTER 8

Pancreas Scanning Protocol

Betty Bates Tempkin

Key Words

Common bile duct (CBD)	Portal splenic confluence
Endocrine	Portal vein
Exocrine	Retroperitoneal
Gastroduodenal artery	Santorini's duct
Pancreas body	Splenic vein
Pancreas head	Superior mesenteric artery
Pancreas neck	Superior mesenteric vein
Pancreas tail	Wirsung's duct
Pancreas uncinate process	

Objectives

At the end of this chapter, you will be able to:

- Define the key words.
- Distinguish the sonographic appearance of the pancreas and the terms used to describe it.
- Describe the transducer options for scanning the pancreas.
- List the various suggested breathing techniques for patients when scanning the pancreas.
- List the suggested patient positions (and options) when scanning the pancreas.
- Describe the patient prep for a pancreas study.
- Distinguish normal variants of the pancreas.
- Name the survey steps and explain how to evaluate the entire length, width, and depth of the pancreas.
- Explain the order and exact locations to take representative images of the pancreas.
- Answer the review questions at the end of the chapter.

Overview

Location

- The pancreas is **retroperitoneal** (located in the *retroperitoneum,* the portion of abdominopelvic cavity posterior to the peritoneal sac). It extends from the second portion of the duodenum, across the midline, to the hilum of the spleen.
- The descriptive portions of the pancreas are located as follows:
  - (a) **Head:** The portion of pancreas immediately anterior to the inferior vena cava; between the medial curve of the second

portion of the duodenum and the **superior mesenteric vein.** Its lateral border is marked anteriorly by the **gastroduodenal artery** and posteriorly by the **common bile duct (CBD).**

(b) **Uncinate process:** A medial extension of the head that lies directly posterior to the superior mesenteric vein. It has been known to extend as far left as the aorta.

(c) **Neck:** The portion of pancreas directly anterior to the superior mesenteric vein.

(d) **Body:** The portion of pancreas that extends left lateral from the neck and lies between the posterior wall of the antrum of the stomach and the superior mesenteric artery. Its left lateral border is generally described as not definite.

(e) **Tail:** The portion of pancreas that typically lies posterior to the stomach, between the left lateral edge of the spine and the hilum of the spleen.

Anatomy

- The pancreas is a nonencapsulated multilobular gland. Its blood supply is from the *superior mesenteric artery, splenic artery,* and *gastroduodenal artery.* Venous drainage is through *splenic* and *superior mesenteric vein tributaries.*

- **Wirsung's duct,** the main pancreatic duct, extends the length of the pancreas and enlarges toward the head up to 3 mm. It meets with the common bile duct at the pancreas head, and joined together or separately, the ducts enter the second portion of the duodenum.

- **Santorini's duct** is a normal variant that serves as an accessory pancreatic duct from the anterior portion of the pancreas head. It enters the duodenum superior to and separate from Wirsung's duct and the common bile duct.

- The size, shape, and lie of the pancreas vary somewhat. The size decreases with age. The shape has been compared to a dumbbell, sausage, and a comma with the larger segment representing the head. The lie or orientation of the pancreas has varying degrees of horizontal oblique.

- The normal adult pancreas is 15 to 20|cm in length.
  - The anterior to posterior dimensions of the head range from 2.0 to 3.0|cm.
  - The anterior to posterior dimensions of the neck range from 1.5 to 2.5|cm.
  - The anterior to posterior dimensions of the body range from 1.5 to 2.5|cm.
  - The anterior to posterior dimensions of the tail range from 1.0 to 2.0|cm.

Physiology

- The pancreas has both endocrine and exocrine functions:
  - Endocrine function: produces the hormone insulin to prevent diabetes mellitus.
  - Exocrine function: produces pancreatic enzymes that, via the pancreatic ducts, aid digestion.

Sonographic Appearance

- Because the pancreas lies at a horizontal oblique in the body, the longitudinal and long axis sections are visualized in an obliqued transverse scanning plane. The following obliqued, transverse scanning plane image shows the long axis of a normal adult pancreas.

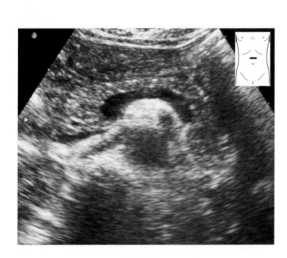 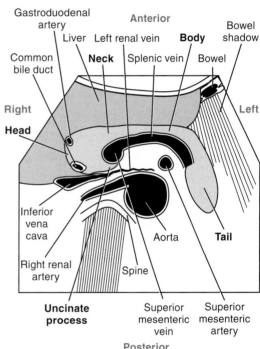

Notice how the pancreas appears midgray, with even texture that is moderately hyperechoic relative to the normal liver (in many cases the pancreas will appear isosonic to the liver). Observe the smooth contour of the pancreas and how it is distinguishable from adjacent structures (the pancreas is non-encapsulated, so it can be infiltrated by retroperitoneal fat making the contour uneven and difficult to evaluate in some cases). The anechoic, longitudinal section of the splenic vein running along the posterior margin of the pancreas *body* serves as an easily recognizable vascular landmark when identifying the pancreas. Notice how the splenic vein (coming from the splenic hilum) courses along the posterior aspect of the pancreas to join with the **superior mesenteric vein** directly behind, or posterior to, the pancreas *neck* (they join to form the portal vein).

The *head* of the pancreas is easily identified as it sits directly in front of, or anterior to, the inferior vena cava and is distinguished by the small anechoic axial sections of the gastroduodenal artery on its anterolateral border and the common bile duct on its posterolateral border. The pancreas *tail* is usually the most difficult part of the pancreas to visualize because it lies behind, or posterior to the stomach; however, it is well demonstrated in this image. Observe how the tail is left lateral to the spine and aorta and more posterior than the pancreas head.

- The axial sections of the pancreas are visualized in sagittal scanning planes (pictured on the facing page). The top scan *A,* is a sagittal scanning plane image showing an axial section of the pancreas *head.* It is easily identified as it sits directly anterior to the anechoic, longitudinal inferior vena cava and is distinguished by the small, anechoic, longitudinal sections of the gastroduodenal artery on its anterior border and the common bile duct on its posterior border.

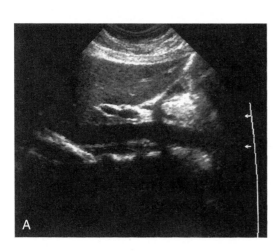

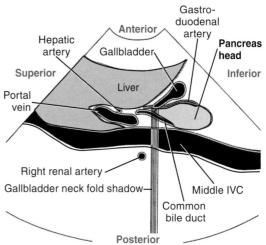

The anatomy in the bottom image *B,* is the same as the anatomy in the top image but the view is different. Now we see a transverse scanning plane image showing a long section of the pancreas; the *head* is clearly distinguished as it sits just anterior to the anechoic, axial inferior vena cava and the anechoic, axial sections of the gastroduodenal artery (anteriorly) and the common bile duct (posteriorly) are easily identified.

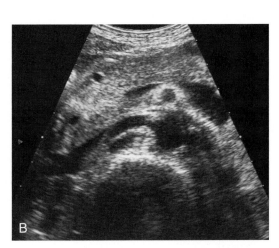

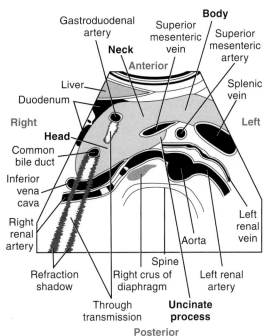

- The next images demonstrate axial and longitudinal views of the pancreas *neck*, *uncinate process*, and the *superior mesenteric vein* that separates them. The top scan *A,* is a sagittal scanning plane image, showing a longitudinal view of the superior mesenteric vein separating axial sections of the pancreas neck (seen anteriorly) and uncinate process (seen posteriorly). The bottom image *B,* is the same as the anatomy in the top image but the view is different. Now we see a transverse scanning plane image showing longitudinal views of the pancreas neck (anteriorly) and uncinate process (posteriorly), clearly separated by the anechoic, round, axial section of the superior mesenteric vein.

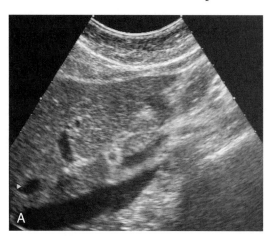
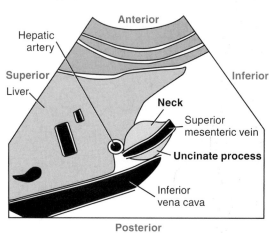

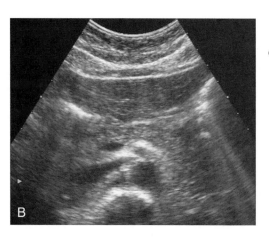
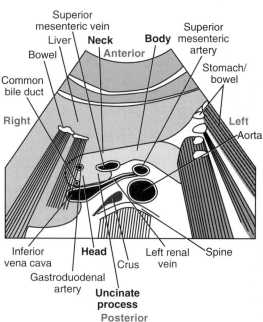

- The splenic vein and superior mesenteric artery serve as vascular landmarks when identifying the *body* of the pancreas. The top scan *A,* is a sagittal scanning plane image demonstrating an axial view of the pancreas body. Observe how the body is seen directly anterior to the anechoic, axial section of the splenic vein, which lies just anterior to the anechoic superior mesenteric artery seen in longitudinal section as it branches from the aorta. The splenic artery marks the superior edge of the pancreas body. Two anechoic, round, axial sections of the splenic artery are easily identified in this image. The anatomy in the bottom transverse scanning plane image *B,* is the same as the anatomy in the top image but the view is different. Now we see a longitudinal view of the pancreas body. Notice how the body sits just anterior to an anechoic, long section of the splenic vein, which is just anterior to the anechoic, round, axial section of the superior mesenteric artery.

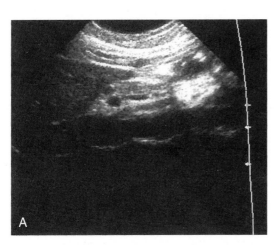
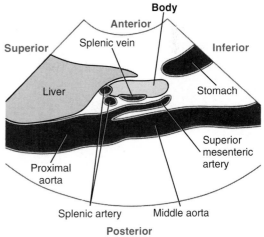
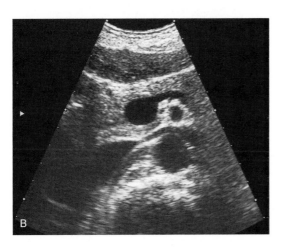
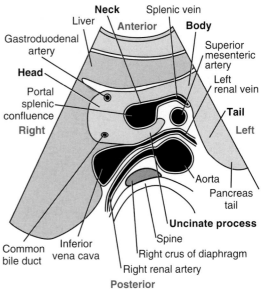

- The splenic vein also serves as a vascular landmark when identifying the *tail* of the pancreas. The left kidney is helpful when locating the tail as well (pictured below). The top scan *A*, is a sagittal scanning plane image, showing an axial section of the pancreas tail seen anterior to the anechoic, long splenic vein section and left kidney. The bottom scan *B*, is a transverse scanning plane image demonstrating the same anatomy as the top image but the view is different. Now we see a longitudinal view of the pancreas tail clearly anterior to the anechoic, axial splenic vein section, left lateral to the spine and posterior to the stomach. Note the left kidney directly posterior to the splenic vein.

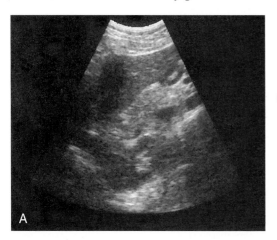
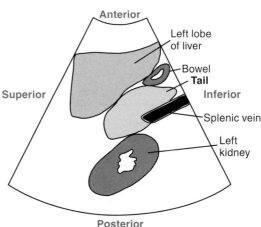

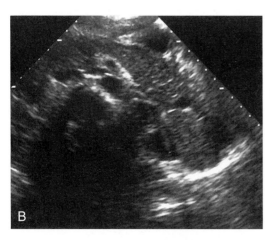
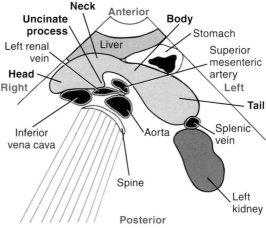

- *Wirsung's duct* (or the pancreatic duct) is commonly seen and most frequently in the body portion of the pancreas. It appears anterior to the anechoic, long splenic vein sections either as a long, thin, bright line or as an anechoic, longitudinal section bordered by thin, bright walls as seen in the following image:

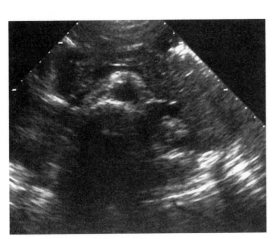
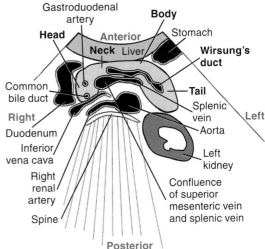

Normal Variants
- The size, shape, and lie of the pancreas are normally variable.
- The duct of Santorini is a normal variant accessory duct.

Preparation

Patient Prep
- The patient should fast for 8 to 12 hours before the study. This reduces the amount of stomach and bowel gas anterior to the pancreas and ensures normal gallbladder and biliary tract dilatation, which is significant because the pancreas and biliary tract are interdependent systems.
- If the patient has eaten, still attempt the examination because in some cases, stomach contents can displace gas and serve as a "window" for the sound beam. Also, for this reason, the patient can be given 2 to 4 cups of water or noncarbonated drink to provide a sonic window and displace any gas in the stomach that may be obscuring the view of the pancreas. In most cases, this fluid technique works best if the patient is sitting erect.

NOTE: When using a fluid technique, peristalsis can cause the fluid to pass very quickly through the stomach and duodenum not allowing enough time to fully evaluate the area of interest. Therefore, peristaltic-reducing drugs can be administered to the patient to slow down peristaltic action.

Transducer

- Curved array 5.1 MHz or 5.2 MHz.
- 10.4, 8.5 MHz for thin patients.

Breathing Technique

- Deep, held inspiration.

> **NOTE:** Different breathing techniques should be used whenever the suggested breathing technique does not produce the desired results.

Patient Position

- **Supine.**
- Sitting semi-erect to erect, left posterior oblique, left lateral decubitus, or prone as needed.

> **NOTE:** Different patient positions should be used whenever the suggested positions do not produce the desired results.

Pancreas Survey Steps

Pancreas • Longitudinal Survey

Transverse Plane • Transabdominal Anterior Approach

1. Begin scanning with the transducer perpendicular, at the midline of the body, just inferior to the xiphoid process of the sternum. Have the patient take in a deep breath and hold it. Slightly rock the transducer superior to inferior while slowly sliding the transducer inferiorly. Look for the *body* of the pancreas to come into view just inferior to the level of the celiac axis branch of the aorta. You should be able to identify an anechoic, longitudinal section of the splenic vein running along the posterior margin of the pancreas body. Round, anechoic, axial sections of the superior mesenteric artery and the aorta should be seen posterior to the long section of the splenic vein.

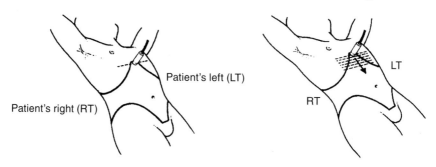

Patient's left (LT)

Patient's right (RT)

LT

RT

2. When the pancreas body is identified, it may be necessary to very slightly twist/rotate the transducer—first one way, then the other—to resolve the long axis of the body. Then, to evaluate the rest of the pancreas body, begin by moving the transducer very slowly superiorly, scanning through and beyond the pancreas margin. Now very slowly slide the transducer inferiorly back onto the body until you scan through and beyond the pancreas. Look for the pancreatic duct(s) running through the center of the body of the pancreas.

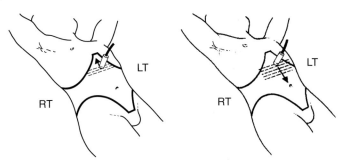

3. To evaluate the *tail,* relocate the long axis of the pancreas body and slightly move the transducer left lateral until you see the pancreas tail in the area between the stomach (anteriorly) and left kidney (posteriorly). As with the pancreas body, long sections or portions of the anechoic splenic vein can be seen along the tail's posterior edge. When the tail is identified, it may be necessary to very slightly twist the transducer—first one way, then the other—to resolve its long axis. Then, to evaluate the rest of the pancreas tail, begin by moving the transducer very slowly superiorly, scanning through and beyond the pancreas margin. Now very slowly slide the transducer inferiorly until you scan through and beyond the tail. Look for the pancreatic duct(s) in the central portion of the tail.

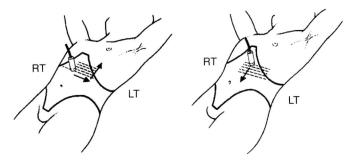

NOTE: If gas from the stomach is obscuring the view of the pancreas tail and the fluid technique cannot be utilized because the patient is restricted from fluids, then you may have to evaluate the tail from an angle or from a posterior approach. The angled view is obtained by relocating the pancreas body then angling the transducer toward the patient's left at varying degrees until the pancreas tail is identified. Once located, finish evaluating the tail from that angle. (If any images are taken from an angle it must be noted as part of the documentation.) When using a posterior approach, the patient may sit erect or lie prone. It is usually helpful to begin by locating the superior pole of the left kidney (just lateral to the spine) then look for the tail in the area directly anterior to the superior pole.

4. To evaluate the *neck* of the pancreas, relocate the long axis of the pancreas body and *very* slightly move the transducer right lateral. Look for the pancreas neck to appear either directly anterior to the anechoic, round axial section of the superior mesenteric vein or the anechoic **portal splenic confluence** at its inferior portion. Very slightly twisting/rotating the transducer can help resolve the longitudinal margins of the neck. To evaluate the rest of the pancreas neck, begin by moving the transducer very slowly superiorly, scanning through and beyond the pancreas margin. Now slowly slide the transducer inferiorly until you scan through and beyond the neck. You may see a portion of the pancreatic duct in the central portion of the neck.

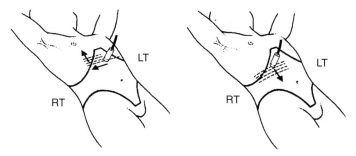

NOTE: If gas is obscuring the view of the pancreas neck and the fluid technique cannot be utilized because the patient is restricted from fluids, then you may have to evaluate the neck from an angle. The angled view is obtained by relocating the pancreas body then angling the transducer toward the patient's right at varying degrees until the pancreas neck is identified. Once located, finish evaluating the neck from that angle. (If any images are taken from an angle it must be noted as part of the image labeling.)

5. To evaluate the *head* and *uncinate process* of the pancreas, relocate the long axis of the neck and *very* slightly move the transducer inferior and right lateral. Look for the head and uncinate process to appear directly anterior to the round or oval anechoic, axial section of the inferior vena cava (IVC). The uncinate process will be just posterior to the anechoic, axial superior mesenteric vein section. Very slightly twisting/rotating the transducer can help resolve the longitudinal margins of the head and uncinate. To evaluate the rest of the pancreas head and uncinate begin by moving the transducer very slowly superiorly, scanning through and beyond the pancreas margin. Now very slowly slide the transducer inferiorly until you scan through and beyond the level of the head and uncinate. In the head, look for the small, round, anechoic, axial sections of the common bile duct at the posterolateral edge and the gastroduodenal artery at the anterolateral edge. In the central portion of the head, try to identify the pancreatic duct.

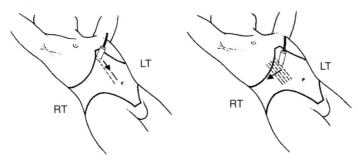

NOTE: If gas is obscuring the view of the pancreas head and uncinate process and the fluid technique cannot be utilized because the patient is restricted from fluids, then you may have to evaluate the head and uncinate from an angle. The angled view is obtained by relocating the pancreas body, moving to a level just inferior to the body, then angling the transducer toward the patient's right at varying degrees until the pancreas head and uncinate are identified. Once located, finish evaluating the head and uncinate from that angle. (If any images are taken from an angle it must be noted as part of the image labeling.)

6. To find the *long axis of the pancreas* you must visibly connect the head, neck, body and tail. Begin by relocating the long axis of the pancreas body. Next, *very* slowly twist the transducer—first one way then the other—to oblique the scanning plane according to the exact lie of the pancreas. At the same time, it may be necessary to barely slide the transducer a little superior or inferior to resolve the long axis.

Pancreas • Axial Survey
Sagittal Plane • Transabdominal Anterior Approach

1. Start the axial survey with the pancreas *head*. Begin scanning with the transducer perpendicular, at the midline of the body, just inferior to the xiphoid process of the sternum. Locate the anechoic, distal, long portion of the IVC. Slowly slide the transducer inferiorly along the IVC. Look for a long section of the anechoic portal vein anteriorly. You should be able to identify the head of the pancreas at the inferior margin of the portal vein section.

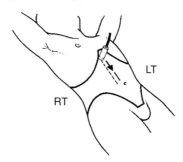

2. When the head of the pancreas is identified, slowly move the transducer toward the patient's right, scanning through the head until you are beyond it. Now slowly move the transducer toward the patient's left, until the head portion reappears. As you evaluate the head, an anechoic, long section of the common bile duct should appear anterior to the portal vein, running inferiorly toward the posterior margin of the head. In some cases, the anechoic long section of the gastroduodenal artery can be identified anterior to the common bile duct, running inferiorly toward the anterior margin of the pancreas head.

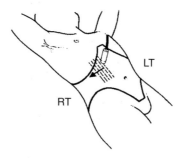

3. Continue by slowly moving the transducer slightly left lateral to evaluate the *uncinate process* and *neck* of the pancreas. Look for the anechoic, long section of the superior mesenteric vein that runs between the pancreas neck (anteriorly) and the uncinate process (posteriorly). Generally the uncinate lies directly anterior to the IVC, but it can extend as far left to lie anterior to the aorta.

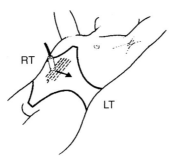

4. Scan left lateral through and beyond the neck and uncinate process and onto the pancreas *body*. It can be helpful to resolve the long axis of the aorta and superior mesenteric artery and look for the pancreas body anterior to them. Other vascular landmarks helpful when identifying the pancreas body include anechoic, axial sections of the splenic artery seen at its superior margin and anechoic, axial sections of the splenic vein seen along its posterior edge.

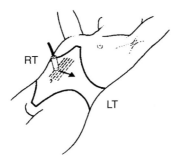

5. Continue to slowly scan left lateral, through and beyond the pancreas body onto the *tail* of the pancreas. In most cases this will be the area left lateral to the aorta. Like the pancreas body, the tail is bordered superiorly by the splenic artery and posteriorly by the splenic vein. Look for the tail between the stomach (anteriorly) and longitudinal sections of the left kidney (posteriorly). Scan left lateral through and beyond the tail of the pancreas.

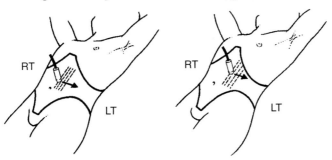

NOTE: If gas from the stomach is obscuring the view of the pancreas tail and the fluid technique cannot be utilized because the patient is restricted from fluids, then you may have to evaluate the tail from a posterior approach. When using a posterior approach, the patient may sit erect or lie prone. It is usually helpful to begin by locating the superior pole of the left kidney (just lateral to the spine) then look for the tail in the area directly anterior to the superior pole.

Pancreas Required Images

NOTE: The required images are a small representation of what a sonographer visualizes during a study. Therefore, the images should provide the interpreting physician with the most telling and technically accurate information available.
NOTE: Measurements of the normal pancreas are not required.
NOTE: If the pancreas cannot be visualized because of overlying stomach or bowel gas, and the patient is restricted from fluids, and every effort has been made to image the pancreas, take the required images in the designated areas to demonstrate nonvisualization and add "area" to the image label.

Pancreas • Longitudinal Images
Transverse Plane • Transabdominal Anterior Approach

1. Image of the **PANCREAS LONG AXIS** to include as much head, uncinate, body, tail, and pancreatic duct as possible.

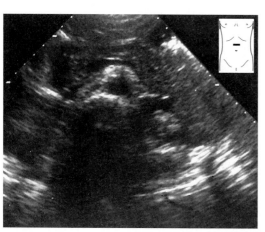
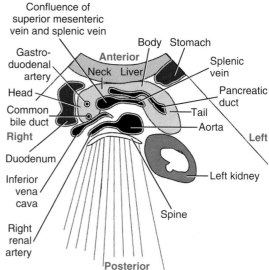

Labeled: **PANCREAS TRV LONG AXIS**

2. Longitudinal image of the **PANCREAS BODY** and **NECK** to include the splenic vein.

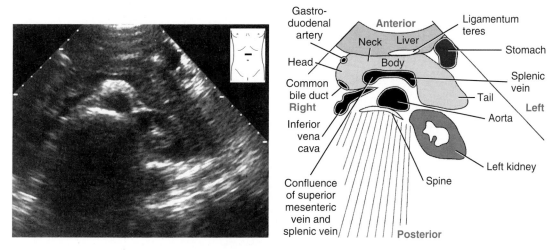

Labeled: **PANCREAS TRV BODY/NECK**

3. Longitudinal image of the **PANCREAS TAIL.**

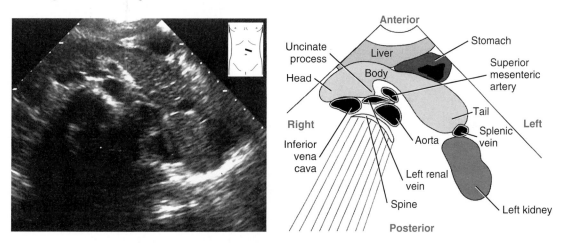

Labeled: **PANCREAS TRV TAIL**

4. Longitudinal image of the **PANCREAS HEAD** to include the uncinate process and common bile duct (if bile filled).

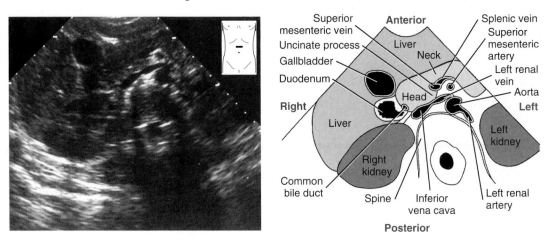

Labeled: **PANCREAS TRV HEAD**

Pancreas • Axial Images
Sagittal Plane • Transabdominal Anterior Approach

5. Axial image of the pancreas head to include the **COMMON BILE DUCT (CBD)** (if bile filled).

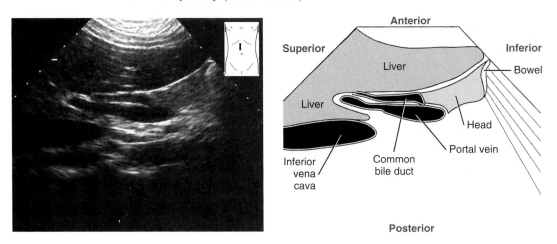

Labeled: **PANCREAS SAG HEAD**

6. Axial image of the **PANCREAS NECK** and **UNCINATE PROCESS** to include the superior mesenteric vein.

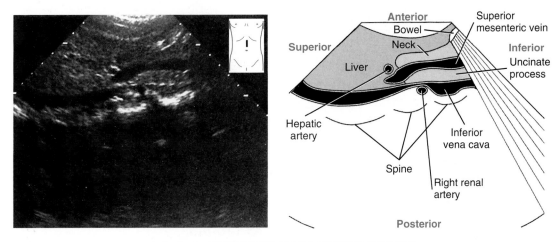

Labeled: **PANCREAS SAG NECK/UNCINATE**

7. Axial image of the **PANCREAS BODY** to include the splenic vein.

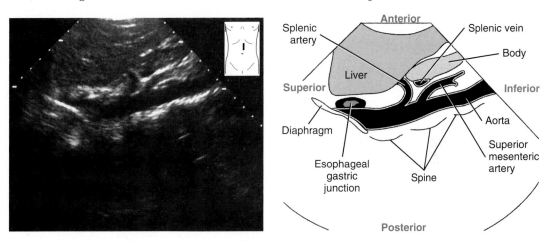

Labeled: **PANCREAS SAG BODY**

8. Axial image of the **PANCREAS TAIL.**

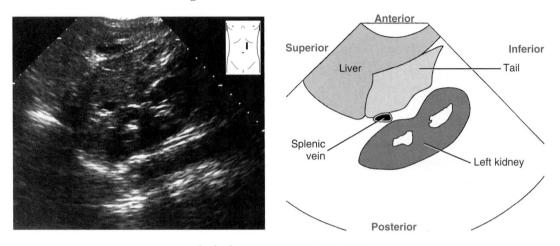

Labeled: **PANCREAS SAG TAIL**

Required Images When the Pancreas is Part of Another Study

Pancreas • Longitudinal Images
Transverse Plane • Transabdominal Anterior Approach

1. Long axis image of the **PANCREAS** to include as much head, uncinate, body, tail, and pancreatic duct as possible.

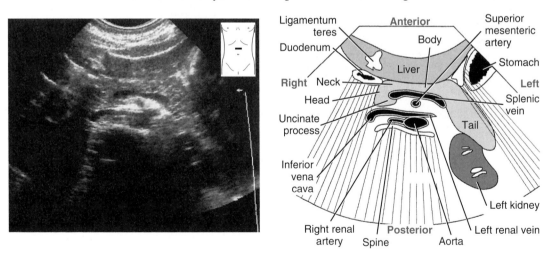

Labeled: **PANCREAS TRV LONG AXIS**

2. Longitudinal image of the **PANCREAS HEAD** to include the uncinate process and common bile duct (CBD) (if bile filled).

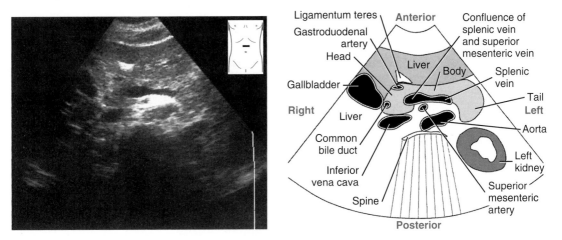

Labeled: **PANCREAS TRV HEAD**

Pancreas • Axial Image
Sagittal Plane • Transabdominal Anterior Approach

3. Axial image of the **PANCREAS HEAD** to include the common bile duct (CBD) (if bile filled).

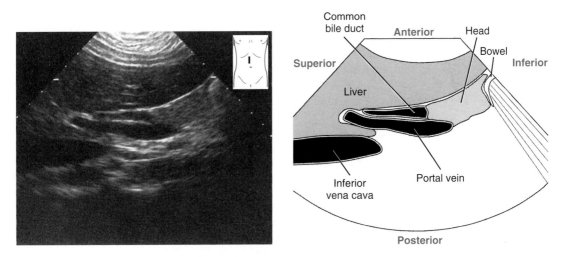

Labeled: **PANCREAS SAG HEAD**

Review Questions

Answers on page 629.

1. The sonographic appearance of the pancreas is described as
   a) heterogeneous and hyperechoic relative to the liver.
   b) heterogeneous and isosonic relative to renal parenchyma.
   c) homogeneous and hypoechoic relative to the liver.
   d) homogeneous and hyperechoic relative to the liver.

2. The contour of the normal pancreas
   a) appears smooth and even.
   b) may be difficult to evaluate due to retroperitoneal fat infiltration.
   c) appears uneven.
   d) may be difficult to evaluate because there are no fat interfaces to distinguish it from adjacent structures.

3. A longitudinal view of Wirsung's duct is
   a) seen in a transverse plane.
   b) seen in a sagittal oblique plane.
   c) too small to distinguish sonographically.
   d) seen only in the head of the pancreas.

4. The long axis of the pancreas is
   a) seen in a transverse plane.
   b) seen in a sagittal oblique plane.
   c) not appreciated sonographically due to the different positions of its various parts.
   d) is an axial portion.

5. The head of the pancreas is
   a) posterior to the liver and stomach, medial to the duodenum, anterior to the IVC.
   b) posterior to the liver, medial to the duodenum, anterior to the SMV.
   c) posterior to the liver, medial to the duodenum, anterior to the IVC.
   d) right lateral to the pancreas body, posterior to the liver, superior to the IVC.

6. The neck of the pancreas is
   a) anterior to the SMA and uncinate process.
   b) posterior to the liver and duodenum.
   c) anterior to the SMV, portal splenic confluence, and uncinate process.
   d) posterior to the liver, duodenum, and hepatic artery.

7. The body of the pancreas is
   a) anterior to the SMV and SMA; inferior to the splenic artery.
   b) anterior to the splenic vein and SMA; inferior to the splenic artery.
   c) posterior to the liver and duodenum; anterior to the SMV.
   d) posterior to the liver and duodenum; just anterior to the portal splenic confluence.

8. The tail of the pancreas is
   a) anterior to the SMA, left renal vein, and left kidney; posterior to the stomach.
   b) anterior to the splenic vein, left renal vein, and left kidney; posterior to the stomach.
   c) lateral to the splenic artery, posterior to the splenic vein and stomach.
   d) just lateral to the spleen, anterior to the splenic vein, and posterior to the stomach.

9. A standard alternative approach for scanning the pancreas tail is
   a) intercostal scanning.
   b) subcostal scanning.
   c) an anterior approach.
   d) a posterior approach.

10. The exocrine function of the pancreas is
    a) accessory storage of bile.
    b) to produce the hormones insulin and cortisone.
    c) to produce the hormone insulin.
    d) to aid digestion in conjunction with the biliary system.

11. What structure is identified at the anterior aspect of the head of the pancreas?
    a) Common bile duct.
    b) Common hepatic artery.
    c) Gastroduodenal artery.
    d) Splenic vein.

12. Which portion of the pancreas is the least commonly visualized by ultrasound?
    a) Uncinate process.
    b) Body.
    c) Neck.
    d) Tail.

13. What is the relationship of the pancreas to the superior mesenteric vein?
    a) Posterior to the tail.
    b) Posterior to the neck.
    c) Lateral to the tail.
    d) Superior to the body.

14. Which part(s) of the pancreas does the duodenum encircle?
    a) Head.
    b) Body.
    c) Neck.
    d) All of the above.

15. The tail of the pancreas is in contact with which structure(s)?
    a) Left kidney.
    b) Splenic flexure of the colon.
    c) Spleen.
    d) All of the above.

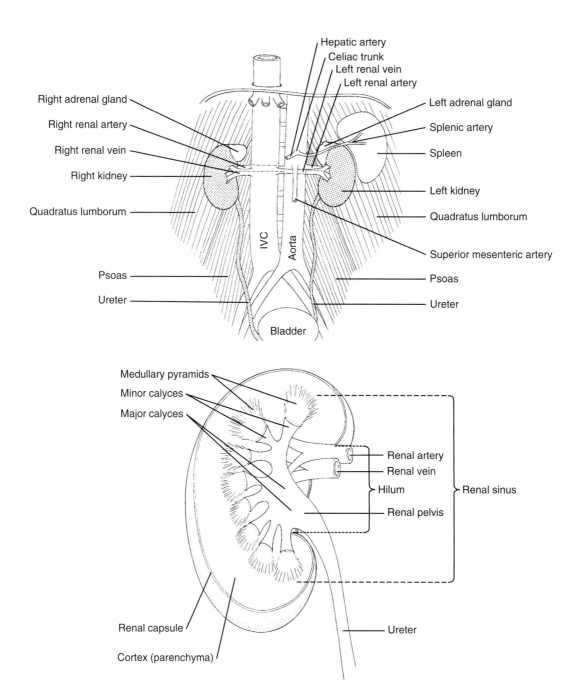

Figure 9-1 *Top,* Location of urinary system. *Bottom,* Kidney anatomy.

CHAPTER 9

Renal Scanning Protocol

Betty Bates Tempkin

Key Words

Adrenal gland	Nephron
Arcuate vessels	Perinephric space
Collecting system	Psoas muscle
Columns of Bertin	Quadratus lumborum muscle
Gerota's fascia	Renal capsule
Heterogeneous	Renal cortex
Homogeneous	Renal hilum
Hypoechoic	Renal parenchyma
Infundibulum	Renal pelvis
Inner medulla	Renal sinus
Major calyces	Retroperitoneum
Medullary pyramid	True capsule
Minor calyces	Ureter
Morison's pouch	

Objectives

At the end of this chapter, you will be able to:

- Define the key words.
- Distinguish the sonographic appearance of the kidneys and urinary system and the terms used to describe them.
- Describe the transducer options for scanning the kidneys.
- List the various suggested breathing techniques for patients when scanning the kidneys.
- List the suggested patient positions (and options) when scanning the kidneys.
- Describe the patient prep for a renal study.
- Distinguish normal renal variants.
- Name the survey steps and explain how to evaluate the entire length, width, and depth of the aorta and its branches.
- Explain the order and exact locations to take representative images of the kidneys.
- Answer the review questions at the end of the chapter.

Overview

Location

- The kidneys lie in the retroperitoneum (portion of abdominopelvic cavity posterior to the peritoneal sac) in the abdomen on each side of the spine, anterior to the psoas and quadratus lumborum muscles

in the area between the twelfth thoracic and fourth lumbar vertebrae. The psoas muscle is posterior and medial to the kidneys. The quadratus lumborum muscle is posterior and lateral to the kidneys.
- The right kidney is normally situated lower than the left kidney.
- The right kidney is posteroinferior to the liver and gallbladder.
- The left kidney is inferior and medial to the spleen.
- Located immediately superior, anterior, and medial to each kidney is an adrenal gland.

Anatomy
- The kidneys are described as having a superior and inferior pole, medial and lateral margins, and an anterior and posterior surface.
- The kidneys are encapsulated by a fibrous renal or true capsule."
- Fat surrounds the encapsulated kidneys in the perinephric or **perirenal** space (part of the retroperitoneal space within the renal fascia that contains the kidney, perirenal fat, adrenal gland, and proximal ureter).
- Gerota's fascia is a fibrous sheath that encloses each kidney, perinephric fat, and adrenal gland.
- Normal adult kidneys measure 9 to 12|cm long, 2.5 to 3.5|cm thick, and 4 to 5|cm wide.
- Each kidney is composed of two distinct areas, the *renal sinus* and *renal parenchyma*:
    I. Renal sinus: consists of the *renal hilum* and *collecting system*:
        A. Renal hilum:
            1. Medial opening into the renal sinus at the mid portion of the kidney.
            2. Through it passes the renal arteries, veins, nerves, lymphatic vessels, and ureter.
        B. Collecting system: consists of the *infundibulum* and *renal pelvis*:
            1. The infundibulum is composed of *minor* and *major calyces*:
                a. 8 to 18 minor calyces, which receive urine from the medullary pyramids (Figure 9-1).
                b. 2 or 3 major calyces, which receive urine from the minor calyces then dump it into the renal pelvis.
            2. The renal pelvis is a urine reservoir formed by the expanded superior end of the ureter. It receives urine from the major calyces before it is transported down the ureter to the urinary bladder.
    II. Renal parenchyma: consists of the *inner medulla* and *outer cortex*:
        A. Inner medulla:
            1. 8 to 18 medullary pyramids that pass urine to the minor calyces in the renal pelvis. The *bases* of the pyramids form

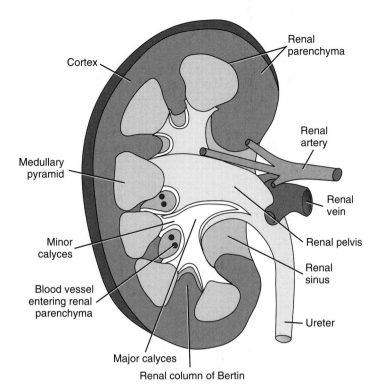

Figure 9-2 Section of internal kidney anatomy. Observe how the ureter begins in the kidney as the renal pelvis. Notice how the number of medullary pyramids equals the number of minor calyces. Note the columns of Bertin separating each medullary pyramid.

a margin with the renal cortex. The *apices* of the pyramids project into the bottom or side of the renal sinus and into the minor calyces. The pyramids are separated from each other by bands of cortical tissue referred to as the col-umns of Bertin, which extend inward to the renal sinus (Figure 9-2).

B. Outer cortex: The outer renal cortex lies between the medulla and outer renal capsule. It contains millions of nephrons; the microscopic functional units of the kidney that form urine.

Physiology
- As part of the excretory system, kidneys function to get rid of meta-bolic wastes.
- Kidneys purify the blood by excreting urine (excess water, salt, toxins).

Sonographic Appearance
- As seen in the following transverse scanning plane image of an axial section of the midportion of the right kidney, the overall sonographic appearance of the normal adult kidney is described as heterogeneous (mixed echo pattern) due to the contrast in

appearance of the renal cortex and renal sinus. The *renal cortex* appears midgray and **homogeneous** (uniform echo pattern) with a smooth contour, whereas the *renal sinus* presents as bright with irregular borders and, in this case, interrupted with anechoic, urine-filled medullary pyramids and blood-filled vessel.

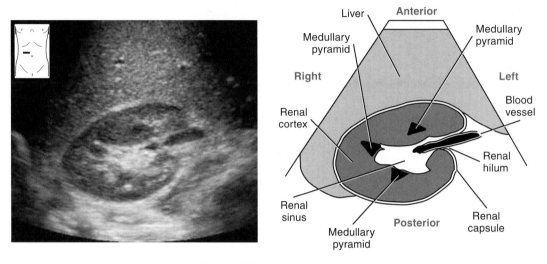

(Courtesy Ultrasoundpaedia.com.)

As this image demonstrates, the kidneys are easily identified by the highly reflective appearance of the surrounding *renal capsule.* It appears as a bright, thin continuous line seen along the periphery of the kidney, adjacent to the renal cortex. This image also shows why the kidney (cortex) is described as **hypoechoic** (less echogenic) compared to the adjacent normal liver.

- Since the orientation of each kidney is vertically obliqued in the body; therefore, longitudinal and long axis views are seen in oblique sagittal scanning planes and oblique coronal scanning planes as demonstrated in the image on the facing page, which was taken in a coronal oblique scanning plane; it shows the long axis of a normal left kidney. Notice how the longitudinal section of the kidney appears elliptical in shape. Observe how the bases of the anechoic, urine-filled medullary pyramids form a margin with the renal cortex. In some cases, the **arcuate vessels** can be visualized at this corticomedullary junction as bright, echogenic dots. Note how the renal sinus appears highly reflective with variable contour due to the fat it contains.

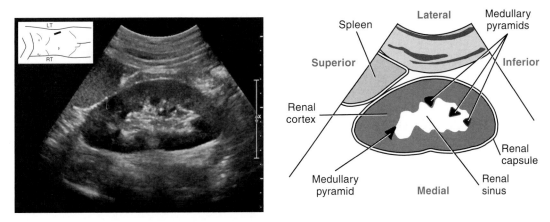

(Courtesy the University of Virginia's Imaging Center, Charlottesville, Virginia.)

- The image below shows an axial section of the mid portion of the right kidney taken in a transverse scanning plane. The renal cortex appears homogeneous, with midgray echoes that are hypoechoic relative to the normal liver. Observe how axial sections of the kidney appear rounded and broken medially by the renal hilum. In this case, we can observe an anechoic, long section of the right renal vein exiting the renal hilum on its course to the inferior vena cava (IVC). Note the anechoic medullary pyramid. The pyramids appear anechoic or hypoechoic relative to the renal cortex depending on the amount of urine they contain. The pyramids as well as the infundibulum and renal pelvis are only visualized when they contain urine. The ureters are not normally visualized. This image also demonstrates Morison's pouch, a peritoneal space that appears as a bright curvilinear line between the right kidney and the liver. This space is important as it is a potential site for abnormal collection of fluid.

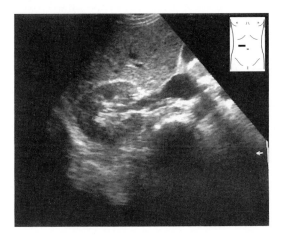

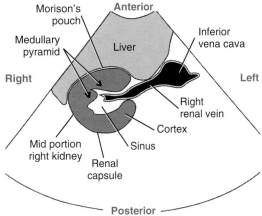

Normal Variants

- **Dromedary humps:**
  - Cortical bulge(s) on the lateral border of the kidney that appear the same as normal renal cortex.
- **Hypertrophied column of Bertin:**
  - Enlarged columns of renal cortex that vary in size and indent the renal sinus.
  - They appear the same as normal renal cortex.
- **Double collecting system:**
  - The renal sinus is divided by a hypertrophied column of Bertin.
  - The appearance is the same as normal renal cortex and two normal renal sinuses.
- **Horseshoe kidney:**
  - The kidneys are connected, usually at the lower poles.
  - Except for their connection, the kidneys appear otherwise normal.
- **Renal ectopia:**
  - One or both kidneys may be found outside the normal renal fossa.
  - Other locations include the lower portion of the abdominal or pelvic cavities, and in rare cases they may be found in the intrathoracic area. Except for the location, the kidney(s) appears otherwise normal.

Preparation

Patient Prep
- None.

Transducer
- **3.0 MHz or 3.5 MHz.**
- 5.0 for very thin patients.

Breathing Technique
- **Deep, held inspiration.** Deep inspiration causes the kidneys to descend, making them easier to visualize sonographically.

> **NOTE:** Different breathing techniques should be used whenever the suggested breathing technique does not produce the desired results.

Patient Position
Right Kidney
- **Supine.**
- Left posterior oblique, left lateral decubitus, and prone as needed.

Left Kidney
- **Right lateral decubitus.**
- Prone as needed.

> **NOTE:** Different patient positions should be used whenever the suggested position does not produce the desired results.

Renal Survey Steps

Right Kidney • Longitudinal Survey
Sagittal Plane • Transabdominal Anterior Approach

1. Begin scanning with the transducer perpendicular, just inferior to the most lateral edge of the right costal margin.

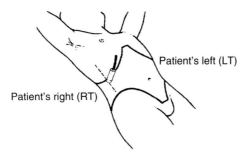

Patient's left (LT)

Patient's right (RT)

2. Have the patient take in a deep breath and hold it. The longitudinal section of the kidney should come into view. If the kidney is not seen here, move the transducer small degrees in medial and inferior sections with the patient holding his or her breath, until the kidney is identified.

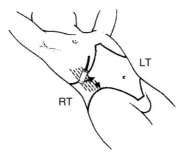

LT

RT

> **NOTE:** Deep inspiration causes the kidneys to descend, making them easier to visualize sonographically.

3. When the kidney is located, very slightly twist/rotate the transducer first one way, then the other (to oblique the scanning plane according to the vertical oblique lie of the right kidney) to resolve the long axis of the right kidney.

4. Once the long axis is determined, very slightly rock the transducer superior to inferior while slowly sliding the transducer medially, scanning through the kidney until you are beyond it.
Evaluate the perirenal region as you scan through it.

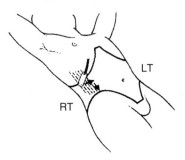

5. Move the transducer back onto the kidney. Slowly rocking and sliding scan right lateral, through and beyond the kidney.
Evaluate the perirenal region as you scan through it.

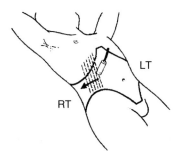

NOTE: The longitudinal survey of the right kidney can be performed from a coronal plane, right lateral approach. This approach can be performed with the patient supine, but it is usually easier to scan with the patient in a left lateral decubitus position.

1. Begin scanning with the transducer perpendicular, midcoronal plane, just superior to the iliac crest. Have the patient take in a deep breath and hold it as you move or angle the transducer superior to inferior or scan intercostally if necessary to locate the kidney.

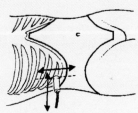

2. When the kidney is identified, resolve the long axis, then very slightly rock the transducer superior to inferior while sliding the transducer anteriorly (toward the patient's front), scanning through and beyond the kidney margin.
   Evaluate the perirenal region as you scan through it.
3. Move the transducer back onto the kidney. Slowly rocking and sliding move posteriorly (toward the patient's back), scanning through and beyond the right kidney.
   Evaluate the perirenal region as you scan through it.

Right Kidney • Axial Survey
Transverse Plane • Transabdominal Anterior Approach

1. Still in the sagittal scanning plane, relocate the long axis of the right kidney. Slowly rotate the transducer 90 degrees into the transverse plane. The rounded, axial section of the kidney will come into view.

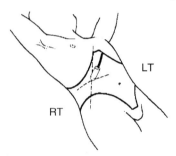

NOTE: As an alternative, you can start the axial survey in the transverse plane. Begin scanning with the transducer perpendicular, just inferior to the costal margin of the medial angle of the ribs. With the patient holding his or her breath, move the transducer in right lateral and inferior sections until the kidney is located.

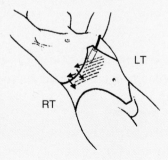

2. When the kidney is identified, slowly move the transducer slightly superior and medial, or inferior and lateral, to locate the mid portion of the kidney and visualize the renal hilum. It may be necessary to very slightly twist/rotate the transducer, first one way then the other, to slightly oblique the scanning plane to adequately resolve the hilum.

3. From the hilum, slightly rock the transducer side to side while slowly sliding the transducer superior and medial through and beyond the superior pole of the kidney.
Evaluate the perirenal region as you scan through it.

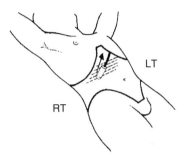

4. Continue rocking, and move the transducer back onto the superior pole. Slowly slide the transducer inferior and right lateral through the mid portion and the inferior pole of the kidney. Scan through and beyond the inferior pole.
Evaluate the perirenal region as you scan through it.

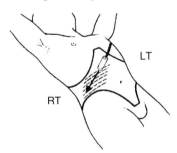

NOTE: The axial survey of the right kidney can be performed from a transverse plane, right lateral approach. This approach can be performed with the patient supine, but it is usually easier to scan with the patient in a left lateral decubitus position.

1. Begin scanning with the transducer perpendicular, at the midline and just superior to the iliac crest. Have the patient hold his or her breath while you move or angle the transducer superior to inferior or scan intercostally if necessary to locate the kidney.

2. When the kidney is identified, resolve the renal hilum, then very slightly rock the transducer side to side while sliding the transducer superiorly through and beyond the kidney margin. Evaluate the perirenal region as you scan through it.
3. Move the transducer back onto the kidney. Slowly rocking and sliding move inferiorly, scanning through and beyond the right kidney.
    Evaluate the perirenal region as you scan through it.

Left Kidney • Longitudinal Survey
Coronal Plane • Left Lateral Approach

NOTE: Although this approach can be performed with the patient supine, it is generally easier with the patient in the right lateral decubitus position. Imaging quality might be improved by placing a sponge or rolled towel under the patient's right side to open up the rib spaces on the patient's left.

1. Begin scanning with the transducer perpendicular, midcoronal plane, just superior to the iliac crest.

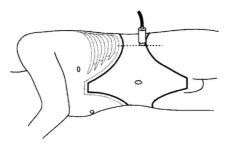

NOTE: If the kidney is not seen in the midcoronal plane, try approaches just to the right and left of the midline.

2. Have the patient take in a deep breath and hold it while you move or angle the transducer superior to inferior to locate the kidney. When the kidney is located, very slightly twist/rotate the transducer, first one way then the other (to oblique the scanning plane according to the vertical oblique lie of the right kidney), to resolve the long axis.

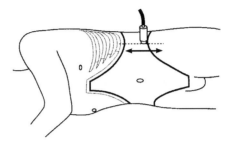

3. Once the long axis is determined, very slightly rock the transducer superior to inferior while slowly sliding the transducer anteriorly (toward the patient's front), scanning through and beyond the kidney margin.
   Evaluate the perirenal region as you scan through it.

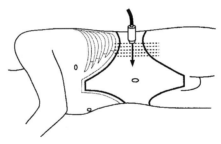

4. Move the transducer back onto the kidney. Slowly rocking and sliding, move posteriorly (toward the patient's back), scanning through and beyond the left kidney.
   Evaluate the perirenal region as you scan through it.

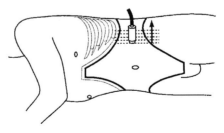

NOTE: The longitudinal survey of the left kidney may have to be performed intercostally, depending on body habitus and the position of the kidney. Begin with the transducer perpendicular, midcoronal plane, in the first inferior intercostal space. Have the patient hold his or her breath while you move superiorly through the adjacent intercostal spaces to evaluate the entire kidney. Varying respiration and angling the transducer within the intercostal spaces can aid evaluation. In some cases, only the superior pole will have to be evaluated intercostally.

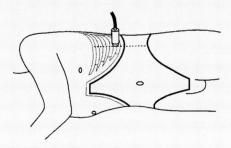

Left Kidney • Axial Survey
Transverse Plane • Left Lateral Approach

1. Still in the coronal scanning plane, relocate the long axis of the left kidney. Slowly rotate the transducer 90 degrees into the plane. The round to oval axial section of the kidney will come into view.

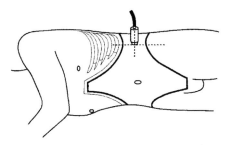

NOTE: As an alternative, you can start the axial survey in the transverse plane. Begin scanning with the transducer perpendicular, at the midline and just superior to the iliac crest. Have the patient hold his or her breath while you move the transducer superior to inferior to locate the kidney.

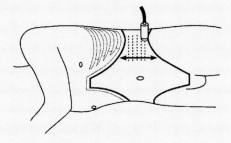

2. When the kidney is identified, slowly move the transducer slightly medial, then very small movements superior and inferior to locate the midportion of the kidney and visualize the renal hilum. It may be necessary to very slightly twist/rotate the transducer, first one way then the other, to oblique the scanning plane to adequately resolve the hilum.

3. From the hilum, slightly rock the transducer side to side while slowly sliding the transducer superior and through and beyond the superior pole of the kidney.

Evaluate the perirenal region as you scan through it.

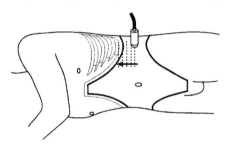

4. Continue rocking, and move the transducer back onto the superior pole. Slowly slide the transducer inferiorly through the mid portion and the inferior pole of the kidney. Scan through and beyond the inferior pole.

Evaluate the perirenal region as you scan through it.

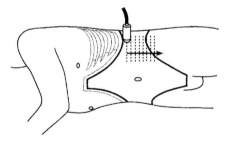

NOTE: The axial survey of the left kidney may have to be performed intercostally, depending on body habitus and the position of the kidney. Begin with the transducer perpendicular, at the midline, in the first inferior intercostal space. Have the patient hold his or her breath while you move superiorly through the adjacent intercostal spaces to evaluate the entire kidney. Varying respiration and angling the transducer within the intercostal spaces can aid evaluation. In some cases, only the superior pole will have to be evaluated intercostally.

Kidneys Required Images

> **NOTE:** The required images are a small representation of what a sonographer visualizes during a study. Therefore, the images should provide the interpreting physician with the most telling and technically accurate information available.

Right Kidney • Longitudinal Images
Sagittal Plane • Transabdominal Anterior Approach

1. Image of the right kidney **LONG AXIS** *with superior to inferior measurement.*

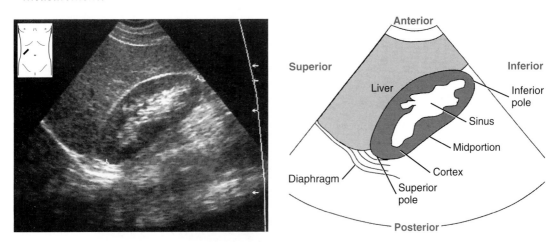

Labeled: **RT KID SAG LONG AXIS**

2. Same image as number 1 *without calipers.*

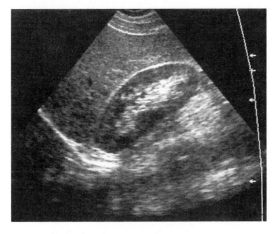

Labeled: **RT KID SAG LONG AXIS**

3. Image of the right kidney **LONG AXIS** *with superior to inferior measurement.*

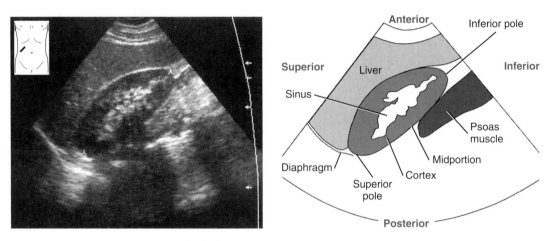

Labeled: **RT KID SAG LONG AXIS**

4. Same image as number 3 *without calipers.*

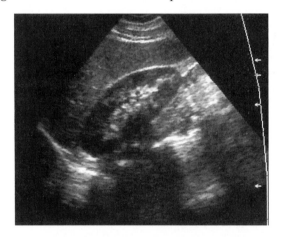

Labeled: **RT KID SAG LONG AXIS**

NOTE: In many cases superior and/or inferior pole definition is sacrificed to achieve the long axis. If so, take those images here and label accordingly.

5. Longitudinal image of the right kidney **SUPERIOR POLE.**

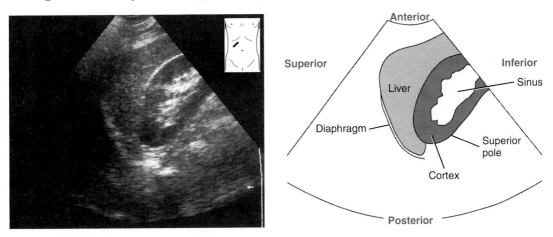

Labeled: **RT KID SAG SUP POLE**

6. Longitudinal image of the right kidney **INFERIOR POLE.**

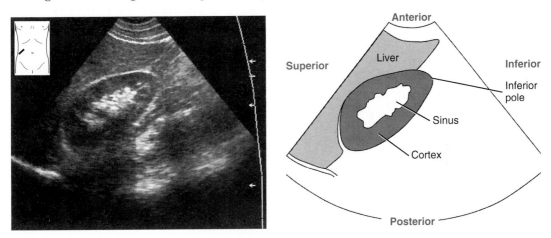

Labeled: **RT KID SAG INF POLE**

7. Longitudinal image of the right kidney **JUST MEDIAL TO THE LONG AXIS.**

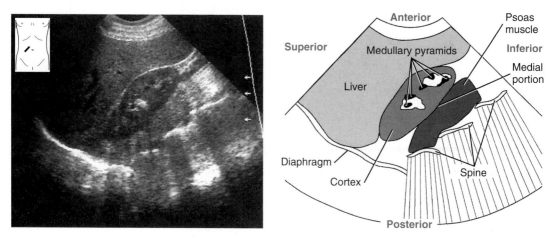

Labeled: **RT KID SAG MED**

8. Longitudinal image of the right kidney **JUST LATERAL TO THE LONG AXIS** to include part of the liver for parenchyma comparison.

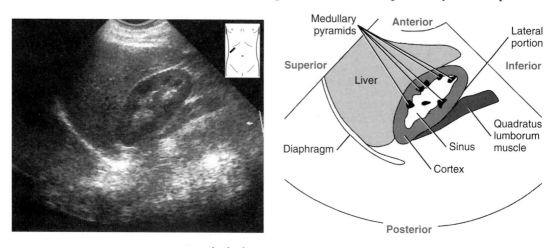

Labeled: **RT KID SAG LAT**

Right Kidney • Axial Images
Transverse Plane • Transabdominal Anterior Approach
9. Axial image of the right kidney **SUPERIOR POLE.**

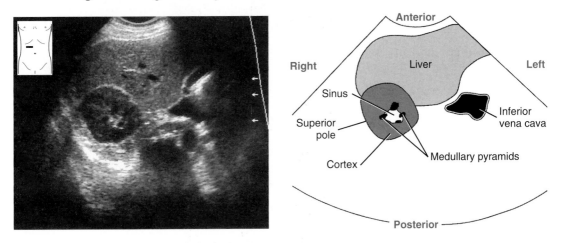

Labeled: **RT KID TRV SUP POLE**

10. Axial image of the right kidney **MID PORTION** to include the
hilum *with anterior to posterior measurement.*

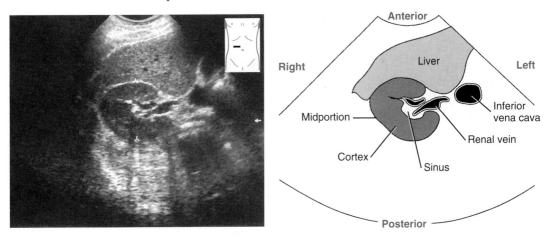

Labeled: **RT KID TRV MID**

11. Same image as number 10 *without calipers.*

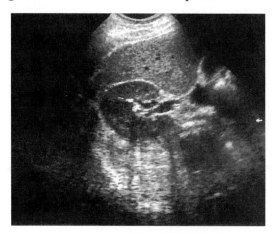

Labeled: **RT KID TRV MID**

12. Axial image of the right kidney **INFERIOR POLE.**

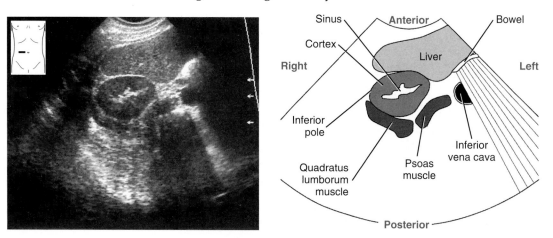

Labeled: **RT KID TRV INF POLE**

Left Kidney • Longitudinal Images
Coronal Plane • Left Lateral Approach

1. Image of the left kidney **LONG AXIS** *with superior to inferior measurement.*

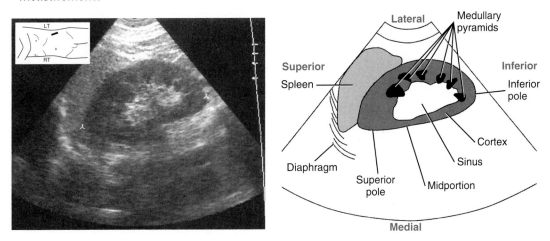

Labeled: **LT KID COR LONG AXIS**

2. Same image as number 1 *without calipers.*

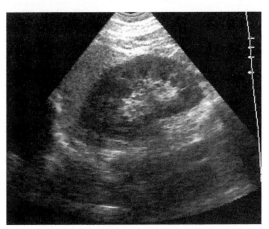

Labeled: **LT KID COR LONG AXIS**

3. Image of the left kidney **LONG AXIS** *with superior to inferior measurement.*

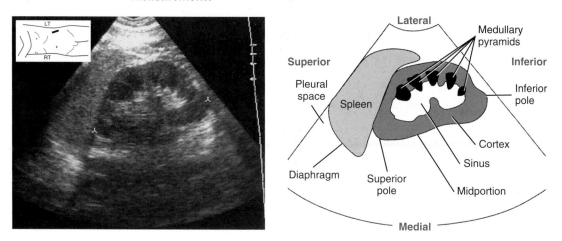

Labeled: **LT KID COR LONG AXIS**

4. Same image as number 3 *without calipers.*

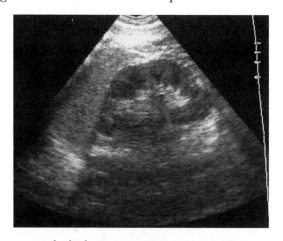

Labeled: **LT KID COR LONG AXIS**

NOTE: In many cases superior and/or inferior pole definition is sacrificed to achieve the long axis. If so, take those images here and label accordingly.

NOTE: One of the long axis images or, if applicable, the superior pole image must include part of the spleen for parenchyma comparison.

5. Longitudinal image of the left kidney **SUPERIOR POLE.**

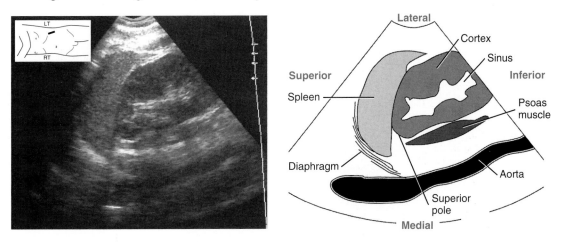

Labeled: **LT KID COR SUP POLE**

6. Longitudinal image of the left kidney **INFERIOR POLE.**

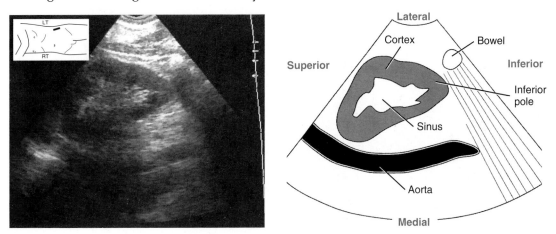

Labeled: **LT KID COR INF POLE**

7. Longitudinal image of the left kidney **JUST ANTERIOR TO THE LONG AXIS.**

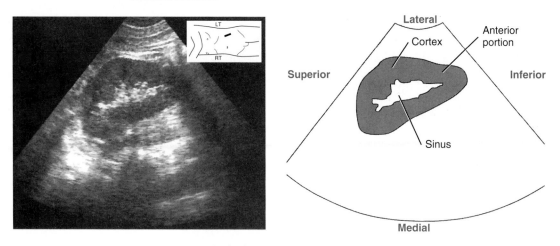

Labeled: **LT KID COR ANT**

8. Longitudinal image of the left kidney **JUST POSTERIOR TO THE LONG AXIS.**

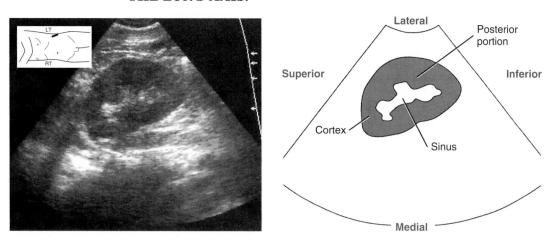

Labeled: **LT KID COR POST**

Left Kidney • Axial Images
Transverse Plane • Left Lateral Approach
9. Axial image of the left kidney **SUPERIOR POLE.**

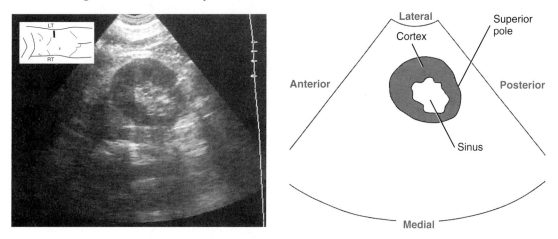

Labeled: **LT KID LT TRV SUP POLE**

10. Axial image of the left kidney **MID PORTION** to include the hilum *with anterior to posterior measurement.*

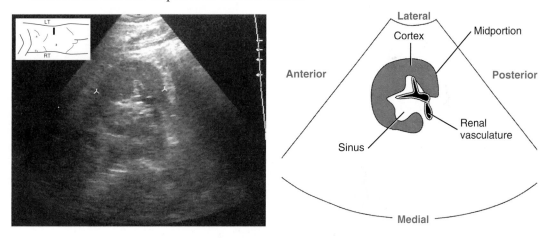

Labeled: **LT KID LT TRV MID**

11. Same image as number 10 *without calipers.*

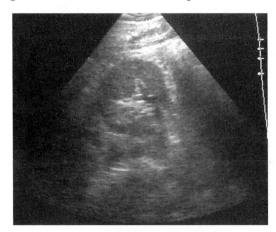

Labeled: **LT KID LT TRV MID**

12. Axial image of the left kidney **INFERIOR POLE.**

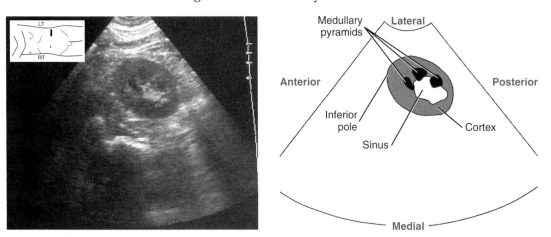

Labeled: **LT KID LT TRV INF POLE**

Required Images When the Kidneys are Part of Another Study

Right Kidney • Longitudinal Images
Sagittal Plane • Transabdominal Anterior Approach
1. Image of the right kidney **LONG AXIS.**

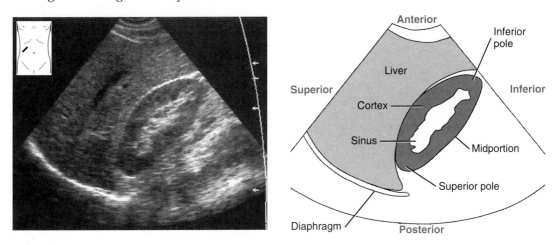

Labeled: **RT KID SAG LONG AXIS**

NOTE: Take additional images of the superior and/or inferior poles if they are not clearly defined in the long axis image and label accordingly.

Right Kidney • Axial Image
Transverse Plane • Transabdominal Anterior Approach
2. Axial image of the right kidney **MID PORTION** to include the hilum.

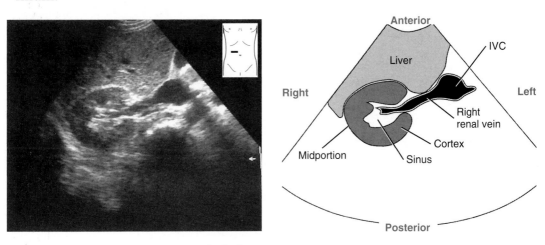

Labeled: **RT KID TRV MID**

Left Kidney • Longitudinal Image(s)
Coronal Plane • Left Lateral Approach

3. Image of the left kidney **LONG AXIS.**

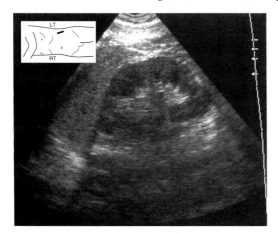 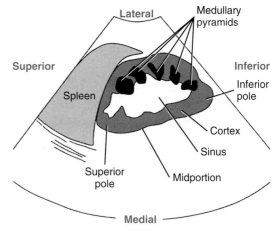

Labeled: **LT KID COR LONG AXIS**

NOTE: Take additional images of the superior and/or inferior poles if they are not clearly defined in the long axis image and label accordingly.

Left Kidney • Axial Image
Transverse Plane • Left Lateral Approach

4. Axial image of the left kidney **MID PORTION** to include the hilum.

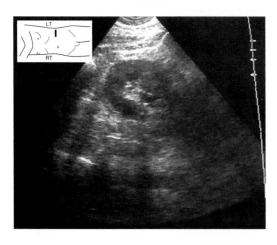 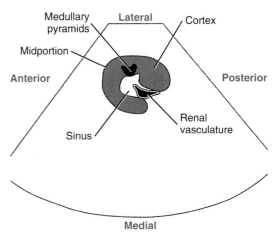

Labeled: **LT KID LT TRV MID**

Review Questions

Answers on page 629.

1. In most cases, the long axis of the left kidney is most easily resolved from which scanning plane?
   a) Coronal transverse scanning plane
   b) Transabdominal sagittal oblique scanning plane
   c) Coronal scanning plane
   d) Coronal oblique scanning plane

2. The overall sonographic appearance of the kidneys can be described as
   a) hyperechoic relative to the liver.
   b) heterogeneous.
   c) hypoechoic relative to the liver.
   d) highly reflective.

3. The sonographic appearance of normal renal cortex is
   a) hyperechoic relative to the liver.
   b) heterogeneous.
   c) hypoechoic relative to the liver.
   d) highly reflective.

4. The sonographic appearance of the normal renal sinus is
   a) homogeneous.
   b) heterogeneous.
   c) hypoechoic relative to the liver.
   d) highly reflective.

5. The medullary pyramids are
   a) not sonographically distinguishable.
   b) abnormal if visualized sonographically.
   c) hypoechoic or anechoic relative to renal cortex depending on the amount of urine they contain.
   d) referred to as the major and minor calyces.

6. The renal pelvis
   a) is formed by the expanded superior end of the ureter where it divides into the medullary pyramids; not visualized sonographically when collapsed.
   b) is another term for the renal hilum.
   c) is formed by the expanded superior end of the ureter where it divides into the infundibula; not visualized sonographically when collapsed.
   d) can be visualized sonographically at the corticomedullary junction when urine-filled.

7. The normal contour of the kidney
   a) can be seen indenting the renal sinus.
   b) appears smooth and even on ultrasound.
   c) is formed by the arcuate vessels.
   d) appears hypoechoic relative to renal cortex.

8. The infundibula
   a) can be seen sonographically at the corticomedullary junction as bright dots.
   b) appears sonographically as triangular or round anechoic urine-filled structures in the cortex.
   c) surrounds the renal sinus.
   d) are the major and minor calyces.

9. The psoas and quadratus lumborum muscles
   a) appear sonographically as the low-gray structures posterior to the kidneys.
   b) form the bright interface between the right kidney and the liver.
   c) are support structures for the kidney that are not appreciated sonographically.
   d) are the low-gray structures seen directly inferior to the kidneys.

10. Which sentence describes the normal echogenicity of the renal cortex?
    a) The normal kidney is never isoechoic with the liver.
    b) The kidney is normally hyperechoic in comparison to the spleen and liver.
    c) The normal kidney echogenicity is frequently isoechoic with the liver and spleen
    d) The echogenicity of the kidney varies and should not be compared to the liver.

11. The normal range in size of the kidney is _____.
    a) 4 to 7 cm
    b) 7 to 9 cm
    c) 9 to 14 cm
    d) 13 to 17 cm

12. Which sentence is true regarding the normal anatomy of the kidneys?
    a) The kidneys are retroperitoneal in location.
    b) The right kidney is located slightly superior compared to the left.
    c) The superomedial aspect of the right kidney does not come in contact with the adrenal gland.
    d) Each kidney is perfectly aligned on either side of the spine.

13. Periodic ureteral "jets" are a sign of _____.
    a) ureteral stone
    b) ureteral spasm
    c) ureteral compression
    d) normality

14. Which of the following is *not* part of the urinary tract?
    a) Kidneys
    b) Uterus
    c) Ureters
    d) Urinary bladder

15. Label the following:

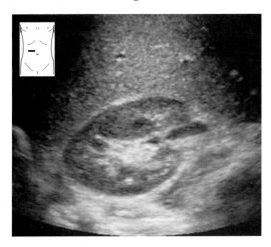 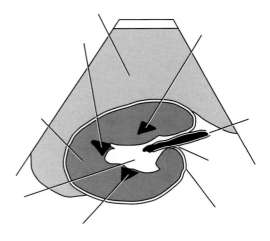

16. Label the following:

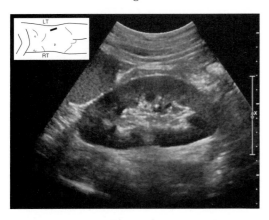 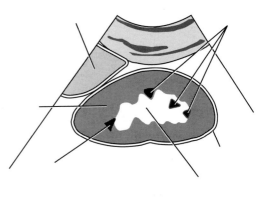

17. Label the following:

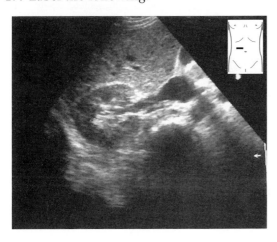 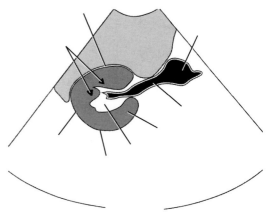

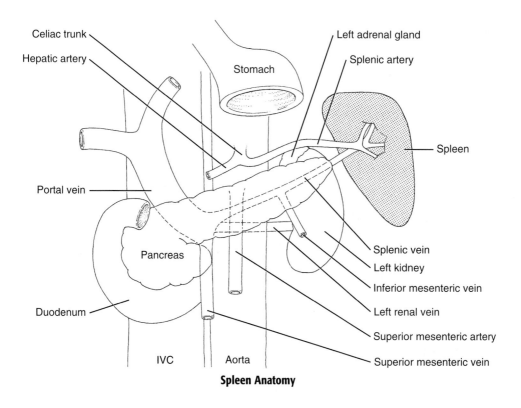

Celiac trunk

Hepatic artery

Stomach

Left adrenal gland

Splenic artery

Spleen

Portal vein

Pancreas

Splenic vein

Left kidney

Inferior mesenteric vein

Left renal vein

Duodenum

Superior mesenteric artery

IVC   Aorta

Superior mesenteric vein

Spleen Anatomy

CHAPTER 10

Spleen Scanning Protocol

Betty Bates Tempkin

Key Words

Accessory spleen
Anemia
Asplenia
Hematopoiesis
Intraperitoneal
Lymphatic tissue

Portal-splenic confluence
Reticuloendothelial system
Splenic artery
Splenic flexure
Splenic hilum
Splenic vein

Objectives

At the end of this chapter, you will be able to:

- Define the key words.
- Distinguish the sonographic appearance of the spleen and the terms used to describe it.
- Describe the transducer options for scanning the spleen.
- List the various suggested breathing techniques for patients when scanning the spleen.
- List the suggested patient positions (and options) when scanning the spleen.
- Describe the patient prep for a splenic study.
- Distinguish normal variants of the spleen.
- Name the survey steps and explain how to evaluate the entire length, width, and depth of the spleen.
- Explain the order and exact locations to take representative images of the spleen.
- Answer the review questions at the end of the chapter.

Overview

Location

- Except for its medial hilum, the spleen is intraperitoneal (enclosed in the sac formed by the parietal peritoneum) in the posterolateral section of the left upper quadrant (or left hypochondrium), beneath the ninth to eleventh intercostal spaces.
- The spleen lies posterior and lateral to the tail of the pancreas, fundus and body of the stomach, and posterior to the splenic flexure (sharp bend between the transverse and descending colon in the left upper quadrant, anterior to the spleen).

- The medial portion of the spleen is superior and lateral to the left kidney.
- The spleen lies inferior and adjacent to the diaphragm, putting it in close proximity to the left pleural cavity.

Anatomy

- The size of the spleen is variable, but is considered normal when it appears about the same size as the adjacent left kidney. Generally, it should be no longer than 12 or 13 cm and no deeper (anteroposteriorly) than 7 or 8 cm. The correct measurement caliper placement is demonstrated in Figure 10-1.
- The shape of the spleen is variable, but it is basically ovoid and may resemble a half moon or crescent. Thus, its superoposterior surface (adjacent to the diaphragm) is convex and smooth and its inferomedial surface (in contact with the stomach, left kidney, splenic flexure, pancreas tail) is concave and indented or nodulous. The **splenic hilum** (entry and exit route for the arterial, venous, and lymphatic vessels and nerves) is located within this concavity. Note that if the spleen becomes enlarged, it loses its concave appearance and becomes more round.
- The **splenic vein** exits the hilum and heads across the body toward the midline, running behind (posterior to) the tail and body of the pancreas to join the superior mesenteric vein at a point just posterior to the pancreas neck to form the portal vein. This location is commonly referred to as the **portal-splenic confluence.**
- The spleen receives blood from the **splenic artery** that branches from the celiac trunk of the abdominal aorta and runs left lateral and just superior to the body and tail of the pancreas, to enter the splenic hilum. In many cases, the artery may divide into two or three smaller branches before entering the spleen.

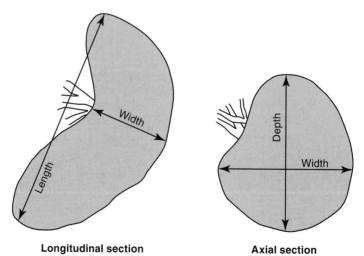

Longitudinal section   **Axial section**

Figure 10-1 Spleen Measurements. Correct caliper placement for measuring the spleen.

Physiology

- Although not essential to life, the spleen filters foreign material from the blood and forms antibodies.
- The spleen is a large mass of **lymphatic tissue** (reticular connective tissue) that is part of the **reticuloendothelial system**, an essential part of the immune system. It is composed of phagocytic cells capable of consuming substances, such as bacteria and viruses, making them incapable of causing harm to the body. They also engulf old cells and abnormal cells, clearing the body of their harmful presence.
- The spleen also breaks down hemoglobin, is a blood reservoir, and is important for **hematopoiesis** (red blood cell formation) in the fetus or when there is severe **anemia** (marked loss of the number of red blood cells produced in bone marrow; symptoms may include fatigue, shortness of breath, irregular heartbeat).

Sonographic Appearance

- The normal adult spleen appears homogeneous, with medium-level echoes and even texture that is described as isosonic or slightly hypoechoic when compared to the normal liver, and hyperechoic relative to kidney parenchyma. In some cases, small vascular branches can be seen interspersed within the spleen. They appear as anechoic, round or tubular structures. Arterial walls usually appear brighter than venous walls; however, the larger venous structures can clearly be distinguished from the smaller arterial branches at the level of the splenic hilum. Occasionally, small, bright reflections may be visualized throughout the spleen that represent calcified granulomatous inclusions or calcifications of small arterial walls.
- The orientation of the spleen is vertically obliqued in the body, therefore longitudinal and long axis views are seen in oblique sagittal scanning planes and oblique coronal scanning planes as demonstrated in the image on the following page. This normal spleen appears crescent in shape and hyperechoic compared to the adjacent left kidney. Notice the spleen's smooth outer convexity and its relationship to the diaphragm and pleural space superiorly.

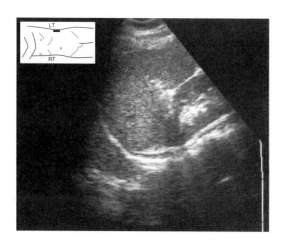

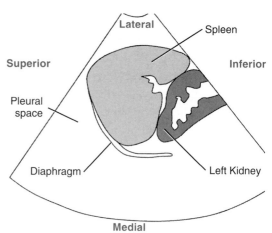

- Axial sections of the spleen are visualized in transverse scanning planes. The following is a transverse scanning plane image from a left lateral approach. It demonstrates an axial section of the spleen that includes the splenic hilum. Note the normal homogeneous appearance and even texture of the spleen.

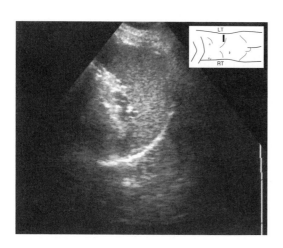

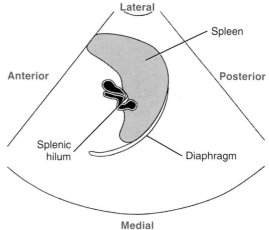

Normal Variants

- Accessory spleen:
  - Splenic tissue found separate from the organ, most often at the splenic hilum. Sonographic appearance is the same as normal splenic tissue.
- Asplenia:
  - Rare absence of the spleen, often associated with congestive heart disease.

Preparation

Patient Prep
- None.

Transducer
- **5.0 MHz for intercostal or lateral subcostal scanning approaches.**
- 3.0 or 3.5 MHz for anterior or posterior scanning approaches.

Breathing Technique
- **Deep, held inspiration.** Deep inspiration causes the spleen to descend, making it easier to visualize sonographically.

> **NOTE:** Different breathing techniques should be used whenever the suggested breathing technique does not produce the desired results.

Patient Position
- **Right lateral decubitus.**
- Supine, sitting semierect to erect, and prone as needed.

> **NOTE:** Different patient positions should be used whenever the suggested position does not produce the desired results.

Spleen Survey Steps

Spleen • Longitudinal Survey
Coronal Plane • Left Lateral Approach

> **NOTE:** Although this approach can be performed with the patient supine, it is generally easier with the patient in the right lateral decubitus position. Imaging quality might be improved by placing a sponge or rolled towel under the patient's right side to open up the rib spaces on the patient's left.
>
> **NOTE:** Rib shadows are a consequence of intercostal scanning and may obscure part of the spleen. In most cases, angling the transducer within the intercostal space toward the unseen area or moving to an adjacent rib space will aid visualization.

1. Begin scanning with the transducer perpendicular, midcoronal plane, in the most inferior intercostal space. Have the patient take in a deep breath and hold it. The superior and inferior margins of the spleen will usually come into view. How much of the normal spleen you see, however, will depend on its shape and the patient's body habitus. If the spleen is not seen in the inferior intercostal space, move the transducer to the adjacent superior intercostal space(s).

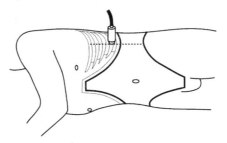

2. When the spleen is located, very slowly rotate/twist the transducer, first one way then the other, to slightly oblique the scanning plane according to the lie of the spleen and to resolve its long axis. Notice the diaphragm and adjacent pleural space superiorly and the left kidney and perinephric space inferiorly. The splenic hilum may also be visualized medially. Very slightly rotating/twisting the transducer can help resolve the hilar structures.

3. While visualizing the long axis of the spleen, slightly move or angle the transducer within the intercostal space toward the patient's front, scanning through and beyond the anterior portion of the spleen.

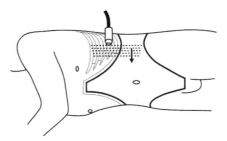

4. Move the transducer back onto the long axis of the spleen. While visualizing the long axis, slightly move or angle the transducer within the intercostal space toward the patient's back, scanning through and beyond the posterior portion of the spleen.

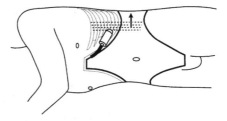

Spleen • Axial Survey
Transverse Plane • Left Lateral Approach

1. Still in the coronal scanning plane, relocate the long axis of the spleen. Slowly rotate the transducer 90 degrees into the transverse scanning plane. Move into adjacent intercostal spaces as necessary and also slightly rotate/twist the transducer, first one way then the other, until the anterior and posterior margins of the spleen are resolved and the hilum is visualized anteromedially.

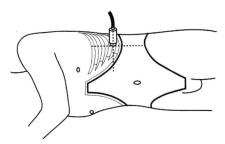

2. Now move or angle the transducer superiorly, scanning through and beyond the superior margin of the spleen. Note the adjacent pleural space.

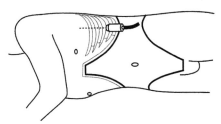

3. Move back onto the spleen and move or angle the transducer inferiorly, scanning through and beyond the inferior margin of the spleen.

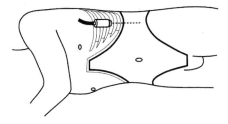

Spleen Required Images

> **NOTE:** The required images are a small representation of what a sonographer visualizes during a study. Therefore, the images should provide the interpreting physician with the most telling and technically accurate information available.

Spleen • Longitudinal Images
Coronal Plane • Left Lateral Approach
1. **LONG AXIS** image of the spleen.

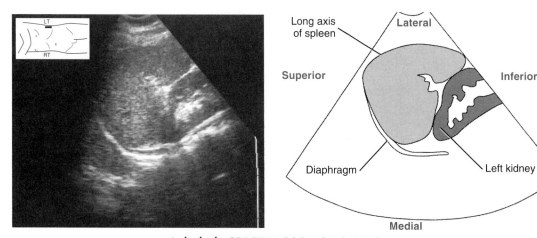

Labeled: **SPLEEN COR LONG AXIS**

2. **SUPERIOR LONGITUDINAL** image of the spleen (to include the adjacent pleural space).

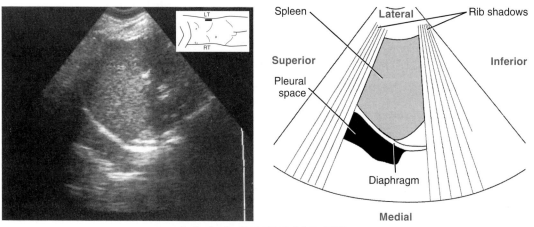

Labeled: **SPLEEN COR SUP**

3. **INFERIOR LONGITUDINAL** image of the spleen (to include part of the left kidney for parenchyma comparison).

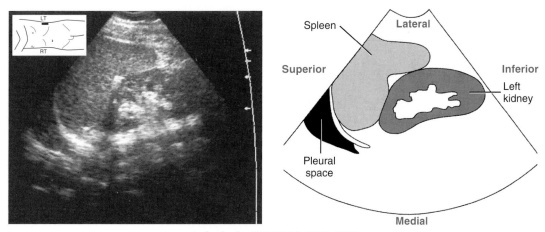

Labeled: **SPLEEN COR INF**

Spleen • Axial Images
Transverse Plane • Left Lateral Approach

4. **AXIAL** image of the spleen (to include both anterior and posterior margins).

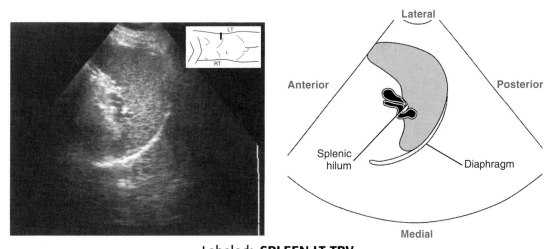

Labeled: **SPLEEN LT TRV**

5. **AXIAL** image of the spleen (to include the anterior margin and splenic hilum).

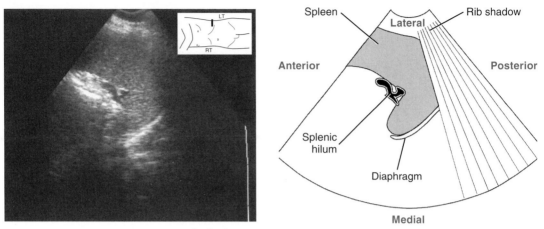

Labeled: **SPLEEN LT TRV ANT**

6. **AXIAL** image of the spleen (to include the posterior margin).

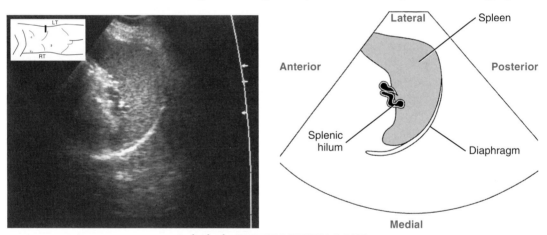

Labeled: **SPLEEN LT TRV POST**

Required Images When the Spleen is Part of Another Study

The required images are the same as the above *except* that:

1. The longitudinal images of the spleen that include the adjacent pleural space and part of the left kidney may be combined into one image if all of the structures are clearly seen. If so, label the image:

   SPLEEN COR

   In some cases these structures may also be seen on the long axis image. If so, label the image:

   SPLEEN COR LONG AXIS

2. Only one axial image of the spleen is necessary as long as the anterior and posterior margins of the spleen are well visualized. If so, label the image:

   SPLEEN LT TRV

Review Questions

Answers on page 629.

1. The sonographic appearance of the normal spleen is
   a) heterogeneous, midgray, interrupted by multiple anechoic vascular branches.
   b) homogeneous, midgray, isosonic or hypoechoic relative to the liver.
   c) homogeneous, midgray, isosonic or hyperechoic relative to the liver.
   d) homogeneous, midgray, lobular outer contour.

2. The spleen is
   a) anterior to the pancreas tail, lateral to the stomach, splenic vein and splenic artery.
   b) retroperitoneal in the left hypochondrium.
   c) intraperitoneal in the left hypochondrium.
   d) lateral to the pancreas tail, anterior to the stomach, anterior to the left kidney.

3. The long axis of the spleen
   a) is only resolved from a posterior approach.
   b) is seen in a left coronal oblique plane.
   c) is seen in a transverse plane.
   d) cannot be resolved intercostally.

4. In most cases, the best patient position to visualize the spleen is
   a) right posterior oblique.
   b) left lateral decubitus.
   c) right lateral decubitus.
   d) left posterior oblique.

5. Accessory spleen is
   a) not sonographically distinguishable.
   b) splenic tissue found separate from the spleen.
   c) abnormal if visualized sonographically.
   d) a rare duplicate spleen.

6. The spleen is part of the reticuloendothelial system and is
   a) a large mass of lymphatic tissue.
   b) essential to life.
   c) the body's largest manufacturer of insulin cells.
   d) responsible for hormone production.

7. The splenic artery
   a) runs directly anterior to the splenic vein.
   b) is visualized longitudinally in a sagittal oblique plane.
   c) is visualized longitudinally in a left coronal plane.
   d) runs superior and slightly anterior to the splenic vein.

8. A scanning technique to help resolve the structures at the splenic hilum is to
   a) use very light pressure within the intercostal space.
   b) angle the transducer anteriorly while the patient performs the Valsalva maneuver.
   c) very slightly rotate/twist the transducer, first one way and then the other.
   d) angle the transducer superiorly while the patient performs the Valsalva maneuver.

9. The spleen is
   a) ovoid with a convex superior surface and concave inferomedial surface.
   b) ovoid with lobulated surfaces.
   c) ovoid with a concave superior surface.
   d) ovoid with a convex inferior surface.

10. The major functions of the spleen are
    a) red blood cell and platelet destruction, defense, hematopoiesis, blood reservoir.
    b) defense, hematopoiesis, red blood cell production, blood reservoir.
    c) defense, insulin production, blood reservoir.
    d) red blood cell and platelet destruction, defense, hormone production, blood reservoir.

11. When scanning near the splenic hilum, what structure will you encounter?
    a) Left kidney
    b) Left lobe of the liver
    c) Splenic vein
    d) Duodenum

12. What vein does the splenic vein drain into?
    a) Portal vein
    b) Left renal vein
    c) IVC
    d) Inferior mesenteric vein

13. The splenic vein joins the SMV and forms the _____.
    a) hepatic vein
    b) gastric vein
    c) portal vein
    d) inferior mesenteric vein

14. This is a coronal scanning plane image of the spleen. Label the accompanying illustration.

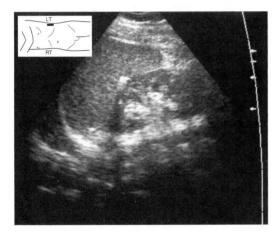

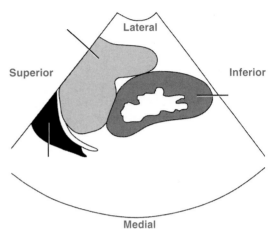

15. This is a transverse left lateral approach image of the spleen. Label the accompanying illustration.

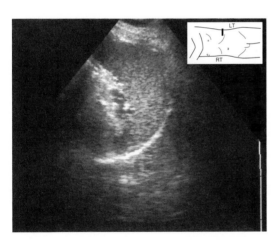

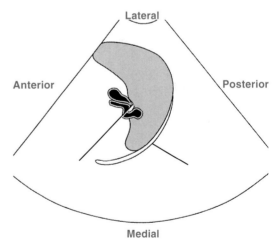

16. This is a coronal scanning plane image of the spleen. Label the accompanying illustration.

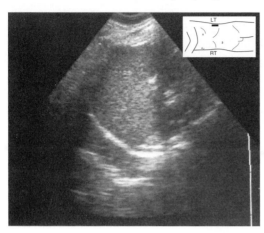

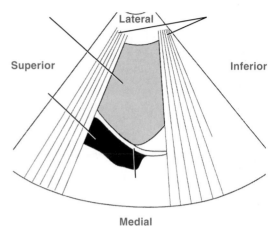

PART IV

PELVIC SCANNING PROTOCOLS

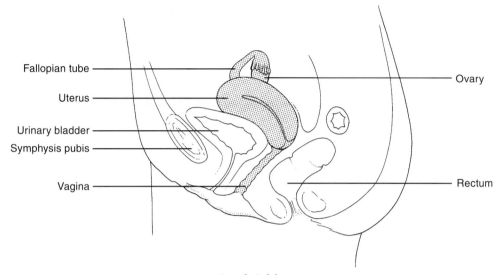

Female Pelvis

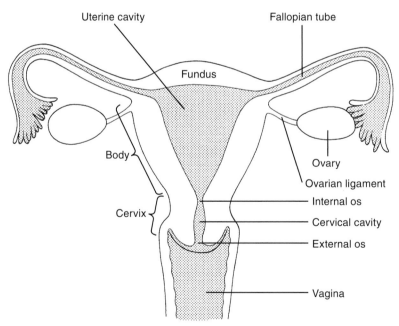

Anatomy of Uterus, Uterine Tubes, Ovaries, and Vagina

CHAPTER 11

Female Pelvis Scanning Protocol

Betty Bates Tempkin

Key Words

Adnexa
Ampulla
Anteflexed
Anterior cul-de-sac
Anteverted
Basal layer
Bicornate uterus
Body
Broad ligaments
Cervix
Corpus
Corpus albicans
Corpus luteum
Didelphia uterus
Endocervical canal
Endometrial canal
Endometrial cavity
Endometrial stripe
Endometrium
Estrogen
External os
False pelvis
False pelvis musculature
Female pelvis
Follicle-stimulating hormone
  (FSH)
Follicles
Follicular phase
Functional layer
Functional zone
Fundus
Genital tract
Hypogastric region
Iliopsoas muscles
Infundibulum
Internal os
Interstitial segment
Left iliac region
Linea alba
Linea terminalis
Luteal phase
Luteinizing hormone (LH)
Menses
Menstrual cycle
Myometrium
Obturator internus muscles
Ovaries
Ovulation
Ovum
Parametrium
Pelvic diaphragm
Pelvis
Piriformis muscles
Pituitary gland
Posterior cul-de-sac
Primary ovarian follicles
Progesterone
Proliferative phase
Psoas muscles
Rectum
Rectus abdominus muscles
Retroflexed
Retroverted
Right iliac region
Secondary ovarian follicles
Secretory phase
Serosa
Sigmoid colon
Space of Retzius
Transverse abdominus muscles
True pelvis
True pelvis musculature
Ureters
Urinary bladder
Uterine canal
Uterine cavity
Uterine cornua
Uterine isthmus
Uterine tube isthmus
Uterine tubes
Uterus
Vagina
Vaginal canal

Objectives

At the end of this chapter, you will be able to:

- Define the key words.
- Distinguish the sonographic appearance of the structures in the female pelvis and the terms used to describe them.
- Describe the transducer options for scanning the female pelvis.
- List the various suggested breathing techniques for patients when scanning the female pelvis.
- List the suggested patient position (and options) when scanning the female pelvis.
- Describe the patient prep for a female pelvis study.
- Distinguish normal variants of female pelvic structures.
- Name the survey steps and explain how to evaluate the entire length, width, and depth of the female pelvis and its structures.
- Explain the order and exact locations to take representative images of the female pelvis and its structures.
- Answer the review questions at the end of the chapter.

Overview

Anatomy

- The **pelvis** is that part of the peritoneal cavity extending from the iliac crests superiorly to the pelvic diaphragm inferiorly.
- The **female pelvis** consists of the **genital tract** (vagina, uterus, and uterine tubes), ovaries, urinary bladder, a portion of the ureters and intestinal tract, pelvic musculature, ligaments, and peritoneal spaces.

True Pelvis and False Pelvis

The descriptive compartments of the pelvic cavity are the true pelvis and false pelvis:

- The true and false pelves are based on an oblique plane in the pelvis defined by the **linea terminalis**, an imaginary line drawn from the symphysis pubis around to the sacral promontory, marking the dividing plane.
  - The **true pelvis** ("lesser pelvis" or "pelvis minor") is the region deep to the linea terminalis.
  - The **false pelvis** ("greater pelvis" or "pelvis major") is the area superior to the linea terminalis and inferior to the iliac crests.

Pelvic Regions

Right Iliac, Hypogastric, and Left Iliac

The descriptive regions of the pelvic cavity *(right iliac, hypogastric, left iliac)* are subdivisions of the **hypogastrium:**

- The **right iliac region** contains the cecum of the colon, appendix, distal end of the right ureter, and right ovary.

- The **hypogastric region** includes the distal end of the ileum, urinary bladder, and uterus.
- The **left iliac region** contains the sigmoid colon, distal end of the left ureter, and left ovary.

Vagina

The **vagina** is a reproductive organ that is part of the genital tract:
- Located in the midregion of the true pelvis between the urinary bladder (anteriorly) and the rectum (posteriorly), the vagina extends from the external genitalia to the cervix of the uterus.
- The vagina is a muscular, tubular organ. The walls are composed of 3 layers:
  1. Inner mucosal lining of epithelial cells
  2. Middle thin, smooth muscle wall
  3. Outer adventitia
- The linings of the vagina and uterus enclose a continuous cavity or channel through which the fetus passes at birth. The inner epithelium encloses a centrally located **vaginal canal** that is approximately 9 cm long.

Uterus

Fundus, Corpus, Isthmus, Cervix (Internal and External Os), Endometrium, Myometrium, and Serosa

The **uterus** is a reproductive organ that is part of the genital tract. It is a muscular, hollow organ where the fertilized ovum embeds and the developing embryo and fetus are nourished:
- The uterus is typically located in the midline of the true pelvis between the urinary bladder (anteriorly) and the rectum (posteriorly). It may also lie just to the right or left of the midline. Its central cavity opens into a uterine (or fallopian) tube on either side and into the vaginal cavity below.
- Uterine walls are composed of 3 layers:
  1. **Endometrium**: inner mucosal layer that encloses the **uterine cavity** (also called the "endometrial cavity," "endometrial canal," or "uterine canal") that is continuous with vaginal epithelium inferiorly. The thickness of the endometrium varies. Just before the onset of menses it measures 8 mm. Following menses it measures 1 mm. The endometrium consists of 2 layers:
     a. Superficial ("**functional layer**" or "**functional zone**"): increases in size during the menstrual cycle and partially sloughs off during menses.
     b. Deep ("**basal layer**"): composed of dense stroma and mucosal glands; it is not significantly influenced by the menstrual cycle.

    2. **Myometrium**: middle, smooth muscle layer that forms the bulk of the uterus.

    3. **Serosa**: outer peritoneal layer is a thin membrane that completely covers the myometrium.

- The uterus is pear-shaped and descriptively divided into 4 parts:
  1. **Fundus**: widest and most superior segment that is continuous with the uterine corpus.
  2. **Corpus or body**: largest part of the uterus that is continuous with the uterine cervix.
  3. **Uterine isthmus:** the slightly constricted portion of the uterus where the uterine body meets the uterine cervix.
  4. **Cervix**: lower cylindrical portion of the uterus that projects into the vagina. The cervical portion of the endometrial canal or the **endocervical canal** extends 2 to 4 cm from its **internal os** (or opening), at approximately the same level as the ithmus, where it joins the endometrial canal to its **external os**, which projects into the vaginal canal.

- The *size* of the uterus is variable and described 4 different ways depending on patient parity and age:
  1. *Prepubertal* size is approximately 2.5 to 3 cm long, 2 cm wide and 1 cm thick. The cervix comprises a significantly greater proportion of the organ.
  2. *Postpubertal, nulliparous* size is usually 7 to 8 cm long, 3 to 5 cm wide, and 3 to 5 cm thick.
  3. *Multiparous* size is usually 8.5 to 9 cm long and 5 cm wide.
  4. *Postmenopausal* size depends on parity but the uterus significantly decreases in size and assumes a prepubertal shape where the cervix comprises the greater portion of the uterus.

- *Uterine position* can be variable but the uterus normally tilts forward, resting on the dome of the bladder. Due to its peritoneal connections and ligaments, there is considerable mobility of the uterus within the true pelvis that affords minimal displacement of the uterus with the filling of the urinary bladder or rectum, as well as marked displacement of the uterus during pregnancy. Further, the flexibility of the uterine support structures affords considerable variations in normal uterine position that are described in 4 different ways as:
  1. **Anteverted** when the bladder is empty; the vagina and cervix form a 90-degree angle and the body and fundus of the uterus are *tilted anteriorly* toward the pubic bone. The uterus is typically anteverted (see illustration **A** on the facing page).
  2. **Anteflexed** when the bladder is empty; the vagina and cervix form a 90-degree angle and the body and fundus of the uterus are *bent anteriorly* toward the pubic bone until the fundus points inferiorly and rests near the cervix (see illustration **B** on the facing page).

3. **Retroverted** when the bladder is empty; the body and fundus of the uterus are *tilted posteriorly* toward the sacrum until the cervix and vagina are linearly oriented (see illustration **C** below).

4. **Retroflexed** when the bladder is empty; the corpus and fundus are *bent posteriorly* toward the sacrum until the fundus points inferiorly and rests near the cervix. The cervix and vagina are linearly oriented (see illustration **D** below).

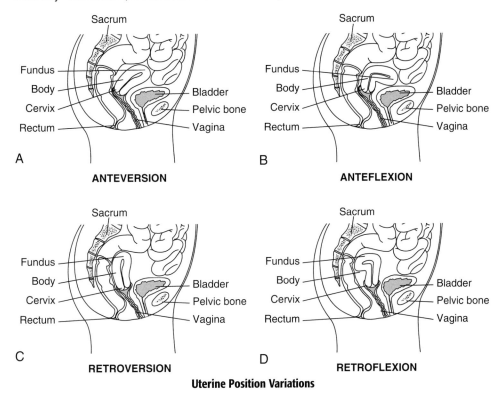

Uterine Position Variations

Uterine Tubes (Fallopian Tubes or Oviducts)
Interstitial Segment, Isthmus, Ampulla, and Infundibulum
The **uterine tubes** are reproductive organs that are part of the genital tract. They are coiled, muscular tubes that emerge from the superolateral margins of the uterus referred to as the **uterine cornua**, then run laterally within the peritoneum along the superior free margin of the *broad ligaments* until they reach the ovaries. Uterine tubes are responsible for directing mature **ovum** (egg cell) from the ovaries to the uterus through gentle peristalsis of its smooth muscle walls:
- Length of the tubes varies from 7 to 12 cm. Their widest diameter is approximately 3 mm.
- Uterine tubes are descriptively divided into 4 segments:
    1. **Interstitial** *or intramural* is the narrowest segment, which is enclosed by the uterus.

2. **Uterine tube isthmus** is the segment adjacent to the uterine wall, connected to the interstitial segment. The isthmus is a short, straight, narrow portion of the tube that widens laterally, to form the ampullary and infundiblular segments.
3. **Ampulla** is the coiled and longest segment where fertilization usually occurs.
4. **Infundibulum** is the widest and funnel-shaped end of the tube that opens into the peritoneal cavity adjacent to the ovary. Fringelike extensions of the infundibulum called fimbria overlie the ovary and direct the released ovum into the tube.

Ovaries

Ovaries are paired, bilateral, almond-shaped, female reproductive organs in which ova are formed. The ovaries contain numerous **follicles**, fluid-filled sacs that contain developing eggs (oocytes).

- The ovaries are located in the **adnexa** (the peritoneal cavity spaces located posterior to the broad ligaments) within the true pelvis. Each ovary is anterior to a ureter and internal iliac artery.
- The *position* of the ovaries is variable:
  - Typically the ovaries lay lateral or posterolateral to the uterus against the pelvic sidewalls when the uterus is characteristically anteverted and lies at the midline of the pelvis.
  - The ovaries never move in front of (or anterior to) the uterus or broad ligaments.
  - If the uterus is retroverted, the ovaries tend to lay superolateral, adjacent to the fundus of the uterus.
  - When the uterus lies to one side of the midline (a normal variation), the ovary on that same side is often displaced from its typical position to lie superior to the fundus of the uterus.
  - If the uterus is enlarged, the ovaries are shifted superolaterally.
  - After a hysterectomy (surgical removal of the uterus), the ovaries shift toward the midline, superior to the vagina.
- The *size* of the ovaries varies and is described 3 ways depending on patient age, phase of the menstrual cycle, and menstrual status:
  1. *Prepubertal* ovaries are relatively large at birth, then between the ages of 2 and 6 ovarian size remains relatively stable with a volume of 2.3 cm^3 or less. Between the ages of 6 and 7, age-related growth associated with cystic functional changes begin and continue through puberty.
  2. *Postpubertal* ovarian size is approximately 4 to 5 cm long, 3 cm wide, and 2 cm thick. Volume measurements are generally 9.8 cm^3 but may be higher during the preovulatory phase and lower during luteal phases.
  3. *Postmenopausal* ovaries are approximately 2 cm long, 1 cm wide, and 0.5 cm thick. Volume measurements are usually 5.8 cm^3. It should be noted that ovarian atrophy takes place gradually.

Urinary Bladder

The **urinary bladder** is a symmetrical, hollow, muscular organ. It is part of the urinary system and serves as a reservoir for the urine that is formed in the kidneys.

- The urinary bladder is fixed inferiorly at its base in the true pelvis, directly posterior to the symphysis pubis and anterior to the uterus and vagina. As the bladder fills with urine, the dome can extend superiorly into the false pelvis.
- Bladder shape is variable depending on distention. The bladder can hold as much as 16 to 18 ounces of urine.
- The normal distended urinary bladder wall measures 1 cm or less.

Ureters

The **ureters** are muscular tubes that are the part of the urinary system that convey urine from the kidneys to the urinary bladder.

- Normally each kidney has one ureter that travels inferiorly through the retroperitoneum for 10 to 12 inches from the renal hilum to the posterior portion of the bladder. They are less than 1.4 inches wide and decrease in diameter as they course to the bladder.
- In the true pelvis the ureter runs between the internal iliac artery (posteriorly) and the ovary (anteriorly), then courses anteromedially to enter the trigone of the urinary bladder just anterior to the vagina.
- Ureters are clinically significant in the female pelvis because pelvic pathologic conditions can cause obstruction of the ureter(s) and ultimately affect the kidney(s).

Colon

Sigmoid and Rectum

The *sigmoid colon* and *rectum* are the parts of the gastrointestinal system located within the true pelvis.

- The **sigmoid colon** is continuous with the descending colon in the left lower quadrant of the pelvis and is loosely secured to the posterior pelvic wall. It descends toward the rectum in the inferoposterior aspect of the pelvis at the level of the third sacral vertebra.
- The **rectum** is fixed in its position posterior to the vagina and is largely retroperitoneal.

Musculature

Psoas Muscles, and False Pelvis and True Pelvis Musculature

Pelvic musculature is part of the musculoskeletal system. The pelvic muscles serve as support and protection:

- **Psoas muscles** are the paired major muscles on either side of the spine that extend from the lateral aspects of the lower thoracic vertebrae anterolaterally across the posterior wall of the abdominopelvic cavity to the iliac crests.

- False pelvis musculature: *iliopsoas, rectus abdominus, transverse abdominus.*
  - Each psoas muscle joins an iliacus muscle at the level of the iliac crests to form the **iliopsoas muscles** that travel anteroinferiorly to insert into the lesser trochanter of the femur.
  - The large pair of **rectus abdominus muscles** extend from the sixth ribs and xiphoid process of the sternum down to the pubic symphysis.
  - Each **transverse abdominus muscle** forms the anterolateral borders of the abdominopelvic cavity. The muscular sheath surrounding each rectus abdominus muscle fuses with the transverse abdominus muscles to form the tendinous **linea alba** at the midline.
- True pelvis musculature: *obturator internus, piriformis, pelvic diaphragm (pubococcygeus, iliococcygeus [levator ani], coccygeus).*
  - The **obturator internus muscles** line the lateral walls of the true pelvis.
  - **Piriformis muscles** are situated in the posterior region of the true pelvis behind the uterus. They are often misidentified as enlarged ovaries.
  - The **pelvic diaphragm** is a group of muscles lining the floor of the true pelvis to support the pelvic organs. Each pubococcygeus muscle extends from the pubic bones to the coccyx, encircling the rectum, vagina, and urethra. The iliococcygeus muscles are located lateral to each pubococcygeus muscle. Together these muscles form a hammock across the pelvic floor and are termed the levator ani muscles. Each coccygeus muscle extends from the ischial spine to the sacrum and coccyx. They are the most posterior muscle pair of the pelvic diaphragm.

Ligaments
Broad, Round, Cardinal, Uterosacral, Infundibulopelvic, Ovarian, Pubovesical, and Lateral

The broad ligaments are the only pelvic ligaments routinely identified sonographically. Pelvic ligaments are part of the musculoskeletal system. They are peritoneal connections that provide flexibility and mobility of pelvic organs:

- **Broad ligaments:** each broad ligament extends between the uterine cornu and ovary. Each uterine (or fallopian) tube, round ligament, ovarian ligament, and vascular structures of the uterus and ovaries are positioned between the 2 layers of the broad ligaments. These structures are surrounded by fat and connective tissue called the **parametrium.**

Pelvic Spaces

Anterior Cul-de-Sac, Posterior Cul-de-Sac, and Space of Retzius

Differentiation of the 3 pelvic peritoneal spaces is significant because of the potential abnormalities that can invade them:

1. Anterior cul-de-sac, or vesicouterine pouch, is a shallow peritoneal space located between the anterior wall of the uterus and the urinary bladder. This space all but disappears as the urinary bladder fills with urine.
2. Posterior cul-de-sac, rectouterine pouch, or pouch of Douglas is the most posterior and dependent portion of the peritoneal sac. It is located between the rectum and the uterus.
3. Space of Retzius, or prevesical or retropubic space, is a fascial space between the anterior bladder wall and pubic symphysis.

Physiology

Female Reproductive System

Between puberty and menopause, the female reproductive system undergoes monthly cyclical changes referred to as the menstrual cycle. The menstrual cycle usually follows a 28-day course, during which a single ovum reaches maturity and is released into the genital tract. The pituitary gland (part of the brain that oversees all hormonal activity) and ovaries secrete hormones that control changes in the ovaries and the uterine endometrium throughout the menstrual cycle. The changes in the ovaries correlate to the changes in the endometrium.

- **Days 1 to 14 of the menstrual cycle correspond to the "follicular phase" of the ovaries and menses and the "proliferative phase" of the uterine endometrium.**
  - By the onset of menses (menstrual flow or monthly discharge of blood from the uterus of nonpregnant women), each ovary contains thousands of undeveloped follicles, each composed of a single primary oocyte. During the ovarian follicular phase (days 1 to 14 of the menstrual cycle), follicle-stimulating hormone (FSH) is released by the pituitary gland to initiate the development of several primary ovarian follicles. As each primary follicle grows, its oocyte reaches a mature size (ovum). At this stage of development, the ovum and surrounding structures are referred to as secondary ovarian follicles.
  - Menses generally occurs during days 1 to 5 of the menstrual cycle. The thickened, superficial layer of the endometrium is shed when fertilization of an ovum does not occur.
  - Following menses, the endometrium goes into the proliferative phase that lasts until day 14 of the menstrual cycle. During the proliferative phase, ovarian follicles contain cells that begin to release the hormone estrogen, which initiates thickening and

swelling of the endometrium in preparation for implantation by a fertilized ovum.

- **Day 14 of the menstrual cycle is when *ovulation* usually occurs.**
  - Although many follicles develop, only one matures completely and will release a mature ovum at ovulation. When the follicle ruptures and the mature ovum is expelled into the peritoneal cavity, the fimbria of the uterine tube draw the released egg into the infundibulum.
- **Days 15 to 28 of the menstrual cycle correspond to the "luteal phase" of the ovaries and "secretory phase" of the uterine endometrium.**
  - Following ovulation, the ruptured follicle fills with blood and is called the corpus luteum. This begins the ovarian luteal phase and the endometrial secretory phase of the menstrual cycle (days 15 to 28). The corpus luteum transforms into an endocrine gland and secretes the hormone progesterone, which promotes glandular secretions of the uterine endometrium further preparing it for implantation by a fertilized ovum.
  - Simultaneously, throughout the menstrual cycle, luteinizing hormone (LH) has been released by the pituitary gland to stimulate the ovaries to secrete estrogen and progesterone. The concentration of estrogen and progesterone promote continued thickening and swelling of the endometrium. The maximum anteroposterior diameter of the endometrium during this secretory phase is 14 to 16 mm. In addition, exocrine glands of the endometrial lining produce glycogen-rich mucus to help prepare a suitable environment for implantation.
  - The corpus luteum depends on LH to continue to produce progesterone but ironically, progesterone levels inhibit LH production. Consequently, the corpus luteum regresses and only a fibrous tissue mass, called the corpus albicans, remains in the ovary.
  - In the absence of fertilization, estrogen and progesterone levels diminish, and a new menstrual cycle starts on day 1 with menses of the endometrium and the beginning of the ovarian follicular phase.

Sonographic Appearance
Vagina, Uterus, Uterine Tubes, Ovaries, Urinary Bladder, Ureters, Sigmoid Colon, Rectum, Pelvic Musculature, Broad Ligaments, and Pelvic Peritoneal Spaces

- *Uterine tubes* are not routinely identified sonographically unless they become outlined by free intraperitoneal fluid or are abnormal.
- The *urinary bladder* cavity is not seen if it is collapsed; distended with urine, it appears anechoic with bright, reflective walls.

- *Ureters* are not routinely identified sonographically.
- The appearance of the *rectosigmoid colon* varies according to content, but typically the sigmoid colon and the rectum contain gas and fecal material that cast a posterior acoustic shadow. Collapsed bowel can mimic an ovary; however, the observation of peristalsis allows differentiation.
- *Pelvic ligaments* are not routinely identified sonographically unless they become outlined by free intraperitoneal fluid. The *broad ligaments* may also be identified when the uterus is retroverted. They are best viewed longitudinally from a transverse plane and appear thin, linear, and midgray.
- The *muscles* of the pelvis appear hypoechoic relative to pelvic organs and exhibit the same characteristic low-gray sonographic muscular pattern seen from other muscles throughout the rest of the body.
- It is normal to visualize a small amount of free fluid in the *posterior cul-de-sac*. Any fluid found in the *anterior cul-de-sac, lateral pelvic recesses* or a large collection of fluid in the posterior cul-de-sac is considered abnormal. The *space of Retzius* is not significant sonographically unless the urinary bladder appears to be displaced posteriorly. This is a characteristic feature of masses in the space of Retzius because other pelvic masses typically displace the bladder anteriorly or inferiorly.
- Since the *uterus* and *vagina* are vertically orientated in the body, their longitudinal and long axis views are seen in transabdominal, sagittal scanning planes as shown in the image on the following page. It demonstrates the long axis of the uterus and vagina. The uterus is well visualized and although the appearance of the uterine endometrium is altered by menstrual cycle changes, the intermediate layer of the *myometrium* and bulk of the normal uterus consistently exhibit a low-gray, homogeneous texture as seen in the image. The only notable sonographic characteristic of the outer serosa layer of the uterus is its smooth contour. It is otherwise indistinguishable. Notice how the central *endometrium* looks thick and appears to be in the secretory phase (days 15 to 28) of the menstrual cycle where the basal layer, functional zone, and canal become isosonic. The vagina appears tubular, its muscular walls are isosonic/isoechoic to and continuous with the uterine myometrium. The bright stripe representing the centrally located *endocervical* and *endovaginal canals* is well delineated. Note the small amount of anechoic free fluid in the *posterior cul-de-sac* (between the rectum and the cervix). Note how the normal *bladder wall* appears thin, smooth, and bright.

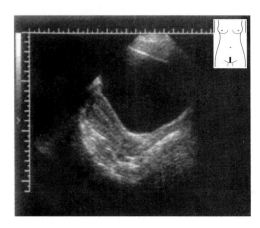

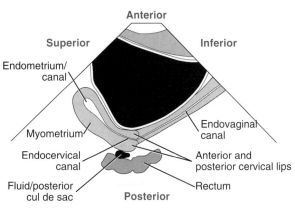

- The central, linear, opposing surfaces of the endometrium that form the *endometrial canal* present sonographically as a bright, thin, midline strip, referred to as the **endometrial stripe**. As the thickness of the endometrium changes cyclically with the menstrual cycle so does its sonographic appearance:
  - During the *menstrual phase* the endometrium appears thin and bright as the superficial layer is sloughed off.
  - During the early *proliferative phase* (days 5 to 9) the endometrium appears as a thin, bright line that normally measures 4 to 8 mm.
  - During the *later proliferative phase* (days 10 to 14), just before ovulation, the functional zone becomes thicker due to increased levels of estrogen, and the endometrium exhibits a multilayered appearance. The bright stripe of the endometrial canal is surrounded by the thick functional zone, which appears hypoechoic relative to the bright basal layer that is surrounded by the hypoechoic inner layer of the myometrium. At this stage, the endometrium will normally measure 6 to 10 mm.
  - During the *secretory phase* (days 15 to 28) the endometrium can normally measure 7 to 14 mm as the functional zone becomes even thicker and edematous due to increased levels of progesterone and the secretion of a glycogen-rich mucous, which together cause the functional zone to appear brighter and become isoechoic to the basal layer and canal.
- The next image shows an axial section of the fundus of the uterus taken in a transabdominal transverse scanning plane. In this image all of the *myometrial layers* are distinguishable. Notice how the outer and inner fibrous layers appear hypoechoic compared to the low-gray appearance of the intermediate layer. The inner layer has been described as a thin, very low gray, hypoechoic halo surrounding the endometrium.

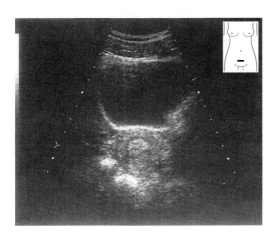

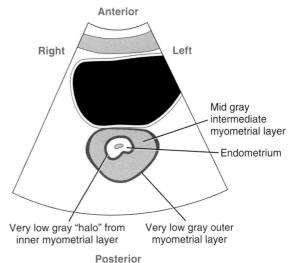

- The arrows in the following image taken in a transabdominal transverse scanning plane are pointing to the fascia around the *broad ligament,* which extends from the uterine cornu to the ovary. Each broad ligament and the uterine tubes that run along the broad ligaments are not appreciated sonographically unless they are abnormal or there is a collection of free fluid in the lateral pelvic recesses making them viewable. The axial sections of the uterus and right ovary normally appear low gray and homogeneous as seen here. Notice how the sidewall *musculature* is hypoechoic compared to the uterus and ovary. Note that the shape of the anechoic, distended bladder varies but it may appear somewhat squared, as it does in this image, when viewed in a transverse scanning plane.

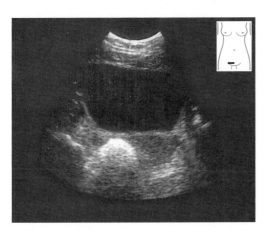

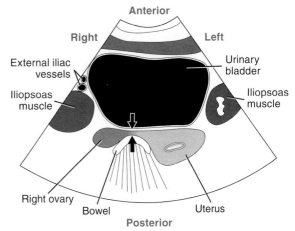

• The next image taken in a transabdominal transverse scanning plane shows axial sections and the general lateral position of the *ovaries* relative to the uterus. Notice how the ovaries appear mid to low gray and homogeneous except for the interruption of the small, anechoic follicles (a common finding during reproductive years). Note that ovarian follicles will vary in size and number.

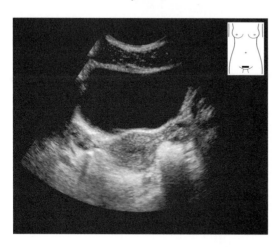

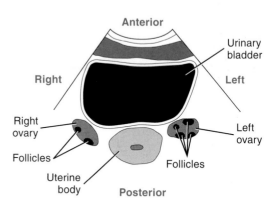

• This endovaginal image demonstrates a normal *ovary* with follicles. Note how the periphery of the ovary appears hypoechoic compared to the midgray parenchyma of the ovary.

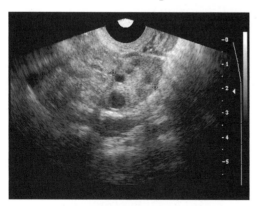

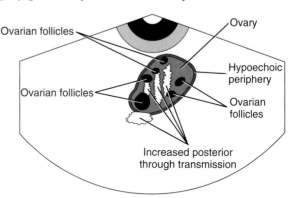

Normal Variants

• Uterine position:
  • As previously discussed, the normal variations in uterine position include anteversion, anteflexion, retroversion, and retroflexion. Sonographic appearance is the same as that of the normal uterus, cervix, and vagina.
• Uterine location:
  • As previously noted, the typical anteflexed uterus usually lies at the midline of the pelvis; however, it is not uncommon for it to

lie just to the right or left of the midline. Sonographic appearance is the same as that of the normal uterus. It is important to note that when the uterus does lie to one side of the midline, the ovary on that same side is often displaced from its typical position (posterolateral to the uterus) to lie superior to the fundus of the uterus.

- Didelphia uterus:
  - Developmental variant causing *2 uterine bodies, 2 cervices, and 2 vaginas*. Sonographic appearance is the same as that of the normal uterus, cervix, and vagina, but the anatomy is duplicated. May occur in any uterine position or location.
- Bicornate uterus:
  - Developmental variant causing *2 uterine bodies (divided)* or *2 uterine horns (septated)* with 1 or 2 cervices and 1 vagina. Sonographic appearance is the same as that of the normal uterus, cervix, and vagina, with duplication of the uterus. May occur in any uterine position or location.

Preparation

Patient Prep

- Before the examination of the female pelvis, a patient history should be taken to include the date of the first day of the patient's last period, parity, gravidity (pregnancy test results if available), symptoms, pelvic examination results, and any history of pelvic surgery. Most sonography departments have standard forms where this information is recorded.
- For transabdominal scanning, the patient must have a full urinary bladder. This moves bowel out of the way and serves as a sonic "window" for visualizing pelvic structures. One hour before the examination, 32 to 40 ounces of clear fluid should be ingested and finished within a 15- to 20-minute time period.
- If for any reason the patient cannot have fluids, sterile water can be used to fill the bladder through a Foley catheter.

> **NOTE:** An overfilled bladder can actually push the pelvic organs out of view. If this occurs, have the patient partially void.
> **NOTE:** Normal bowel can mimic a pathologic condition. To distinguish between the two, the patient can be given a water enema to differentiate the bowel.

Transducer

- **3.0 MHz or 3.5 MHz.**
- 5.0 MHz for thin patients.

Breathing Technique
• **Normal respiration.**

Patient Position
• **Supine.**

Female Pelvis Survey

> **NOTE:** Survey of the female pelvis begins with the longitudinal and axial surveys of the vagina, uterus, and pelvic cavity followed by longitudinal and axial surveys of the ovaries.

Vagina, Uterus, and Pelvic Cavity Survey Steps

Vagina, Uterus, and Pelvic Cavity • Longitudinal Survey
Sagittal Plane • Anterior Approach

1. It is easiest to survey the longitudinal sections of the vagina and uterus when they are visualized together; therefore, finding their long axis is the best way to begin. Start scanning with the transducer perpendicular, at the midline of the body, just superior to and directly against the symphysis pubis. In most cases, the long sections of the vagina and cervix will be visualized here and possibly the body and fundus of the uterus depending on their position. Look for the vagina inferiorly, in the area between the anechoic bladder (seen anteriorly) and the bright rectum (seen posteriorly). If the vagina and cervix are not visualized, move the transducer a little to the right and/or left of midline, or slightly angle the transducer inferiorly, or use a combination of both until the vagina and cervix come into view. If the body and fundus of the uterus are not seen in the same scanning plane with the vagina and cervix, then oblique the plane by slowly rotating/twisting the transducer varying degrees until the body and fundus come into view and visually "connect" to the cervix. Further adjust (oblique) the scanning plane until the long axis of the uterus and vagina and endometrial, endocervical, and vaginal canals are visualized together.

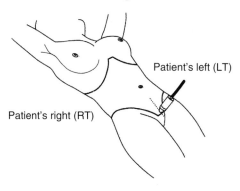

Patient's left (LT)

Patient's right (RT)

2. Once the long axes of the uterus and vagina are determined, slowly move the transducer to the patient's right, scanning through and beyond the lateral margins of the uterus, vagina, adnexa, and pelvic sidewalls. Note the location of the right ovary if it is visualized.

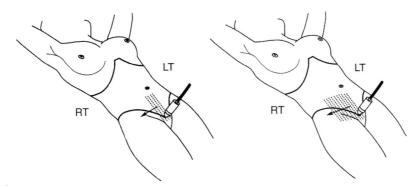

3. Relocate the long axis of the uterus and vagina. Now slowly move the transducer to the patient's left, scanning through and beyond the lateral margins of the uterus, vagina, adnexa, and pelvic sidewalls. Note the location of the left ovary if it is visualized.

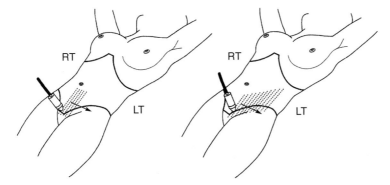

Vagina, Uterus, and Pelvic Cavity • Axial Survey
Transverse Plane • Anterior Approach

1. Still in the sagittal scanning plane, relocate the long axis of the uterus and vagina. Focus on the vagina, then rotate the transducer 90 degrees into the transverse scanning plane until a small, oval, axial section of the vagina comes into view in the area between the bladder (seen anteriorly) and the rectum (seen posteriorly). Slightly rotate/twist the transducer as necessary to resolve the centrally located vaginal canal.

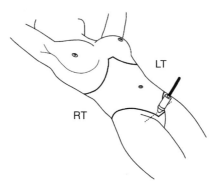

2. Now very slowly angle the transducer inferiorly to scan through and beyond the margins of the vagina and pelvic cavity. Very slowly straighten the transducer back up to perpendicular, scanning into the pelvis and back onto the vagina. Note the pelvic sidewalls.

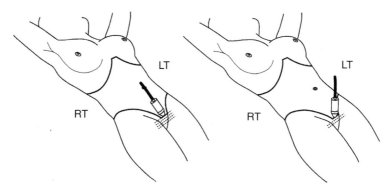

3. Keep the transducer perpendicular and very slowly slide superiorly, scanning through and beyond the margins of the vagina and onto the cervix. Look for the small axial section of the cervix to appear slightly larger than the vagina and to come into view in the area between the bladder (seen anteriorly) and the posterior cul-de-sac (seen posteriorly). Slightly rotate/twist the transducer as necessary to resolve the centrally located endocervical canal. Note the pelvic sidewalls.

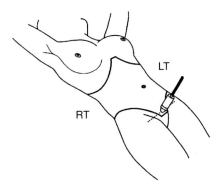

4. Keep the transducer perpendicular and very slowly slide superiorly, scanning through and beyond the cervix and onto the body of the uterus. Look for the body to appear significantly larger than the cervix. Slightly rotate/twist the transducer as necessary to resolve the centrally located endometrial canal. One or both ovaries may come into view laterally or posterolaterally to the body of the uterus. Note the pelvic sidewalls.

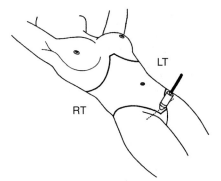

5. Continue to move the transducer superiorly, slowly scanning through the body of the uterus and onto the fundus. Look for the axial section of the fundus to appear slightly larger than the body. Slightly rotate/twist the transducer as necessary to resolve the centrally located endometrial canal. Scan superiorly through the fundus and urinary bladder walls all the way to the level of the umbilicus. As you scan beyond the bladder, the bowel will come into view. Adjust technique according to bowel content. One or both ovaries may be visualized posterior and lateral to the fundus. Note the pelvic sidewalls.

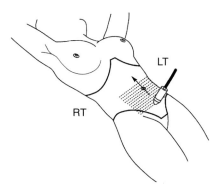

Ovaries Survey Steps

NOTE: The location and lie of the ovaries is quite variable; therefore, they can be a challenge to locate and the long axis can lie in either scanning plane. Ovaries tend to be lateral to the body or fundus of the uterus but may be found tucked in close to the side of the uterus. Other locations include far posterior or even superior to the uterus. If the ovaries are not identified during the following surveys, every effort must be made to locate them, including endovaginal sonography (see Chapter 12).

Right Ovary • Longitudinal Survey
Sagittal Plane • Anterior Approach

For the sake of instruction, this assumes that the ovary long axis is visualized in a sagittal plane.

1. Begin with the transducer perpendicular, at the midline of the body, just superior to the symphysis pubis. Slowly move the transducer to the patient's right, scanning just beyond the right lateral margin of the uterus. Look for the ovary to appear in the area lateral to the uterus between the external iliac vein and/ or urinary bladder (seen anteriorly) and the external iliac artery (seen posteriorly). It may be necessary to twist the transducer varying degrees as you move right laterally to bring the ovary

into view. Once the ovary is identified, very slightly rotate/twist the transducer, first one way and then the other, to resolve its long axis.

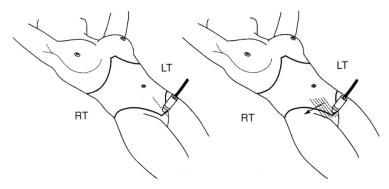

NOTE: If the ovary cannot be seen because of overlying bowel, angle the transducer right lateral toward the right ovary from the midline of the pelvic cavity or just to the left of the midline.

2. Now very slowly move or angle the transducer toward the patient's right, scanning through and beyond the right lateral margin of the ovary. Move back onto the ovary and very slowly move or angle the transducer toward the midline of the pelvic cavity, scanning through and beyond the medial margin of the ovary.

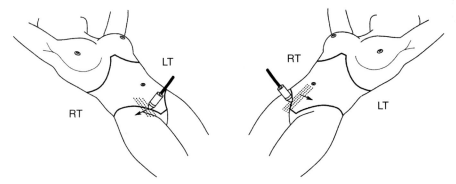

Right Ovary • Axial Survey
Transverse Plane • Anterior Approach

1. Still in the sagittal scanning plane, relocate the long axis of the right ovary then rotate the transducer 90 degrees into the transverse scanning plane until the small, oval, axial section of the ovary comes into view.

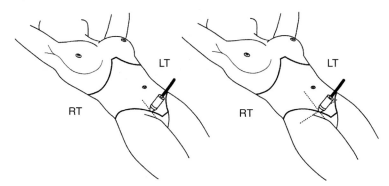

2. Very slowly move or angle the transducer superiorly, scanning through and beyond the superior margin of the ovary. Move back onto the ovary and very slowly move or angle the transducer inferiorly, scanning through and beyond the inferior margin of the ovary.

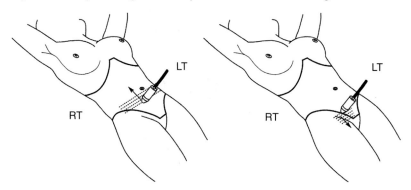

Left Ovary • Longitudinal and Axial Surveys
Use the same survey steps and scanning methods as those used for the right ovary.

Female Pelvis Required Images

NOTE: The required images are a small representation of what a sonographer visualizes during a study. Therefore, the images should provide the interpreting physician with the most telling and technically accurate information available.

Vagina, Uterus, and Pelvic Cavity • Longitudinal Images
Sagittal Plane • Anterior Approach

Longitudinal images begin with representative images of the pelvic cavity followed by a long axis image of the uterus.

1. Longitudinal image of the **MIDLINE** of the pelvic cavity just superior to the symphysis pubis.

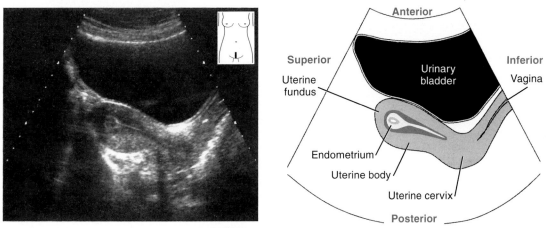

Labeled: **PELVIS SAG ML**

2. Longitudinal image of the **RIGHT ADNEXA** that may include part of the uterus depending on its position.

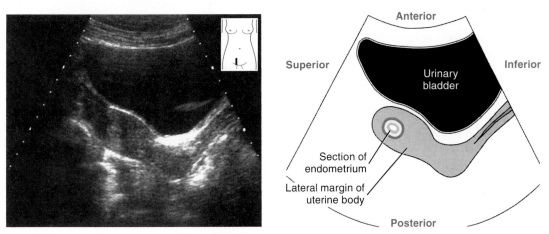

Labeled: **PELVIS SAG R1**

3. Longitudinal image to include the right lateral wall of the **BLADDER** and **PELVIC SIDEWALL.**

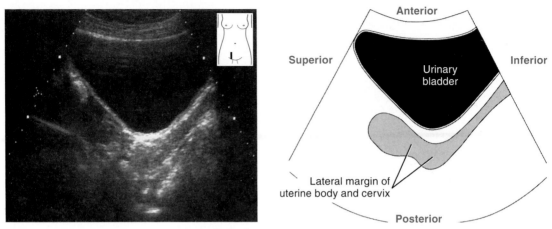

Labeled: **PELVIS SAG R2**

4. Longitudinal image of the **LEFT ADNEXA** that may include part of the uterus depending on its position.

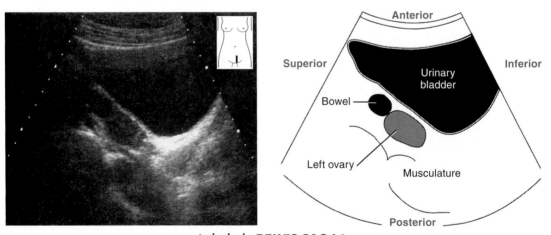

Labeled: **PELVIS SAG L1**

5. Longitudinal image to include the left lateral wall of the **BLADDER** and **PELVIC SIDEWALL.**

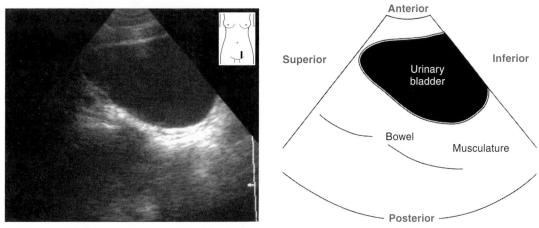

Labeled: **PELVIS SAG L2**

6. **LONG AXIS** image of the uterus to include as much endometrial cavity as possible *with uterine length (superior to inferior) and height (anterior to posterior) measurements.*

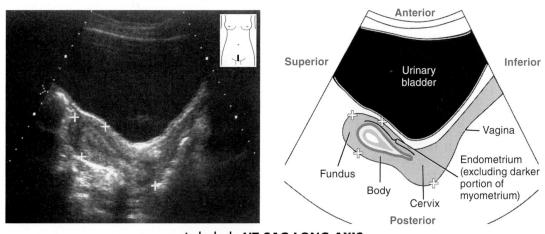

Labeled: **UT SAG LONG AXIS**

7. Same image as number 6 *without calipers.*

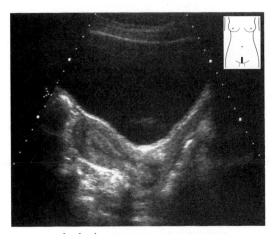

Labeled: **UT SAG LONG AXIS**

> **NOTE:** It may be necessary to take an additional image demonstrating the long axis of the endometrial, endocervical, and vaginal canals. If so label: **UT SAG**

Vagina, Uterus, and Pelvic Cavity • Axial Images
Transverse Plane • Anterior Approach
8. Axial image of the **VAGINA.**

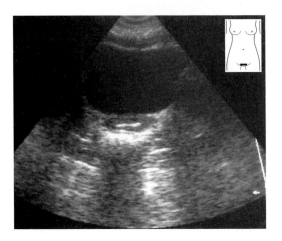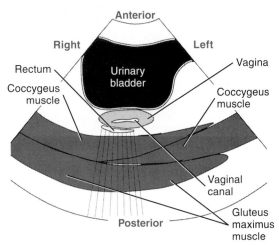

Labeled: **TRV VAG**

9. Axial image of the **CERVIX.**

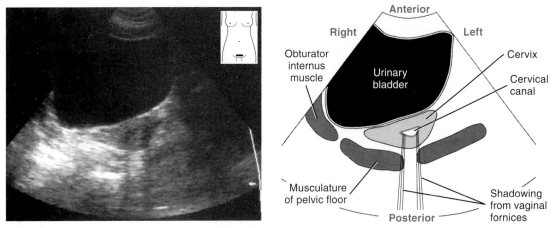

Labeled: **TRV CERX**

10. Axial image of the **UTERUS BODY.**

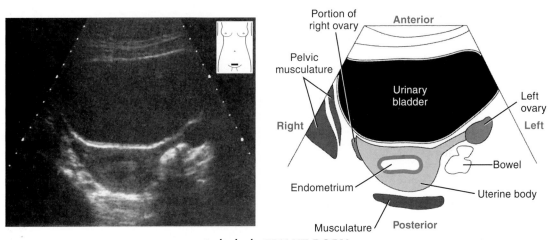

Labeled: **TRV UT BODY**

11. Axial image of the **UTERUS FUNDUS** *measuring uterine width (right to left).*

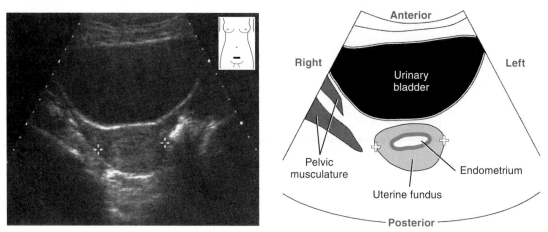

Labeled: **TRV UT FUNDUS**

12. Same image as number 11 *without calipers.*

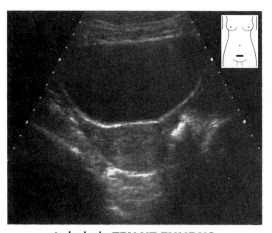

Labeled: **TRV UT FUNDUS**

Right Ovary • Longitudinal Images
Sagittal Plane • Anterior Approach

13. **LONG AXIS** image of the right ovary *measuring length (superior to inferior) and height (anterior to posterior).*

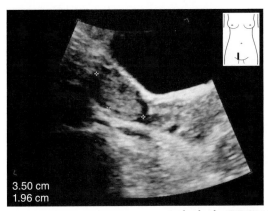 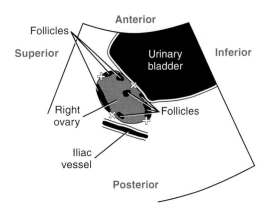

Labeled: **RT OV SAG LONG AXIS**
(Courtesy University of Virginia Health Systems Imaging Center.)

NOTE: If this image of the ovary was angled from midline, then the image is obliqued and must be labeled: **RT OV SAG OBL LONG AXIS**

14. Same image as number 13 *without calipers.*

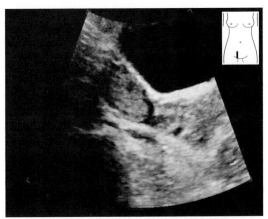

Labeled: **RT OV SAG LONG AXIS**
(Courtesy University of Virginia Health Systems Imaging Center.)

Right Ovary • Axial Images
Transverse Plane • Anterior Approach

15. Axial image of the **RIGHT OVARY** *with width (right to left) measurement.*

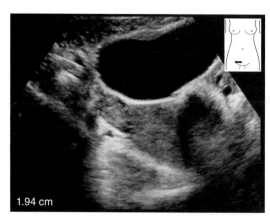

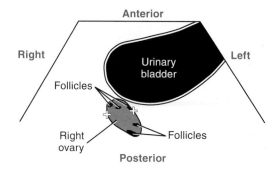

Labeled: **RT OV TRV**
(Courtesy University of Virginia Health Systems Imaging Center.)

NOTE: If this image of the ovary was angled from midline, then the image is obliqued and must be labeled: **RT OV TRV OBL**

16. Same image as number 15 *without calipers.*

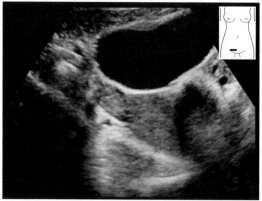

Labeled: **RT OV TRV**
(Courtesy University of Virginia Health Systems Imaging Center.)

Left Ovary • Longitudinal Images
Sagittal Plane • Anterior Approach

17. **LONG AXIS** image of the left ovary *measuring length (superior to inferior) and height (anterior to posterior).*

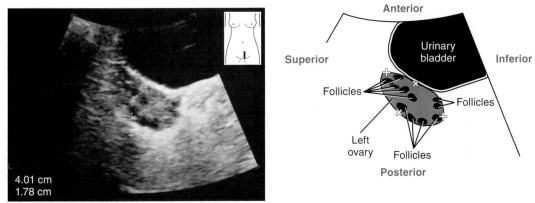

Labeled: **LT OV SAG LONG AXIS**
(Courtesy University of Virginia Health Systems Imaging Center.)

NOTE: If this image of the ovary was angled from midline, then the image is obliqued and must be labeled: **LT OV SAG OBL LONG AXIS**

18. Same image as number 17 *without calipers.*

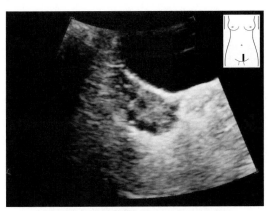

Labeled: **LT OV SAG LONG AXIS**
(Courtesy University of Virginia Health Systems Imaging Center.)

Left Ovary • Axial Images
Transverse Plane • Anterior Approach

19. Axial image of the **LEFT OVARY** *with width (right to left) measurement.*

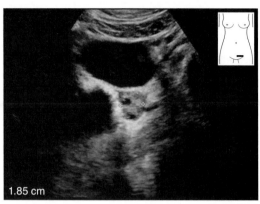

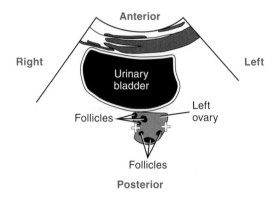

Labeled: **LT OV TRV**

(Courtesy University of Virginia Health Systems Imaging Center.)

> **NOTE:** If this image of the ovary was angled from midline, then the image is obliqued and must be labeled: **LT OV TRV OBL**

20. Same image as number 19 *without calipers.*

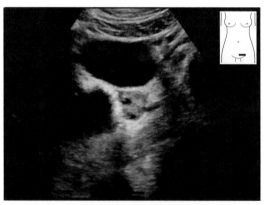

Labeled: **LT OV TRV**

(Courtesy University of Virginia Health Systems Imaging Center.)

Review Questions

Answers on page 630.

1. The linings of the vagina and uterus
   a) are separated by the external os of the cervix.
   b) excrete glycogen-rich mucous during the secretory phase.
   c) are shed during menses.
   d) enclose a continuous cavity or channel through which the fetus passes at birth.

2. The walls of the uterus are composed of
   a) the serosa, basal layer, and endometrium.
   b) outer adventita, middle thin smooth muscle, and inner mucosal lining.
   c) endometrium, myometrium, and basal layer.
   d) endometrium, myometrium, and serosa.

3. What part of the uterus enlarges during the menstrual cycle?
   a) Endometrium
   b) Basal layer
   c) Myometrium
   d) Endometrial canal

4. The functional zone
   a) occurs during the proliferative phase.
   b) is the superficial layer of the endometrium.
   c) is the innermost layer of the myometrium.
   d) is not influenced by the menstrual cycle.

5. The isthmus is the slightly constricted portion of
   a) the uterine body where it meets the uterine cervix.
   b) uterine cervix where it meets the vagina.
   c) the uterine body that is abnormal if visualized sonographically.
   d) a rare duplicate cervix.

6. The normal position of the uterus is described as
   a) anteflexed.
   b) retroverted.
   c) anteverted.
   d) retroflexed.

7. When the urinary bladder is displaced posteriorly
   a) look for a mass in the space of Retzius.
   b) it is considered a normal variant.
   c) the uterus is anteflexed.
   d) the uterus is retroflexed.

8. The luteal phase correlates with
   a) menses.
   b) the proliferative phase.
   c) follicle maturation.
   d) the secretory phase.

9. The follicular phase correlates with
   a) menses.
   b) the proliferative phase.
   c) follicle maturation.
   d) the secretory phase.

10. When does the endometrium exhibit a multilayered appearance?
   a) During menses
   b) During the early proliferative phase
   c) During the late proliferative phase
   d) During the late secretory phase

11. Which muscles are sometimes mistaken for ovaries?
   a) Levator ani
   b) Piriformis
   c) Obturator internus
   d) Coccygeus

12. Which muscles form a hammock across the pelvic floor?
   a) Levator ani
   b) Piriformis
   c) Obturator internus
   d) Coccygeus

13. Just before the onset of menses, the endometrium measures ____.
   a) 1 mm
   b) 12 mm
   c) 4 mm
   d) 8 mm

14. The maximum anteroposterior diameter of the endometrium during the secretory phase is ____.
   a) 14 to 16 mm
   b) 15 to 28 mm
   c) 4 mm
   d) 8 mm

15. It is normal to visualize a small amount of free fluid in the _____.
   a) vesicouterine pouch
   b) anterior cul-de-sac
   c) posterior cul-de-sac
   d) lateral pelvic recesses

16. The pouch of Douglas is also known as the _____.
   a) vesicouterine pouch
   b) anterior cul-de-sac
   c) posterior cul-de-sac
   d) lateral pelvic recesses

17. The rectouterine pouch is also known as the _____.
   a) vesicouterine pouch
   b) anterior cul-de-sac
   c) posterior cul-de-sac
   d) lateral pelvic recesses

18. Label the following:

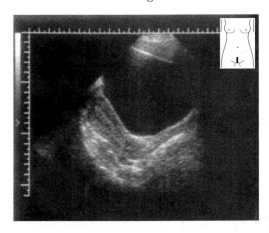 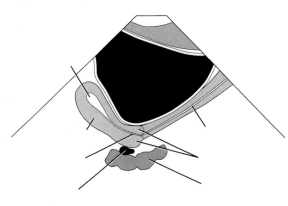

19. Label the following:

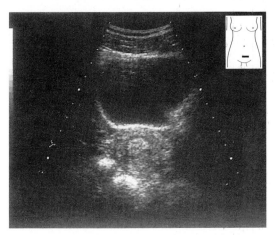 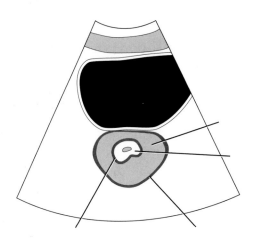

20. Label the following:

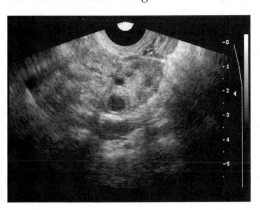 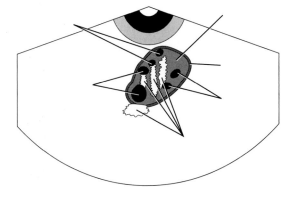

CHAPTER 12

Transvaginal Scanning Protocol for the Female Pelvis

Betty Bates Tempkin

> **NOTE:** In most institutions it is standard practice to begin a sonographic evaluation of the female pelvis with a transabdominal study. If the transabdominal study provides the diagnosis, then the transvaginal scan is not necessary.

Objectives

At the end of this chapter, you will be able to:

- Describe the transducer options for transvaginal scanning.
- List the scanning planes and image orientations for transvaginal scanning.
- List the suggested patient position (and options) for transvaginal scanning.
- Describe the patient prep for transvaginal scanning.
- Name the survey steps and how to evaluate the entire length, width, and depth of the female pelvis and its structures.
- Explain the order and exact locations to take representative images of the female pelvis and its structures.
- Answer the review questions at the end of the chapter.

Overview

Transvaginal sonography is an ultrasound performed inside the vaginal cavity with an endocavital transducer or probe. Most experts feel that transvaginal sonography is a limited and incomplete evaluation of the female pelvis because of its narrow field of view (compared to transabdominal scanning, which has a much wider field of view). Therefore, "trans" or "endo" vaginal sonography is typically used in conjunction with transabdominal sonography when pelvic contents require further evaluation. Resolution of pelvic structures is better with transvaginal imaging than transabdominal imaging because there is less attenuating tissue between the transvaginal transducer and pelvic structures. This provides better anatomic detail than transabdominal sonography because the transvaginal transducer can be placed closer to areas of interest. **Ideally, transabdominal sonography may**

**show the size and location of a pelvic mass, which can then
be better characterized with transvaginal sonography.**

Preparation

Patient Prep

- Verbal or written consent is required from the patient. Explain the details of the examination; inform the patient that the examination is virtually painless, that the inserted transducer feels like a tampon, and the examination is necessary for the interpreting physician to make an accurate diagnosis.
- The examination should be chaperoned by a female health care professional. The initials of the witness should be included as part of the film labeling.
- Empty urinary bladder.
- The patient, sonographer, or physician may insert the transducer.

Patient Position

- Transducer design determines patient position, so ideally having a gynecological examining table and the ability to put the patient in lithotomy position is optimal.
- The patient can be positioned at the end of the examining table or stretcher with the hips elevated by a pillow or foam cushion.

Transducer

- **5.0 MHz** or higher.
- Apply gel to the end of the transducer and then cover it with a condom or disposable sheath. Make sure there are no air bubbles at the tip. Apply additional gel to the outside of the condom or sheath before insertion. If infertility is a consideration, water or nonspermicidal gel may be used.
- Following the examination, the condom or sheath covering the transvaginal probe should be disposed. The probe should be soaked in an antimicrobial solution. Follow the manufacturer's instructions and infectious disease control recommendations for solution type and soak time. If the sheath or condom was torn during the procedure, the probe's fluid channels must be flushed with the antimicrobial solution.

Image Orientation

- Standard transvaginal scanning utilizes sagittal and coronal planes from an inferior approach. Transvaginal image orientations from an inferior approach are described in Figures 12-1 and 12-2. Manipulation of the transducer causes variation from these standard interpretations (Figure 12-3). As a result, image orientation for transvaginal sonography can vary among institutions, authors, and textbooks.

- Proper image orientation is challenging in transvaginal scanning due to the narrow field of view, the inferior scanning approach, and normal positional variations of the reproductive organs. Therefore, it is important to determine proper positioning of the probe prior to insertion at the beginning of the examination. Proper positioning of the probe in the sagittal plane is confirmed when touching the edge of the probe, which is directed toward the ceiling, creates visible motion at the left of the image. From this position, the probe can be rotated 90 degrees counterclockwise in order to scan in the coronal plane.

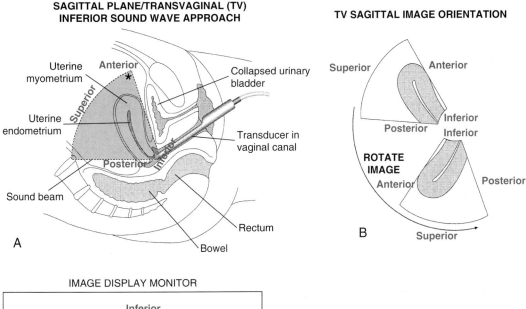

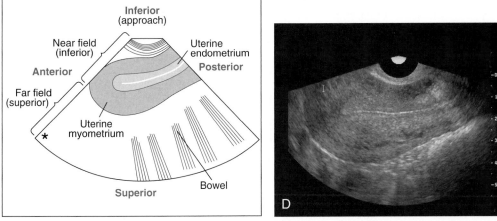

Figure 12-1 Transvaginal (TV) sagittal plane orientation.* **A,** Illustrates the TV transducer position and sagittal plane field of view. **B,** Depicts the rotation of the image as seen on the display monitor. **C,** Illustrates a longitudinal section of the uterus in a TV sagittal plane. The apex of the image on the display monitor corresponds to the anatomy closest to the face of the transducer. In TV sonography, the near field and left side of the sagittal plane image generally correspond to the inferoposterior region of the true pelvis. The far field and right side of the sagittal plane image generally correspond to the anterosuperior region of the true pelvis. **D,** Longitudinal section of the uterus taken in a TV sagittal scanning plane. Note how the section of uterus fills the screen, limiting the overall view of the pelvis but providing increased anatomic detail of the uterus. (*Denotes corresponding locations in **A** and **C.**)

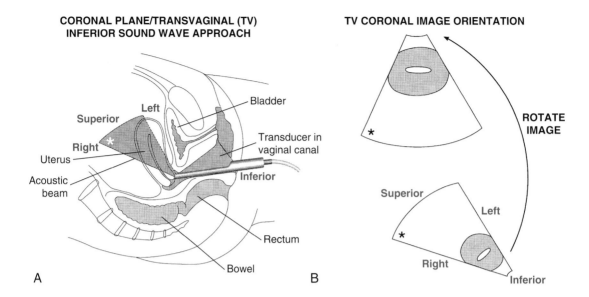

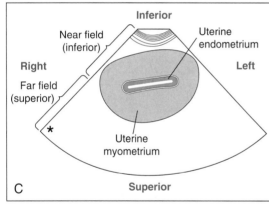

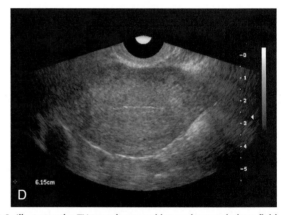

Figure 12-2 Transvaginal (TV) coronal plane orientation.* **A,** Illustrates the TV transducer position and coronal plane field of view. When the bladder is empty, the fundus of the typical anteverted (anteflexed) uterus tilts forward toward the anterior abdominal wall. Therefore, in TV imaging the uterus is seen in short axis from a coronal plane. **B,** Depicts the rotation of the image as seen on the display monitor. **C,** Illustrates an axial or short-axis section of the uterus in a TV coronal plane. The apex of the image on the display monitor corresponds to the anatomy closest to the face of the transducer. In TV sonography, the near field and left side of the coronal plane image generally correspond to the inferolateral region of the true pelvis. The far field and right side of the coronal plane image generally correspond to the superolateral region of the true pelvis. **D,** Axial or short-axis section of the fundus of the uterus taken in a TV coronal scanning plane. Note how the section of uterus fills the screen, limiting the overall view of the pelvis but providing increased anatomic detail of the uterus. (*Denotes corresponding locations in **A, B,** and **C.**)

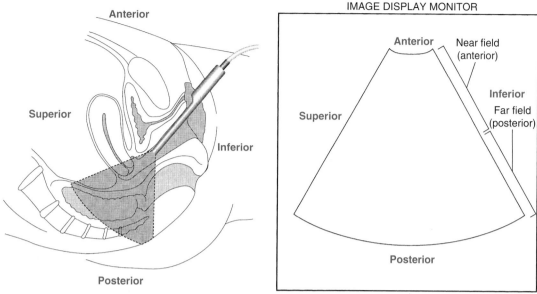

Figure 12-3 Transvaginal imaging: anteroinferior approach. Most TV imaging is performed from the standard inferior approach as explained in Figures 12-1 and 12-2. Alternatively, manipulation of the TV transducer causes variation from the standard TV orientation. For example, these illustrations show that when the transducer is lifted anteriorly, toward the pubic symphysis, the sound beam is directed more posteriorly making the near and far fields of the TV sagittal plane image correspond to anterior and posterior regions of the pelvis instead of inferior and superior regions (from an inferior approach). The left and right sides of the image now correspond more closely to the superior and inferior regions of the pelvis instead of anterior and posterior (from an inferior approach). Utilizing a posterior TV approach also causes significant variation in image orientation. Consequently, image orientation for TV sonography can vary among institutions, authors, and ultrasound texts.

Transvaginal Female Pelvis Survey

NOTE: Because of the limited field of view, the uterus and adnexa are scanned in sections by slightly angling the inserted transducer in different directions.

NOTE: During the transvaginal evaluation, adnexal structures can be brought into view by using one hand to compress the lower abdominal wall while the other hand operates the transducer.

Uterus and Adnexa • Longitudinal Survey
Sagittal Plane • Inferior Approach

1. Begin scanning by slowly lowering the handle toward the floor to view a longitudinal section of the fundus of the uterus. Now move the transducer a little to the right, then to the left to evaluate its lateral margins. Note and evaluate the centrally located endometrial canal. If the bladder contains any urine, it will be seen anteriorly (on the left side of the imaging screen).

2. Withdraw the transducer slightly, and slowly lift the handle toward the ceiling to view the body and cervix of the uterus and the posterior cul-de-sac. Now move the transducer a little to the right,

then to the left to evaluate the lateral margins. Note and evaluate the centrally located endometrial and endocervical canals.

3. After evaluating the uterus, continue the longitudinal survey to the adnexal regions. Very carefully reinsert the partially withdrawn transducer. Keep the transducer straight at the midline and lower the handle to relocate the uterine fundus and then the pelvic cavity region superior to the uterus. Now slowly move the transducer handle toward the patient's left thigh in order to scan through the right adnexa. Return to midline; slowly move the transducer handle toward the patient's right thigh to scan through the left adnexa.

> **NOTE:** For a retroverted uterus, the uterine fundus is visualized by lifting the transducer handle towards the ceiling. It may also be helpful to rotate the probe 180 degrees and invert image orientation.

4. Repeat these lateral sweeps through the adnexal regions at the levels of the uterine body and cervix.

Uterus and Adnexa • Axial Survey
Coronal Plane • Inferior Approach
1. Following the longitudinal survey from the sagittal plane, rotate the transducer 90 degrees counterclockwise into the coronal plane.
2. Begin scanning by slowly lowering the handle of the inserted transducer toward the floor to evaluate the uterine fundus.
3. Withdraw the transducer slightly and slowly lift the transducer handle toward the ceiling to scan through the uterine body, cervix, and posterior cul-de-sac.
4. After evaluating the uterus, continue the axial survey through the adnexa. Moving the transducer handle toward the floor, relocate the uterine fundus. Now slowly move the transducer handle toward the patient's left thigh to visualize the right adnexa, and very slowly move the transducer handle toward the ceiling in order to sweep through the area.
5. Return the transducer to the midline, then slowly move the handle toward the patient's right thigh to visualize the left adnexa. By very slowly moving the transducer handle up and down, sweep through the area.

Right Ovary • Axial Survey
Coronal Plane • Inferior Approach
1. The ovaries are most easily evaluated by beginning in the coronal scanning plane. From initial insertion of the transducer in the sagittal plane, the transducer handle should be rotated 90 degrees counterclockwise into the coronal plane.
2. Begin scanning by putting the transducer in a right oblique position. This is done by slowly moving the transducer handle toward

the patient's left thigh, which angles the beam toward the right adnexa. Find the ovary by slightly moving the transducer handle up and down. Identify the adjacent iliac vessels.

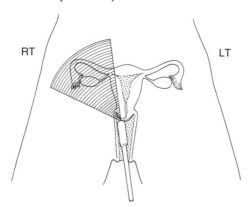

3. When the ovary is located, very slightly move the transducer handle as far up and down as necessary to scan through the ovarian margins.

Right Ovary • Longitudinal Survey
Sagittal Plane • Inferior Approach
1. Still viewing the ovary in the coronal plane, slowly rotate the transducer 90 degrees clockwise to visualize the ovary in the sagittal plane.
2. Begin scanning by very slightly moving the transducer handle to the right and then to the left to scan through the lateral and medial margins of the ovary. Identify the adjacent iliac vessels.

Left Ovary • Axial Survey
Coronal Plane • Inferior Approach
1. Return to the coronal scanning plane by rotating the transducer 90 degrees counterclockwise.
2. Begin scanning by putting the transducer in a left oblique position. This is done by slowly moving the transducer handle toward the patient's right thigh, which angles the beam toward the left adnexa. Find the ovary by slightly moving the transducer handle up and down. Identify the adjacent iliac vessels.

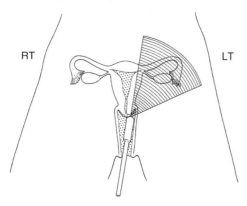

3. When the ovary is located, very slightly move the transducer handle as far up and down as necessary to scan through the ovarian margins.

Left Ovary • Longitudinal Survey
Sagittal Plane • Inferior Approach

1. Still viewing the ovary in the coronal plane, slowly rotate the transducer 90 degrees clockwise to visualize the ovary in the sagittal plane.
2. Begin scanning by very slightly moving the transducer handle to the right and then to the left to scan through the lateral and medial margins of the ovary. Identify the adjacent iliac vessels.

Transvaginal Scanning Protocol for the Female Pelvis
Required Images

Uterus and Adnexa • Transvaginal Longitudinal Images
Sagittal Plane • Inferior Approach

1. **LONGITUDINAL MIDLINE IMAGE.** If the long axis of the uterus is visualized, then *include length and height measurements.*

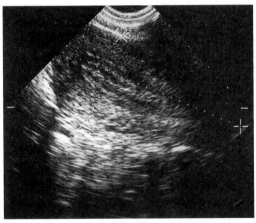
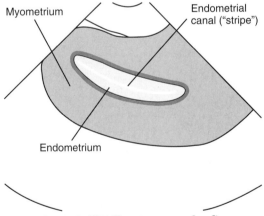

Labeled: **TV SAG ML** *or* **TV SAG ML UT LONG AXIS** ("TV" = transvaginal)

2. Same image as number 1 *without calipers.*

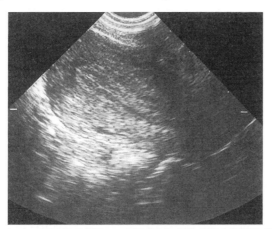

Labeled: **TV SAG ML** *or* **TV SAG ML UT LONG AXIS**

NOTE: If the long axis was not visualized at the midline, it should be taken here and labeled: **TV SAG UT LONG AXIS**

3. **LONGITUDINAL MIDLINE IMAGE** *with anteroposterior measure-ment* of the endometrium.

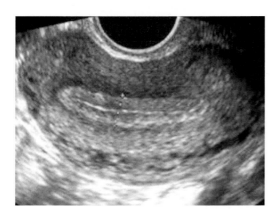
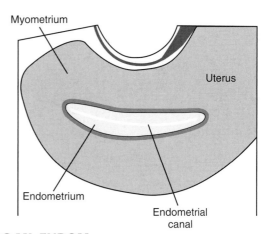

Labeled: **TV SAG ML ENDOM**

NOTE: The measurement of the endometrium should include anterior and posterior portions of the basal endometrium, the thickest echogenic area, from one interface across the endometrial canal to the other inter-face. The adjacent hypoechoic myometrium and any endometrial fluid should not be part of the measurement.

4. Same image as number 3 *without calipers.*

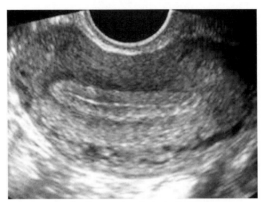

Labeled: **TV SAG ML ENDOM**

5. Longitudinal image of the **UTERUS FUNDUS** to include the endometrial cavity.

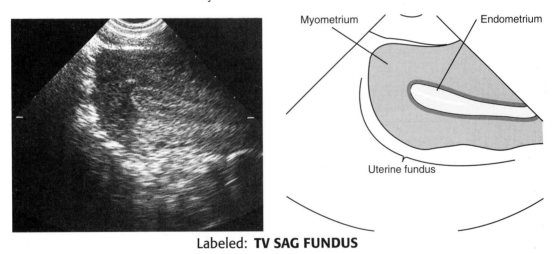

Labeled: **TV SAG FUNDUS**

6. Longitudinal image of the **UTERUS BODY** and **CERVIX** to include the endometrial cavity.

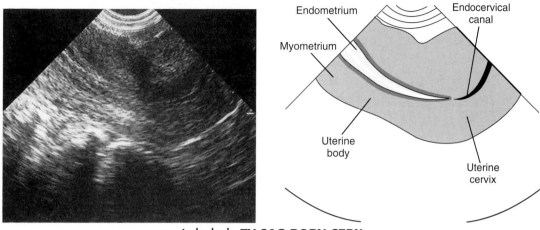

Labeled: **TV SAG BODY CERX**

Uterus and Adnexa • Transvaginal Axial Images
Coronal Plane • Inferior Approach

7. Axial image of the uterine fundus *measuring uterine width.*

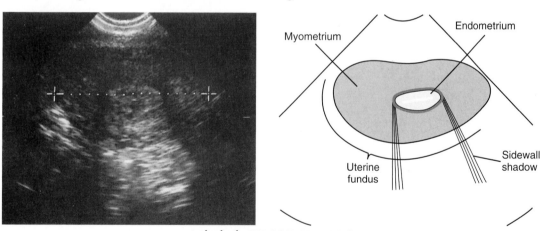

Labeled: **TV COR FUNDUS**

8. Same image as number 7 *without calipers*.

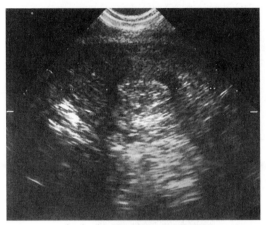

Labeled: **TV COR FUNDUS**

9. Axial image of the **UTERINE BODY.**

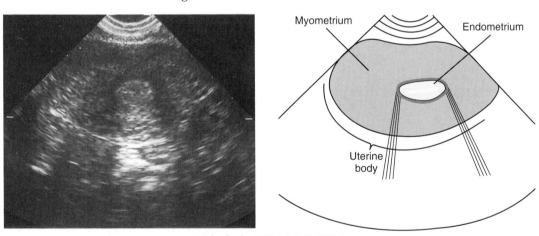

Labeled: **TV COR BODY**

10. Axial image of the **CERVIX.**

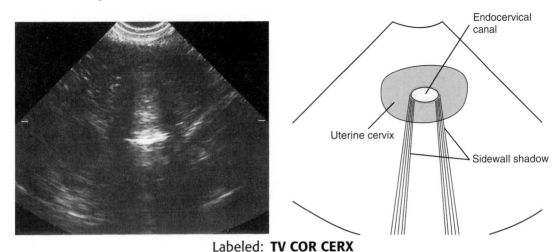

Labeled: **TV COR CERX**

Right Ovary • Transvaginal Axial Images
Coronal Plane • Inferior Approach

For the sake of instruction, this assumes that the ovary long axis is visualized in a sagittal plane.

11. Axial image of the right ovary *measuring ovarian width.*

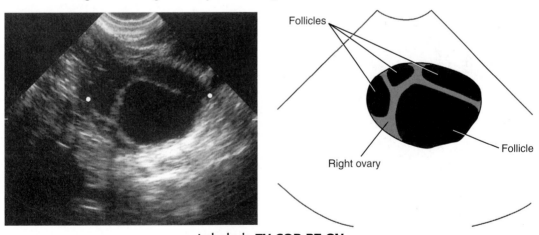

Labeled: **TV COR RT OV**

12. Same image as number 11 *without calipers.*

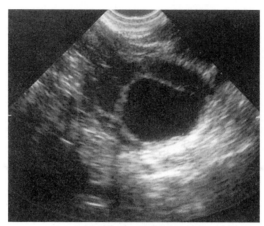

Labeled: **TV COR RT OV**

Right Ovary • Transvaginal Longitudinal Images
Sagittal Plane • Inferior Approach

For the sake of instruction, this assumes that the ovary long axis is visualized in a sagittal plane.

13. **LONG AXIS** image of the right ovary *measuring ovarian length and height.*

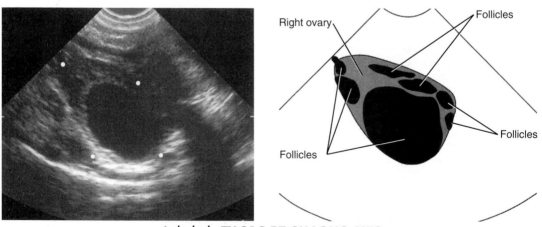

Labeled: **TV SAG RT OV LONG AXIS**

14. Same image as number 13 *without calipers.*

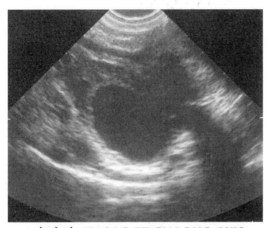

Labeled: **TV SAG RT OV LONG AXIS**

Left Ovary • Transvaginal Axial Images
Coronal Plane • Inferior Approach

For the sake of instruction, this assumes that the ovary long axis is visualized in a sagittal plane.

15. Axial image of the **LEFT OVARY** *measuring ovarian width.*

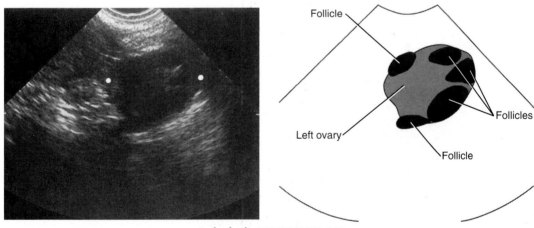

Labeled: **TV COR LT OV**

16. Same image as number 15 *without calipers*.

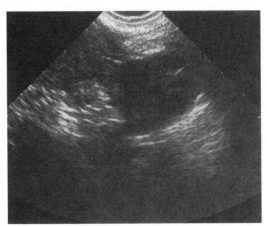

Labeled: **TV COR LT OV**

Left Ovary • Transvaginal Longitudinal Images
Sagittal Plane • Inferior Approach

For the sake of instruction, this assumes that the ovary long axis is visualized in a sagittal plane.

17. **LONG AXIS** image of the left ovary *measuring ovarian length and height.*

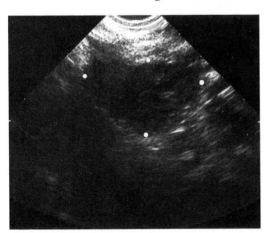 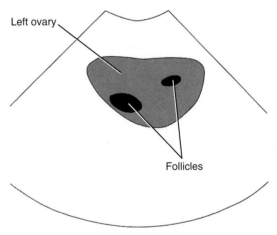

Labeled: **TV SAG LT OV LONG AXIS**

18. Same image as number 17 *without calipers*.

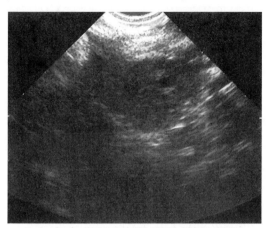

Labeled: **TV SAG LT OV LONG AXIS**

Review Questions

Answers on page 629.

1. In most cases, transvaginal sonography is used
   a) to evaluate ovarian abnormalities.
   b) for ultrasound-guided ova retrieval.
   c) as a complementary study for transabdominal pelvic studies.
   d) in place of transabdominal pelvic sonography.

2. Transvaginal studies must be witnessed by
   a) an immediate family member of the patient.
   b) another sonographer whose initials should be included on all images.
   c) a female health care professional whose initials should be included on all images.
   d) any health care professional whose initials should be included on all images.

3. The sound beam approach for transvaginal sonography is
   a) inferior.
   b) sagittal and coronal.
   c) anterior.
   d) variable.

4. One disadvantage of transvaginal sonography is
   a) transducer placement close to areas of interest.
   b) no requirement for the patient to have a full urinary bladder.
   c) it can be used during surgery.
   d) its narrow field of view.

5. When comparing transabdominal sonography to transvaginal
   a) transabdominal sonography is considered to be better for evaluating the ovaries.
   b) transvaginal sonography is best for demonstrating the size of a pelvic mass.
   c) transabdominal sonography is considered the complementary study.
   d) transvaginal sonography is better at characterizing abnormalities.

6. Transvaginal sonography is also known as _____ and _____ sonography.
   a) endocavital, endovaginal
   b) intrapelvic, endovaginal
   c) endovaginal, endocanal
   d) intra-abdominal, endocavital

7. The limitation of transvaginal sonography is
   a) the amount of distance between the transducer and pelvic structures.
   b) higher frequency transducers.
   c) limited field of view.
   d) not having a full urinary bladder to serve as a "window" for better visualization.

8. Resolution of pelvic structures is better with transvaginal imaging than transabdominal imaging because
   a) there is less attenuating tissue between the transvaginal transducer and pelvic structures.
   b) in most cases, the bladder is empty.
   c) lower frequency transducers are utilized.
   d) transabdominal imaging of the pelvis is outdated.

9. The standard scanning plane(s) utilized in transvaginal imaging are
   a) sagittal and transverse.
   b) coronal.
   c) transverse.
   d) sagittal and coronal.

10. Transvaginal sonography is a sterile procedure.
    a) True
    b) False

11. An anteverted uterus cannot be evaluated transvaginally.
    a) True
    b) False

12. Transvaginal sonography has replaced transabdominal sonography of pelvic structures.
    a) True
    b) False

13. Only the fundal portion of the uterus can be evaluated transvaginally.
    a) True
    b) False

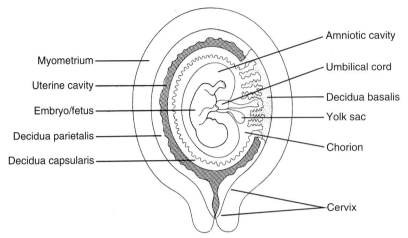

Myometrium

Uterine cavity

Embryo/fetus

Decidua parietalis

Decidua capsularis

Amniotic cavity

Umbilical cord

Decidua basalis

Yolk sac

Chorion

Cervix

First Trimester

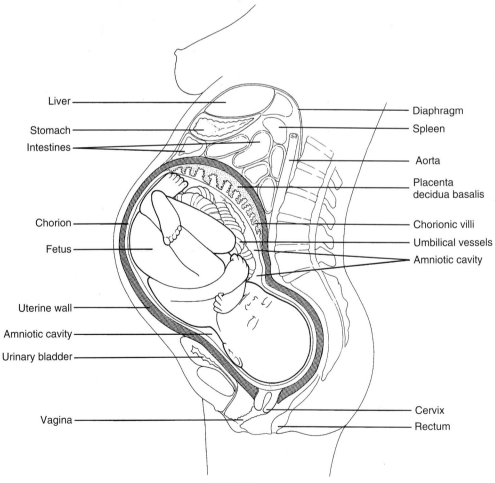

Liver

Stomach

Intestines

Chorion

Fetus

Uterine wall

Amniotic cavity

Urinary bladder

Vagina

Diaphragm

Spleen

Aorta

Placenta
decidua basalis

Chorionic villi

Umbilical vessels

Amniotic cavity

Cervix

Rectum

Third Trimester

CHAPTER 13

Obstetrical Scanning Protocol for First, Second, and Third Trimesters

Betty Bates Tempkin

Key Words

Abdominal circumference (AC)	Foramen ovale
Amnion	Fronto-occipital diameter (FOD)
Amniotic cavity	Gestational sac
Amniotic fluid	Gravid
Amniotic membrane	Human chorionic gonadotropin
Basal layer	(hCG)
Blastocyst	Intradecidual sign
Biparietal diameter	Lacunae
measurement (BPD)	Mean sac diameter (MSD)
Chorionic cavity	Morula
Chorionic membrane	Placenta
Chorionic plate	Placenta previa
Crown rump length (CRL)	Placental grading
Decidua capsularis	Primary yolk sac
Decidua parietalis	Secondary yolk sac
Double bleb sign	Trophoblast
Double sac sign	Umbilical cord
Ectopic pregnancies	Umbilical cord insertion
Embryo	Vitelline duct
Embryoblast	Yolk stalk
Embryonic disk	Zygote
Fertilization	

Objectives

At the end of this chapter, you will be able to:

- Define the key words.
- Distinguish the sonographic appearance and development during the first, second, and third trimesters of pregnancy and the terms used to describe it.
- Distinguish gestational age during the first, second, and third trimesters of pregnancy.
- Distinguish the sonographic appearance of fetal anatomy.
- Describe the transducer options for scanning during the first, second, and third trimesters of pregnancy.
- List the suggested patient position (and options) when scanning during the first, second, and third trimesters of pregnancy.
- Describe the patient prep for the first, second, and third trimesters of pregnancy.

> - Name the survey steps and explain how to evaluate the first, second, and third trimesters of pregnancy.
> - Explain the order and the specifics of taking representative images of the first, second, and third trimesters of pregnancy.
> - Answer the review questions at the end of the chapter.

Overview

Maternal Anatomy and Physiology

- As discussed in Chapter 11, the female pelvis organs include the genital tract (uterus, vagina, and uterine tubes), bilateral ovaries, urinary bladder, a portion of the ureters, and the rectosigmoid colon. The osseous or bony pelvis forms the outer boundaries of the female pelvic cavity, whereas the skeletal muscles which line the pelvic cavity form the inner boundaries. Refer to Chapter 11 for anatomical specifics and sonographic appearance.

- Chapter 11 also discussed how the menstrual cycle prepares the uterus for implantation by a fertilized ovum. If fertilization does not occur, hormone levels decrease and the nonimplanted endometrial lining of the uterus is shed during menses. If fertilization does occur, it usually takes place within 1 day of ovulation, day 15 of the menstrual cycle, at the ampulla portion of the uterine tube. Fertilization is complete when the ova and sperm fuse to form a zygote or cell mass. The cell mass repeatedly divides into the morula, a cluster of 16 or more cells that leave the uterine tube and enter the uterine cavity on the day 18 or 19 of the cycle. The morula is then transformed into a blastocyst. The *outer layer* of the blastocyst, the trophoblast will develop into the chorionic membrane, the fetal component to the placenta (temporary organ joining mother and fetus; oxygen and nutrients are transferred from mother to fetus; waste products are transferred fetus to mother). The *inner layer* of the blastocyst, the embryoblast (or embryonic disk) develops into the primary and secondary yolk sacs (nutrient-filled sacs adjacent to the developing embryo), amnion (innermost layer of developing embryo), embryo (early stages of fetal growth, from conception to the week 8 of pregnancy), and umbilical cord (flexible cord comprised of 2 arteries and 1 vein that arises from the umbilicus and connects the fetus with the placenta). On day 20 or 21 of the cycle, the 1 mm blastocyst starts to implant the decidualized or gravid (pregnant) uterine endometrium. By the day 28 the blastocyst becomes completely imbedded into uterine myometrial tissue and implantation is complete.

First Trimester

Using a 28-day menstrual cycle, most radiologists and obstetricians define the first trimester as the 12 weeks beginning with the first day of the last normal menstrual period. Further, they describe the time span in terms of gestational age (GA) or menstrual age (MA), which are used interchangeably.

Anatomy and Sonographic Appearance During Early First Trimester

Gestational Sac

- The blastocyst is too small to be visualized sonographically, but other intrauterine changes can be detected to confirm a pregnancy during the early first trimester. The following transvaginal image shows an early pregnancy. It is described by sonologists as the gestational sac, a term used to represent the small, round or oval, fluid-filled, anechoic chorionic cavity completely enclosed by bright, echogenic walls that represent developing chorionic villi (fetal portions of the placenta that are fingerlike projections of the trophoblast layer that extend into the endometrium) and the adjacent endometrium.

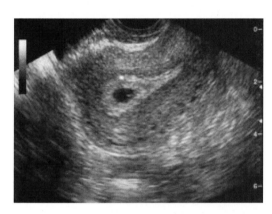
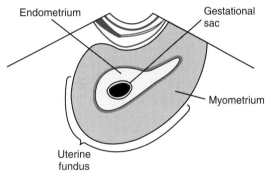

- The first key sonographic finding in an early intrauterine pregnancy is referred to as the "intradecidual sign," which is the location of the early gestational sac right next to the centrally located endometrial cavity at the level of the fundus or body of the uterus. Transvaginal sonography is usually the best choice for visualizing the intradecidual sign, as illustrated below. Note that there should be no displacement or change in size of the endometrial cavity at this early stage.

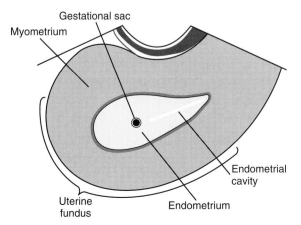

- Although transabdominal transducers are not generally the choice for resolving the intradecidual sign, they can visualize the intrauterine gestational sac as early as 3 to 5 weeks GA when sac diameter is 2 to 4 mm or serum human chorionic gonadotropin (hCG) (hormone secreted by developing placenta to communicate to the rest of the body that a gestation is present within the uterus) levels exceed 1025 mIU/mL. As the gestational sac enlarges, the walls get thicker and markedly hyperechoic relative to the imbedded myometrium.

Determining Gestational Age During the First Half of the First Trimester

Mean Sac Diameter

In the first half of the first trimester, *gestational sac size* is used to date a pregnancy. The method most institutions use to calculate the gestational/menstrual age is the mean sac diameter (MSD) method. As seen in the next image, caliper placement is illustrated between calipers 1 and 2. The three orthogonal dimensions of the chorionic cavity are added together and divided by 3. Alternatively, the length and anteroposterior dimensions can be measured on a long axis section of the gestational sac and width of the sac can be measured on the widest axial section. Notice how the bright rim of choriodecidual reaction is *not* included in the measurement. GA (in weeks) is determined by adding 3 to the MSD (in mm).

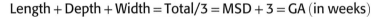

$$\text{Length} + \text{Depth} + \text{Width} = \text{Total}/3 = \text{MSD} + 3 = \text{GA (in weeks)}$$

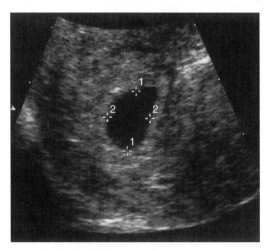

Sonographic Appearance and Development During the First Half of the First Trimester

Double Sac Sign

- This next transabdominal, sagittal scanning plane image shows that with further growth the gestational sac takes on the distinctive sonographic appearance known as the "double sac sign." The 2 bright concentric lines separated by anechoic fluid in the uterine cavity are the decidua capsularis and decidua parietalis (layers of the gravid endometrium). Identification of the double sac sign is *confirmation of the presence of an intrauterine pregnancy before a yolk sac is visualized* and it rules out a pseudosac associated with **ectopic pregnancies** (pregnancies that occur outside the uterus, more often than not in a uterine tube).

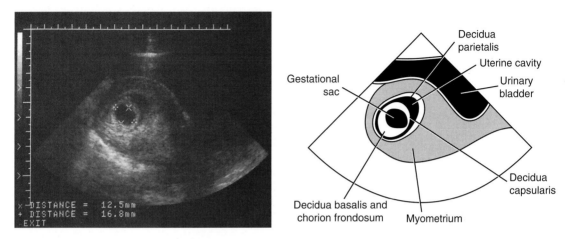

Yolk Sac

- By the end of 4 weeks GA, the primary yolk sac has regressed and is replaced by the secondary yolk sac, which is the first anatomic structure visualized within the gestational sac. The secondary yolk sac provides nutrients to the developing embryo and is the initial site of blood cell development. As illustrated below, the sonographic appearance of the yolk sac is small and round with bright, well-defined walls and an anechoic, fluid-filled center. Identification of the yolk sac is variable; however, it can be detected as early as 5 weeks GA with transvaginal transducers and should be visible by 7 weeks GA using a transabdominal approach. A faint flickering motion seen adjacent to the yolk sac represents the neurologically active heart tissue. From 5 to 10 weeks GA the yolk sac progressively increases to a maximum diameter of 5 to 6 mm. By the end of the first trimester, the yolk sac shrinks and is no longer appreciated sonographically.

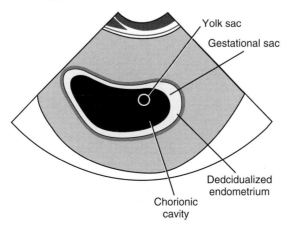

Double Bleb Sign

- When a subtle area is visualized on the periphery of the yolk sac, the embryonic disk has distinguished itself from the embryoblast layer. The *embryonic disk* lies between the *yolk sac* and developing *amniotic membrane*. On occasion, these three structures are visualized together. During the later portion of 5 weeks GA, their sonographic appearance, as illustrated below, has been described as a **"double bleb"** or "double bleb sign" because the embryonic disk is seen lying between the thick yolk sac and thin amniotic membrane. With developmental changes, the double bleb is not detectable after 7 weeks GA.

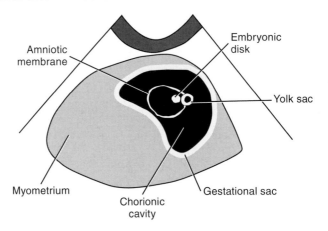

Determining Gestational Age During the Second Half of the First Trimester

Crown Rump Length

- Embryonic development is rapid during 6 to 10 weeks GA. As development continues into the second half of the first trimester, the MSD is replaced by the crown rump length (CRL) measurement that is thought to be the *most accurate assessment of GA during pregnancy*. At 6 weeks + days GA it is not possible to distinguish the crown and rump thus the embryonic disk length is taken for the CRL measurement.

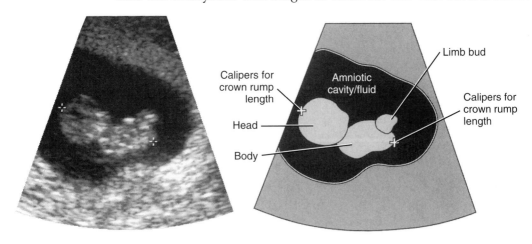

Between 6+ weeks and 8 weeks GA, the embryo's head becomes prominently flexed making the longest axis for measurement from the neck to the rump. As seen in the image and illustration on the facing page, from 8+ weeks to 12 weeks GA the embryo's head extends, making a true crown rump long axis for measurement.

Sonographic Appearance and Development During the Second Half of the First Trimester

Amniotic Sac

- By 6.5 weeks the amniotic membrane and its fluid filled sac or cavity have enlarged enough to surround the embryo. The thin, reflective amniotic membrane encloses the developing echogenic embryo and "bathes" it in the anechoic amniotic fluid within the amniotic sac. As the trimester progresses, not only do the CRL and amniotic sac diameter increase 1 mm per day, but their measurements are equal. Between 12 weeks and 16 weeks GA, the chorionic cavity will be obliterated when the amniotic cavity has enlarged enough for the fusion of the amniotic and chorionic membranes. At this time, it may or may not be possible to distinguish an actual embryo crown (or cephalic pole) from a rump (or caudal pole) but the yolk sac should be seen lying outside the amniotic cavity. The yolk sac and embryo retreat from each other but remain connected by the yolk stalk or vitelline duct that eventually becomes part of the umbilical cord, the 3-vessel connection between the embryo/fetus and mother. Also seen during this time is the tail-like appendage that is often identified at the site of the rump.

Embryonic Heart

- As previously mentioned, the embryonic heart may be detected as early as 5 weeks GA as a flickering motion. As the first trimester progresses the embryonic heart will appear small and pulsatile. The anechoic chambers, echogenic walls, and contour may be discernable by GA weeks 11 or 12.

Skeletal System

- The axial and appendicular skeletons form between the sixth and eighth gestational weeks. The bright reflection of the fetal skeleton indicates the degree of mineralization that has taken place within the developing bones. Ultrasound is able to distinguish how ossified portions of the fetal skeleton appear highly echogenic compared with the midgray appearance of adjacent cartilaginous structures.

Umbilical Cord

- During GA week 8 the embryo assumes a "C" shape, fetal limb buds start to be visible, placental development begins, and the umbilical cord can be visualized. The cord will appear thick and about as long as the embryo. In short axis it presents as 1 large, round, anechoic vein with bright walls, flanked by 2 small, round anechoic arteries with bright, walls. A gelatinous tissue, Wharton's jelly, surrounds the 3 vessels within the cord and prevents it from becoming crushed. The umbilical cord will continue to grow at a rate similar to the embryo.

Tenth Week

The following image demonstrates that by GA week 10 (30 mm CRL, between measurement calipers), limbs are detectable, and normal gut herniation into the base of the umbilical cord is evident. Normal gut herniation should not be seen after GA week 12.

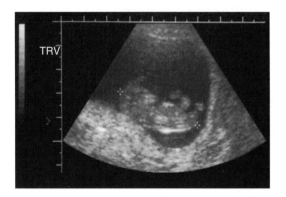 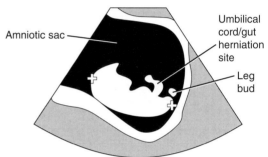

End of the First Trimester

• During GA weeks 11 and 12, individual fingers and toes can be identified as well as anechoic fluid in the stomach and urinary bladder, and the midgray, homogeneous liver. By the end of the first trimester, the oral cavity including hard and soft palates and the tongue are consistently identified. The mid- and distal portions of the esophagus may occasionally be seen as 5 parallel lines anterior to the thoracic aorta. The distal esophagus is nearly impossible to see. The embryonic head and body become proportional and the embryo has developed into a fetus that assumes a distinct humanlike appearance.

Second and Third Trimesters

Using a 28-day menstrual cycle, most radiologists and obstetricians define the second and third trimesters as GA weeks 13 to 42.

Sonographic Appearance and Development During the Second and Third Trimesters

By GA week 13, the majority of organs formed during the first trimester are located in their final anatomic positions. During the second and third trimesters, these organs and their associated organ systems become fully developed as other body structures continue to grow and mature. To grow properly and develop normally, the fetus depends on the placenta and umbilical cord for nutrients, oxygen, and removal of metabolic waste products.

Placenta

- The early placenta appears medium gray with homogeneous echo texture. It darkens slightly during the second and third trimesters and as the gestation advances, the homogeneous appearance of the placenta may be interrupted by bright, echogenic calcium deposits and/or small anechoic lacunae (maternal venous lakes) and/or retroplacental and intraplacental arteries that appear anechoic with bright walls. Anechoic tubular structures on the uterine surface of the placenta representing maternal marginal veins may also be visualized.

Placental Grading

- Many institutions utilize placental grading, a system that classifies placenta maturation according to its sonographic appearance (see Figure 13-1). Basically a *grade 0* placenta appears normal throughout pregnancy. The chorionic plate (sac border) remains smooth; the basal layer (uterine border) is free of calcification, and the parenchyma or bulk of the placenta remains medium gray and homogeneous except for anechoic lacunae. With *grade I,* the chorionic plate shows some subtle indentations, the basal layer becomes hypoechoic or anechoic relative to adjacent structures, and the parenchyma exhibits a few scattered, bright punctate densities (calcifications). These findings are considered normal any time after 34 weeks of development. A *grade II* placenta presents with medium-sized indentations of the chorionic plate, a few small, linear, bright densities are identified at the basal layer, and the parenchyma contains bright, scattered, "commalike" densities. These findings are considered normal any time after 36 weeks of development. With *grade III,* the chorionic plate shows indentations extending as far as the basal layer, dividing the placenta into segments. The basal layer exhibits very long, linear, bright, densities that may, in advanced stages appear as a bright, unbroken line. The placental parenchyma may contain highly echogenic and anechoic areas. The bright echoes represent large calcifications that may cast acoustic shadows. These findings are considered normal any time after 38 weeks of development.

Placenta Previa

The location of the placenta is variable within the uterus and may change as the uterus expands to accommodate the growing fetus. Sonographic evaluation of the placenta includes its position relative to the cervical internal os to rule out placenta previa, a condition where the os is obstructed by overlying placenta. Depending on the

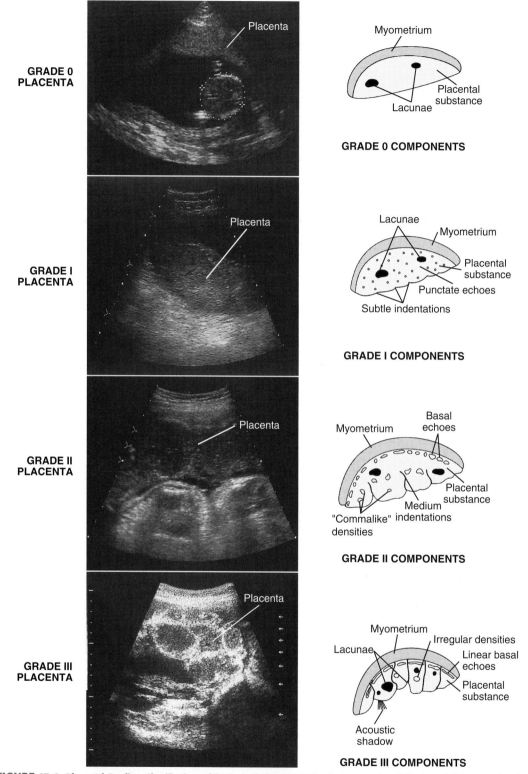

FIGURE 13-1 Placental Grading. Classifications of the "aging" placenta. Notice the increase in calcifications (bright-appearing densities) and changes in contour from grades 0 to III. **Grade 0:** Represents the normal placenta. The placental substance appears homogeneous with medium- to low-level echoes that may be interrupted by anechoic lacunae. **Grade I:** The chorionic plate begins to show some signs of subtle indentations, a few scattered densities are present, and the basal layer appears anechoic. **Grade II:** Medium-sized indentations are evident in the chorionic plate, "commalike" densities are prevalent throughout the placental substance, and a few small linear densities appear in the basal plate. **Grade III:** The chorionic plate contains indentations extending to the basal layer, dividing the placenta into segments. The placental substance appears complex, with both anechoic areas and bright focal areas representing large calcifications that may cast shadows. Long, linear densities are evident in the basal plate. In advanced stages they may appear as an unbroken line.

degree of blockage, it is described as *marginal*, *partial*, or *complete* previa. When there is partial or complete placenta previa the patient may require a cesarean delivery rather than a vaginal delivery that would be dangerous for the fetus and mother. A placenta previa can be ruled out if the placental edge is 2 cm from the internal os. The following image shows an example of partial placenta previa (*PL*, Placenta; *CX*, cervix; *BL*, bladder).

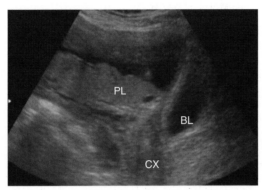

(Courtesy Joe Antony, MD, from www.ultrasound-images.com, and inspired by Ravi Kadasne, MD.)

Umbilical Cord

- The umbilical cord is the vascular connection between the fetus and the placenta where fetal circulation begins. The normal umbilical cord is composed of a single vein flanked by 2 arteries. The vessel lumens appear anechoic; the surrounding walls appear bright. The umbilical cord develops multiple spiral turns as it increases in length; therefore, the 3 vessels are usually easier to distinguish in short axis sections as seen in these images

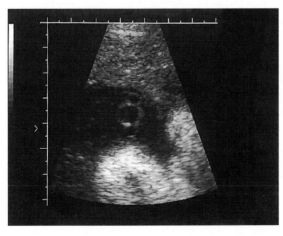

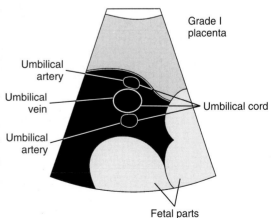

Umbilical Cord Insertion

- The next 2 images show the **umbilical cord insertion** into the placenta and into the fetus. After the first trimester, the fetal surface vessels are routinely visualized. As demonstrated in the top image, they can be traced to the site where the vessels merge and penetrate the placental parenchyma. The bottom image shows that the umbilical cord can be identified where it enters or inserts into the fetus at the umbilicus. The umbilical vein runs cephalically to join fetal portal circulation. The arteries take a caudal course, running on each side of the urinary bladder to meet the iliac arteries.

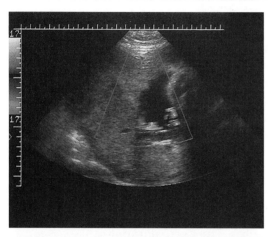
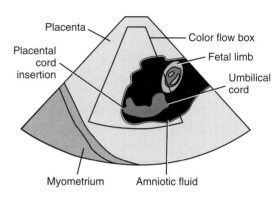

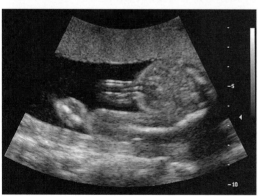
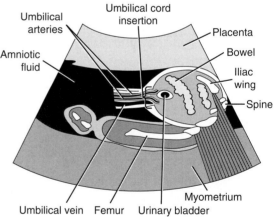

Sonographic Appearance of Fetal Anatomy

- ***Midgray structures:*** *Organ parenchyma and muscles fall into a wide range of midgray shades that provide delineation between the different structures.*
- ***Reflective structures:*** *Bone (ossified), choroid plexus, and the meninges appear highly echogenic with varying degrees of intensity.*
- ***Anechoic structures:*** *Echo-free, fluid-filled anatomy that includes the urinary bladder, stomach, gallbladder, blood vessels, brain ventricles, and heart chambers.*

Skeletal System
Axial Skeleton

- During the second and third trimesters most of the bones of the axial skeleton are routinely visualized. The calvaria of the skull appear highly echogenic and prominent. The contour of the normal fetal head should appear smooth and elliptical in shape. Other identifiable bones include the rib cage in the thorax, mandible, nasal ridge, orbits, and fetal spine. The vertebrae have a highly reflective appearance, making them easy to recognize. The image below shows a longitudinal section of the fetal spine that can be described as 2 rows of closely spaced reflectors on each side of the medium- to low-gray appearance of the spinal cord. The 2 rows are roughly parallel, but wider in the cervical and lumbar regions and narrower in the sacral region. The gaps between the vertebral bodies are composed of nonossified margins of adjoining vertebral bodies and the intervertebral disks. In short axis sections, the vertebral anterior ossification center is seen equidistant from the 2 posterior ossification centers.

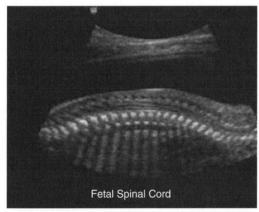

Fetal Spinal Cord

(Image courtesy of Philips. [Philips acquired ATL in 1998.])

Appendicular Skeleton

- During the early to midpart of the second trimester most of the bones of the appendicular skeleton are routinely visualized. This

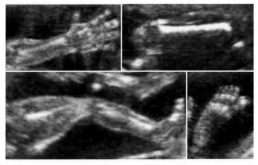

(From Pilu G, Nicolaides KH: *Diagnosis of fetal abnormalities: The 18- to 23-week scan,* Boca Raton, Fla., 1999, CRC Press. Figure 8-1, p. 88.)

includes upper and lower extremities as demonstrated in the previous image. In short axis sections, they appear as bright echogenic foci surrounded by low-gray, homogeneous soft tissue. The longitudinal sections of the bones appear linear, bright, and reflective. The femurs especially, cast a very prominent shadow. The cartilaginous ends of the bones appear homogeneous and low-gray.

Cardiovascular System
Heart

- By 15 weeks GA the 4 chambers of the fetal heart can be visualized. The walls of the heart appear midgray and hyperechoic relative to the anechoic blood in the chambers. The 4 chambers should appear relatively symmetric as demonstrated in the image below. They are divided by the echogenic atrioventricular septa, which will appear "broken" at the foramen ovale (a normal opening between the atria allowing blood to move right to left in the fetal heart). The heart is normally visualized on the left side of the thorax.

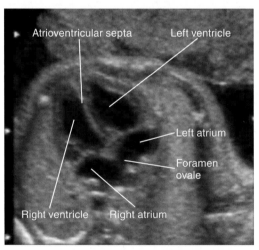

(Image courtesy GE Healthcare.)

Blood Vessels

- Blood vessels in the fetus appear as they do after birth, bright walls and anechoic blood in the lumens. The superior vena cava, thoracic aorta, and pulmonary artery can be visualized in the upper mediastinum during the second trimester. With advanced GA, the brachiocephalic artery, common carotids, left subclavian, and the jugular veins are frequently visualized. The abdominal aorta and inferior vena cava are easy to identify in the posterior portion of the abdomen. The iliac arteries and veins are also often observed. Color Doppler sonography is helpful for resolving small vessel branches such as the celiac axis, superior mesenteric artery, renal arteries, and renal veins.

Respiratory System
Upper Respiratory Tract

- Sonography is able to visualize upper respiratory tract structures such as the nose, nasal cavity and septum, and the palate. The pharynx, hypopharynx, piriform sinuses, and the epiglottis (with advanced fetal age) are easily identified due to anechoic amniotic fluid in portions of the upper tract. The fluid filled trachea can usually be traced from its distal end to the level of the aortic arch. When the hypopharynx contains amniotic fluid the larynx can be identified.

Lungs

- During the first trimester, the lungs are identified more by the structures adjacent to them such as the heart, ribs, diaphragm, and liver. The image below demonstrates that during the second trimester, however, the lungs *(LG rt lung)* become more apparent and appear isosonic/isoechoic to the midgray, homogeneous appearance of the fetal liver *(LIV)*. The muscular diaphragm *(arrow)* separates the thorax from the abdomen and appears hypoechoic relative to the liver and lungs. As GA advances, the lungs become more echogenic.

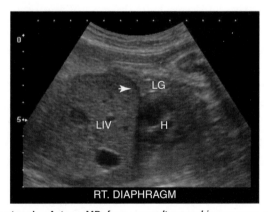

H, Heart. (Image courtesy Joe Antony, MD, from *www.ultrasound-images.com,* and inspired by Ravi Kadasne, MD.)

Gastrointestinal System
Stomach and Gallbladder

- The fetal stomach and gallbladder are readily identified sonographically as they are the only subdiaphragmatic gastrointestinal system structures normally filled with fluid. As seen in the next image, the fluid-filled stomach appears anechoic and is easy to identify on the left side of the fetal abdomen. Size of the stomach varies depending on the amount of amniotic fluid swallowed by the fetus. The bile-filled gallbladder appears anechoic and on the right side of the fetal abdomen. The gallbladder may not be visualized after 32 weeks GA. Some experts believe that the gallbladder contracts, releasing bile, due to initiation of gallbladder function.

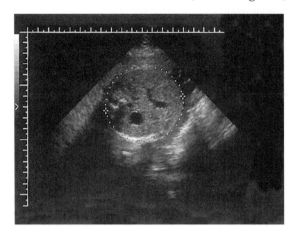
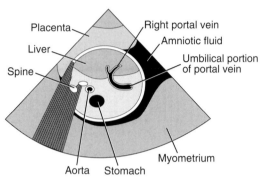

Liver

- The liver is the largest parenchymal organ of the gastrointestinal system and of the body. It is routinely visualized during the second trimester. It appears midgray and homogeneous and fully occupies the right side and much of the rest of the fetal abdomen. The anechoic umbilical vein is routinely identified coursing through a portion of liver parenchyma to reach its point of bifurcation.

Pancreas

- The pancreas is another major parenchymal organ of the gastrointestinal system; it is rarely seen. It may be visualized between the anechoic fluid-filled stomach (posterior wall) and anechoic splenic vein. It appears hyperechoic relative to the fetal liver.

Spleen

- The spleen is not a gastrointestinal organ but is included as part of this discussion because it is associated with the liver by virtue of portal-splenic circulation. Like the fetal liver, the spleen is routinely identified from the second trimester onward. The spleen occupies the left upper quadrant of the fetal abdomen and appears isosonic to the fetal liver.

Small and Large Bowel

- Small bowel loops and large bowel loops can be well distinguished sonographically in the second and third trimesters. The muscle layers of the bowel appear hypoechoic relative to the highly echogenic appearance of the serosa and subserosal linings. By the end of the third trimester it is normal to visualize a small amount of anechoic fluid and bright areas of meconium (fetal waste) within the small bowel.

Genitourinary System

Kidneys

• The fetal kidneys have been identified sonographically as early as 15 weeks GA. At this stage of renal development the sonographic appearance of the kidneys can be difficult to differentiate from adjacent structures. However, after 20 weeks GA, the highly echogenic retroperitoneal fat comes to surround the kidneys, making them easier to identify. Normal fetal renal cortex appears mid- to low-gray or slightly hypoechoic relative to adjacent structures. Unlike adult kidneys, there is very little fat in the fetal renal sinus making it virtually indistinguishable from the cortex. This leads to visualization of urine-filled intrarenal structures (renal pelvis and infundibula) that are not normally appreciated sonographically in adult kidneys. With advanced GA, the renal sinus can become slightly hyperechoic relative to the cortex making the kidneys easier to sonographically distinguish. The distinctive elliptical shape and bright renal capsule assist sonographic identification of the longitudinal sections of the fetal kidneys as seen in image *A* (*arrow* and between calipers). Image *B* shows that the short axis or axial sections of the fetal kidneys can be identified in their normal paraspinal location *(arrows).*

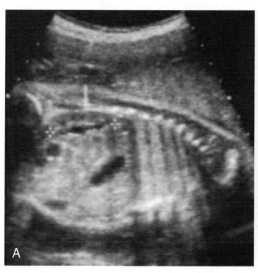 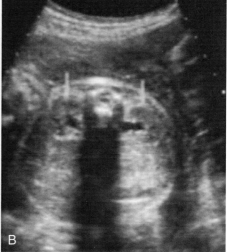

Adrenal Glands

• The fetal adrenal glands are not part of the genitourinary system yet their close proximity to the kidneys makes them a significant sonographic marker. The adrenals appear to cap the upper renal poles. The triangular shaped adrenals present sonographically as low-gray organs that are hypoechoic relative to the liver and renal cortex on the right and the spleen and renal cortex on the left.

Ureters
• Normally, fetal ureters are not visualized sonographically.

Urinary Bladder
• The urine-filled fetal bladder is easily recognized in the fetal pelvis because of its characteristic anechoic appearance and midline position. Another distinction is the thin, bright bladder wall that virtually disappears when the bladder is fully distended. Changes in the volume of the urinary bladder not only confirm normal fetal renal function but also, with time, differentiate the bladder from pathologic structures in the fetal pelvis, such as true cysts that have the same sonographic appearance.

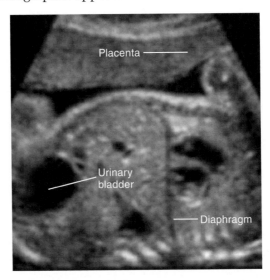

Urethra
• On occasion, the urethra is identified in male fetuses. If the penis is erect, the urethra appears as a bright, reflective line running along the length; otherwise it cannot be identified.

Genitalia
• Fetal gender can be established from the early second trimester by identifying either the male scrotum or the female labia. The penis and scrotum appear homogeneous and mid to low gray. It is not uncommon to identify the testes within the scrotum in the early to mid third trimester. Occasionally, small, bilateral, anechoic testicular hydroceles (fluid collection) will be visualized. The labia have

2 parts that are sonographically distinguishable, the major labia and minor labia. The major labia flank the minor. Both appear homogeneous and midgray but the major labia is hyperechoic relative to the minor. The vaginal cleft lies at the midline between the minor labia; it appears linear and bright. The labia can be identified sonographically as early as 17 or 18 weeks GA.

Intracranial Anatomy

NOTE: Image examples appear under Required Images later in chapter.

Lateral Ventricles
- By 11 weeks GA, the most prominent intracranial structures visualized are the highly echogenic choroid plexus, easily identified within the body of the lateral ventricles. There is a striking contrast between the appearance of the bright choroid plexus and the anechoic appearance of the ventricular chambers filled with cerebrospinal fluid. The walls of the ventricles appear vivid and bright. At this stage, only the ventricular bodies and frontal horns are developed well enough to visualize; the occipital and temporal horns are still rudiments. The outer walls of the lateral ventricles appear as bright linear structures lying the same distance from the interhemispheric fissure. The medial walls of the lateral ventricles are not quite as vivid in appearance as the outer ventricular walls. The appearance of the lateral ventricles changes as development continues. The occipital and temporal horns become visible by 18 to 20 weeks GA and as brain tissue volume increases with normal development, ventricular shape is altered and overall ventricular size decreases. The atria are the sites where the temporal and occipital horns join the body of the lateral ventricles. Ventricular width is normal up to 10 mm. Cerebrospinal fluid flows from the lateral ventricles to the third and fourth ventricles; into the subarachnoid space; then to the dural sinuses where it is absorbed into the venous bloodstream.

Third Ventricle
- The third ventricle lies at the midline of the brain and appears as a highly reflective line parallel to the interhemispheric fissure. Occasionally the third ventricle's cavity fills with cerebrospinal fluid giving it the appearance of an anechoic, midline slit.

Fourth Ventricle
- The fourth ventricle also lies at the midline of the brain, posterior to the third ventricle.

Interhemispheric Fissure and Falx
- The interhemispheric fissure visually separates the cerebral hemispheres. The fissure appears as a single, linear, bright structure at the midline of the brain. The falx cerebri, a fold of dura mater, lies within the interhemispheric fissure, and because they are not sonographically distinguishable from one another, the terms are used interchangeably.

Cerebrum
- The cerebrum is the largest component of the brain. It is almost completely divided anteroposteriorly into two lateral, symmetrical hemispheres by the callosal fissure. It is composed of 5 lobes: parietal, temporal, occipital, frontal, and insula (or isle of Reil), the only lobe not named for an overlying bone. The normal cerebrum appears homogeneous and mid- to low-gray.

Cerebellum
- The cerebellum sits below the cerebrum and superoposterior to most of the brain stem. Like the cerebrum, it is composed of 2 lateral, symmetrical hemispheres. The vermis, a small central lobe relays information between the 2 hemispheres. The normal cerebellum appears mid- to low-gray with low-level echoes that tend to be hypoechoic relative to the cerebrum. In the posterior portion of the brain, the small, round, cerebellar hemispheres are seen on either side of the homogeneous, midgray vermis, which is located at the midline of the brain.

Tentorium Cerebelli
- The tent-shaped tentorium cerebelli separates the cerebellum from the more superior structures.

Brain Stem
- The medulla, pons, midbrain, thalamus, and hypothalamus compose the brain stem, which forms the base of the brain that is continuous with the spinal cord. The components of the brain stem present sonographically as midgray homogeneous structures that vary in their echo level intensity depending on the stage of development. The spinal cord is detectable by 15 or 16 weeks GA. Spinal cord neural tissue appears low-gray with low-level echoes. It is easily identified lying between the highly reflective, bony vertebrae.

Thalamus
- The thalamus can be identified in the center of an axial section of the temporal lobe of the brain. It is composed of 2 ovoid-shaped halves that are primarily composed of brain gray matter. Each half lies on either side of and forms a portion of the lateral walls of the third ventricle. Thalami appear midgray with medium-level echoes.

Cavum Septum Pellucidi
- The cavum septum pellucidi is another anechoic, fluid-filled structure that lies at the midline of the brain. Located superoanterior to the thalamus and third ventricle, it is larger than the third ventricle and subsequently holds more cerebrospinal fluid. It appears as 2 small, bright parallel lines separated at the midline of the brain by cerebrospinal fluid.

Cerebral Peduncles
- The cerebral peduncles are 2 heart-shaped masses that also lie on each side of the midline of the brain. They are similar in shape and texture to the thalami, but are smaller and more rounded. Peduncle parenchyma appears midgray with medium- to low-level echoes.

Meninges
- As the linings of the brain (pia- and dura-arachnoid) become visible, they can be distinguished by their hyperechoic appearance relative to adjacent structures.

Basilar Artery
- The basilar artery can be seen pulsating at the midline of the brain between the anterior portions of the peduncles.

Circle of Willis
- The circle of Willis can be seen pulsating at the midline of the brain anterior to the peduncles.

Cisterns
- Cisterns are varying sizes of enlarged portions of the subarachnoid space (space between the pia mater and arachnoid layer) where cerebrospinal fluid, pia-arachnoid, or a combination of both can accumulate. The largest intracranial cistern for cerebrospinal fluid is the cisterna magnum. It is located in the posterior portion of the brain at the base of the cerebellum and appears anechoic with bright borders. Cisterns filled with pia-arachnoid will appear bright.

Fossae
- The anterior, middle, and posterior fossae appear anechoic and divided from one another by the highly echogenic appearance of the petrous ridges of the skull (posteriorly) and the sphenoid bones (anteriorly). The posterior fossa contains the cerebellum.

Determining GA During the Second and Third Trimesters
The beginning of the second trimester (12 to 13 weeks GA) is the accepted time to make the transition from using CRL measurements to determine GA to using multiple measurement parameters that include biparietal diameter

(BPD), head circumference (HC), abdominal circumference (AC), and long bone measurements.

Biparietal Diameter Measurement

- The biparietal diameter (BPD) can be measured through any plane of section that demonstrates a symmetrical view of the *short axes of the third ventricle and thalami.*
- Measurements cursors may be positioned in 1 of the following 3 ways. The majority of institutions use the first method. Most modern ultrasound equipment computes a GA as soon as the second measurement cursor is placed and charts are available that correlate the BPD measurement with GA.
  1. *Outer* edge of the near calvarial wall *to* the *inner* edge of the far calvarial wall.
  2. *Inner* edge of the near calvarial wall to the outer edge of the far calvarial wall.
  3. Middle of the near calvarial wall *to* the *middle* of the far calvarial wall.

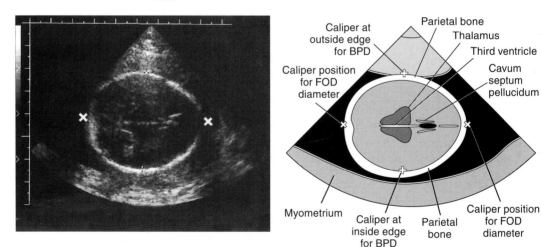

NOTE: Certain conditions such as breech presentations and multiple gestations require an additional measurement to calculate the cephalic index (CI) to assess head shape. The previous image shows how the **fronto-occipital diameter (FOD)** is measured by placing cursors from outer edge to outer edge of the calvaria. Most modern ultrasound machines automatically compute the CI. Normally the CI should be between 0.72 and 0.86. If the CI is greater than 0.86, the head is wider than average or brachiocephalic. If the CI is less than 0.72 the head is dolichocephalic or narrower than average. The cephalic index is calculated as follows:

$$BPD/FOD \times 100 = Cephalic\ index$$

Head Circumference

> **NOTE:** An image example appears later in the chapter under Required Images.

- The **head circumference (HC)** is measured through a single plane of section that demonstrates a symmetrical view of the *third ventricle and thalami* (like the BPD) and the *cavum septum pellucidum* and *tentorium.* Therefore, the HC image section can be used to obtain the BPD as well. Most modern ultrasound equipment computes a GA as soon as the second measurement cursor is placed and charts are available that correlate the BPD measurement with GA.
- Measurements cursors must be positioned from the *outer* edge of the near calvarial wall *to* the *outer* edge of the far calvarial wall.

Abdominal Circumference

> **NOTE:** An image example appears later in the chapter under Required Images.

- The **abdominal circumference (AC)** is measured through a single plane of section that demonstrates where the *umbilical vein branches and the left and right portal veins are continuous with one another.* The fetal abdomen should be an axial section that appears round or nearly round to obtain an accurate AC measurement. If the ultrasound machine is not equipped for tracing or drawing ellipses, the AC can be calculated by adding the anteroposterior and axial diameters of the abdomen (measured skin edge to skin edge) and multiplying the sum by 1.57. Standard reference tables are used to correlate the AC with predicted GA.
- Elliptical measurement cursor must be positioned so the cursor is fit to the skin edge.

Long Bone Measurements

> **NOTE:** An image example appears later in the chapter under Required Images.

- The long axis of the femur and the humerus are used for measurements to determine GA. If both *cartilaginous ends of the long bones* are visualized, this guarantees that the plane of section is the long axis. The measurement is confined to the ossified portions.

Preparation

Patient Prep

Patient Prep for Transabdominal Approach

- Before the examination a patient history should be taken to include the date of the first day of the patient's last period, parity, gravidity (pregnancy test results if available), symptoms, pelvic examination results, and history of pelvic surgery. Most sonography departments have standard forms where this information is recorded.
- The patient must have a full urinary bladder. This moves the bowel out of the way and serves as a sonic "window" for visualizing pelvic structures. Clear fluid (32 to 40 ounces) should be ingested 1 hour before the examination and finished within a 15- to 20-minute time period.
- If for any reason the patient cannot have fluids, sterile water can be used to fill the bladder through a Foley catheter.

> **NOTE:** An overfilled bladder can actually push the pelvic organs out of view. If this occurs, have the patient partially void.
> **NOTE:** Normal bowel can mimic pathology. To distinguish between the two, the patient can be given a water enema to differentiate the bowel.

Patient Prep for Transvaginal Approach

- Verbal or written consent is required from the patient. Explain the details of the examination; inform the patient that the examination is virtually painless, that the inserted transducer feels like a tampon, and the examination is necessary for the interpreting physician to make an accurate diagnosis.
- The examination should be witnessed by a female health care professional. The initials of the witness should be included as part of the film labeling or legal record.
- Empty urinary bladder.
- The patient, sonographer, or physician may insert the transducer.

Transducer

Transducer for Transabdominal Approach

- **3.0 MHz or 3.5 MHz.**
- 2.5 MHz for very large patients. 5.0 MHz for thinner patients or earlier gestational ages.
- Sector, curvilinear, and linear transducers may also be required. It is not unusual to use different transducers during an obstetric ultrasound examination.

Transducer for Transvaginal Approach

- **5.0 MHz to 7.5 MHz**.
- Apply gel to the end of the transvaginal, endocavital transducer, and then cover it with a condom or sheath. Make sure there are no

air bubbles at the tip. Then apply additional gel to the outside of the condom before insertion. If infertility is a consideration, water or nonspermicidal gel may be used.

Patient Position
Patient Position for Transabdominal Approach
- Supine.
- Right lateral decubitus or left lateral decubitus.
- During the third trimester if the fetal head is in the lower uterine segment, it may be helpful to elevate the patient's hips with a pillow or foam cushion.

Patient Position for Transvaginal Approach
- Transducer design determines patient position, so having a gynecological examining table and the ability to put the patient in lithotomy position is optimal.
- The patient can be positioned at the end of the examining table or stretcher with the hips elevated by a pillow or foam cushion.

Obstetrics Survey

Irrespective of the trimester, all obstetrical surveys begin with a survey of the female pelvis (vagina, uterus, and adnexa) in at least two scanning planes followed by a survey of the pregnancy.

Female Pelvis Survey

Vagina • Uterus • Adnexa
Sagittal Plane • Transabdominal Approach
1. Begin scanning with the transducer perpendicular, at the midline of the body, just superior to and directly against the symphysis pubis. In most cases, the longitudinal sections of the vagina and cervix will be visualized here and possibly the body and fundus of the uterus depending on their position according to the trimester. Look for the vagina inferiorly, in the area between the anechoic urinary bladder (seen anteriorly) and hyperechoic rectum (seen posteriorly). If the vagina and cervix are not visualized, move the transducer a little to the right and/or left of midline or slightly angle the transducer inferiorly or use a combination of both until the vagina and cervix come into view. If the body and fundus of the uterus are not seen in the same scanning plane with the vagina and cervix then oblique the scanning plane by slowly rotating/twisting the transducer first one way, then the other, until the body and fundus come into view and visually "connect" to the cervix. Further adjust the scanning plane until the long axis of the uterus, cervix, and vagina and endometrial, endocervical, and vaginal canals are visualized together.

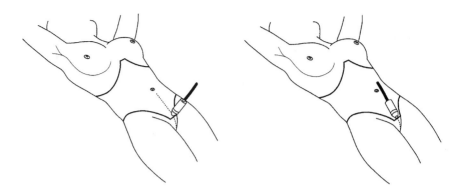

> **NOTE:** During the survey of the uterus look for signs of pregnancy, viability, and whether the pregnancy is single or multiple. If a fetus is visualized, note its presentation. Observe the location of the placenta. Evaluate amniotic fluid volume subjectively; extremes are obvious.

2. Once the long axis of the uterus and vagina are visualized, slowly move the transducer to the patient's right, scanning through and beyond the lateral margins of the uterus, the vagina, the adnexa, and the pelvic sidewalls. Note the location of the right ovary if it is visualized.

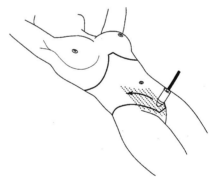

3. Relocate the long axis of the uterus and vagina. Now slowly move the transducer to the patient's left, scanning through and beyond the lateral margins of the uterus, the vagina, through the adnexa, and pelvic sidewalls. Note the location and lie of the left ovary if it is visualized. Keep in mind that the position of the ovaries is variable.

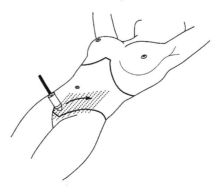

Transverse Plane • Transabdominal Approach

1. Still in the sagittal scanning plane, relocate the long axis of the uterus, cervix, and vagina. Focus on the vagina, then rotate the transducer 90 degrees into the transverse scanning plane until a small, oval, axial section of the vagina comes into view in the area between the bladder (seen anteriorly) and the rectum (seen posteriorly). Rotate/twist the transducer as necessary to resolve the centrally located, hyperechoic vaginal canal.

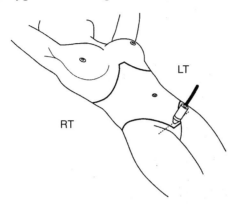

2. Now very slowly angle the transducer inferiorly, as far as necessary to scan through and beyond the margins of the vagina and pelvic cavity. Slowly straighten the transducer back up to perpendicular, scanning back into the pelvis and onto the vagina. Note the pelvic sidewalls.

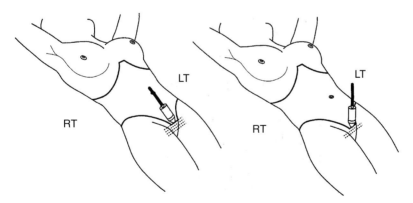

3. Keep the transducer perpendicular and very slowly slide the transducer superiorly, scanning through and beyond the margins of the vagina and onto the cervix. Look for the small axial section of the cervix to appear slightly larger than the vagina and to come into view in the area between the bladder (seen anteriorly) and the posterior cul-de-sac (seen posteriorly). Rotate/twist the transducer as necessary to resolve the centrally located, hyperechoic, endocervical canal. Note the pelvic sidewalls.

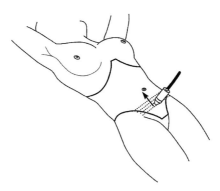

4. Still keeping the transducer perpendicular, slowly slide superiorly, scanning through and beyond the cervix and onto the body of the uterus. Look for the body to appear significantly larger than the cervix. Rotate/twist the transducer as necessary to resolve the centrally located, endometrial canal. One or both ovaries may come into view posterior and slightly lateral to the body of the uterus. Note the pelvic sidewalls.

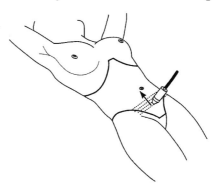

5. Continue to move the transducer superiorly, slowly scanning through the body of the uterus and onto the fundus. Look for the axial section of the fundus to appear a bit larger than the body. Rotate/twist the transducer as necessary to resolve the centrally located endometrial canal. Scan superiorly through and beyond the fundus and urinary bladder wall all the way to the level of the umbilicus. As you scan beyond the bladder, the bowel will come into view. Adjust technique according to bowel content. One or both ovaries may be visualized posterior and lateral to the fundus. Note the pelvic sidewalls.

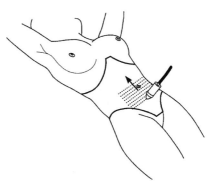

First Trimester Survey

Gestational Sac • Yolk Sac • Embryo
Sagittal Plane • Transabdominal Approach

1. Begin scanning by relocating the long axis of the uterus and locating the gestational sac within. A normal gestational sac will be located in the upper portion of the body of the uterus or in the fundus; embedded into the endometrium; adjacent to the endometrial cavity without displacing it. Look for a small collection of anechoic fluid within the gestational sac surrounded by a rim of highly echogenic tissue.

2. When a gestational sac is present, make sure the transducer is perpendicular when viewing the sac, and then very slowly slide the transducer toward the patient's right, scanning through and just beyond the sac. Then slowly slide the transducer toward the patient's left, moving back through the sac and beyond its margin. Very early in the gestation it is not uncommon for the sac to appear empty.

3. As the gestation progresses, evaluate any contents within the gestational sac. The yolk sac will be the first anatomic structure visualized. It will be joined by the embryonic disk that develops into the embryo. By the beginning of the second half of the first trimester, the crown and rump of the embryo are distinguishable, and by the end of the first trimester the embryo takes on a humanlike appearance as it enters the early fetal stage.

> **NOTE:** When a yolk sac is visualized early in the first trimester, inspect the areas adjacent to the yolk sac for cardiac activity. This may be more apparent than the fetal pole itself. Late in the first trimester, M-Mode or Doppler ultrasound may be used to document viability.

Transverse Plane • Transabdominal Approach

1. Still viewing the gestational sac in the sagittal plane, rotate the transducer 90 degrees into the transverse plane.

2. With the transducer perpendicular, slowly slide the transducer superiorly, toward the patient's head, scanning through and just beyond the sac. Now slowly slide the transducer inferiorly, toward the patient's feet, moving back through the sac and beyond its margin. Very early in the gestation it is not uncommon for the sac to appear empty.

3. As the gestation progresses, evaluate any contents within the gestational sac.

Second and Third Trimester Survey (The Fetus)

When scanning the fetus:

1st: Determine fetal position/presentation

Is the fetus in a cephalic, breech, transverse, or oblique position?

2nd: Decide the plane of view

Is the anatomic structure seen better in a plane parallel to the fetal long axis or perpendicular to it?

3rd: Determine the focal zone

Is the focus portion of the ultrasound beam at an optimal frequency for reaching the correct depth of the anatomic structure?

Determining Fetal Position/Presentation

Fetal presentation is determined by comparing the long axis of the fetus to the long axis of the uterus. Presentation refers to the fetal part closest to the cervix.

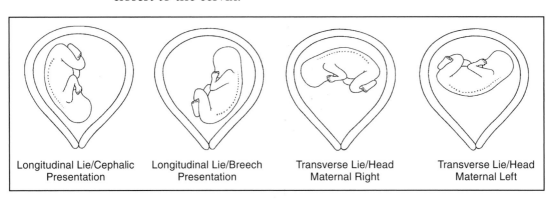

| Longitudinal Lie/Cephalic Presentation | Longitudinal Lie/Breech Presentation | Transverse Lie/Head Maternal Right | Transverse Lie/Head Maternal Left |

Thoracic Cavity • Abdominopelvic Cavity • Fetal Limbs • Fetal Spine • Fetal Cranium

Fetal Long Axis • Transabdominal Approach

Fetal Limbs

1. Begin in the scanning plane where the long axis of the fetus was visualized during the survey of the uterus. Fetal position is variable, so the position of the long axis may change. Change the scanning plane accordingly. Look for long sections of the fetal spine then slightly twist the transducer varying degrees until the entire spine (or largest portion depending on the trimester) comes into view. When the fetal long axis is established, begin the survey at the level of the fetal chest. Look for the distinctive rib cage and heart. Now slowly scan toward the direction of the fetal cranium; identify both fetal arms and hands. When the cranium is identified, scan through and beyond it. Scan back to the level of the fetal chest then through the abdomen and

pelvis, toward the direction of the fetal feet. Identify both legs and feet.

> **NOTE:** When the fetus moves during a study, follow it and reorient the transducer to the optimal plane of view.

2. Return to the level of the fetal chest. Very slowly scan through and beyond each side of the chest. Carefully evaluate the heart for viability. Note the lungs and diaphragm.
3. Move the transducer to the level of the fetal abdomen and pelvis (or the abdomen followed by the pelvis depending on the trimester). Slowly scan through and beyond each side of the abdomen and pelvis. Take note of fetal abdominopelvic contents that include the liver, spleen, kidneys, inferior vena cava, aorta, and bowel. The gallbladder, stomach, and urinary bladder are easily recognized if fluid-filled.

> **NOTE:** The examination is not complete until a significant amount of time has been given to visualize the fetal urinary bladder. Nonvisualization of the fetal urinary bladder may be interpreted as nonfunctioning fetal kidneys.

Fetal Spine
4. Resolve the long axis of the fetal spine. Locate a long section of the fetal spine then very slowly twist the transducer first one way, then the other, until the long axis is visualized. As fetal growth progresses, it may not be possible to visualize the long axis of the entire spine in a single view. In those cases, find the longest visible section. Next, very slowly move down along the spine through the sacral end, and then slowly back up through the cervical end to the skull. Note that the spine narrows at the sacrum and widens at the skull. Any other deviations seen along the "double line" appearance of the spine may indicate an abnormality.
5. Relocate the longitudinal cervical section of the fetal spine. Slowly rotate the transducer 90 degrees until an axial section of the spine comes into view. Look for 3 small, highly reflective areas of ossification that represent portions of the vertebra. One portion is the centrum (or body), and 1 on each side of the posterior neural arch that eventually ossify into the laminae. To ensure that each of the 7 cervical vertebrae are evaluated, slowly move the transducer until the base of the fetal skull comes into view then back onto the first cervical vertebra. Continue to scan inferiorly through each cervical vertebra then each thoracic vertebra. Note the heart, lungs, and diaphragm.

6. Keep scanning inferiorly along the spine and evaluate each lumbar vertebra and then the sacrum until you scan through and beyond the sacral margin.

Fetal Cranium

7. Relocate the long axis of the fetal spine then scan superiorly along the spine to the base of the skull. Slowly scan through the fetal cranium until you are beyond its margins. Note the contour of the cranium, intracranial anatomy, and observe facial features.

8. Return to the base of the skull and rotate the transducer 90 degrees. Again, slowly scan through the fetal cranium until you are beyond it. Note the contour of the cranium, intracranial anatomy, and facial features.

Required Images for Obstetrics

Early First Trimester

NOTE: Depending on how early the gestation is, it may be helpful to magnify the field of view for the gestational sac images.

Sagittal Plane • Transabdominal Approach

1. **LONG AXIS** image of the **UTERUS** showing the location of the gestational sac.

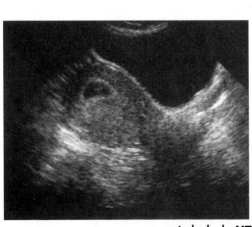
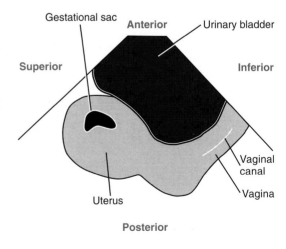

Labeled: **UT SAG LONG AXIS**

NOTE: Gestational sac images are taken whether an embryo is identified or not.

Scanning Plane Determined by Position of Anatomy • Transabdominal Approach

2. Longitudinal image of the **GESTATIONAL SAC** *with length (superior to inferior) and depth (anterior to posterior) measurements (calipers inside wall to inside wall)*

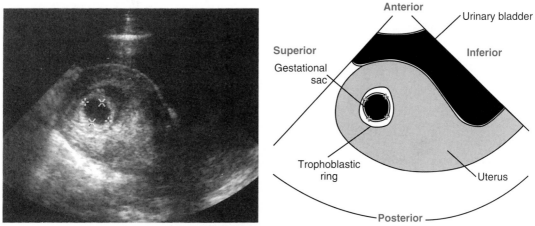

Labeled: **GS SAG or TRV**

3. Same image as number 2 *without calipers.*

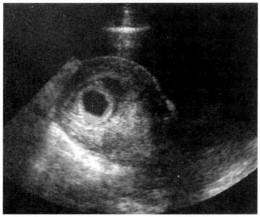

Labeled: **GS SAG or TRV**

4. Axial image of the **GESTATIONAL SAC** *with greatest width (right to left) measurement (calipers inside wall to inside wall).*

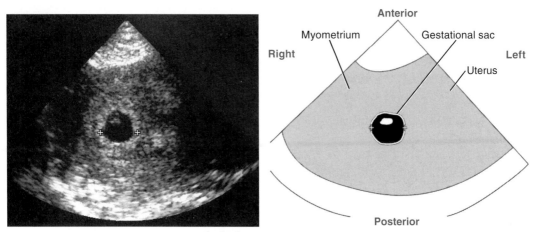

Labeled: **GS SAG or TRV**

5. Same image as number 4 *without calipers.*

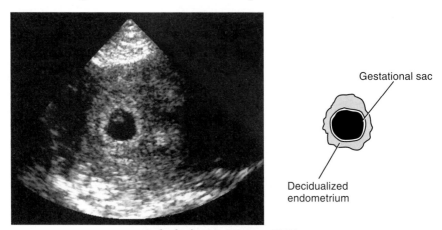

Labeled: **GS SAG or TRV**

NOTE: If the yolk sac and/or embryo are present and have not been clearly demonstrated with the gestational sac measurement images, an additional image of the yolk sac and/or embryo should be taken and labeled accordingly.

6. Image demonstrating the **YOLK SAC** and/or **EMBRYO.**

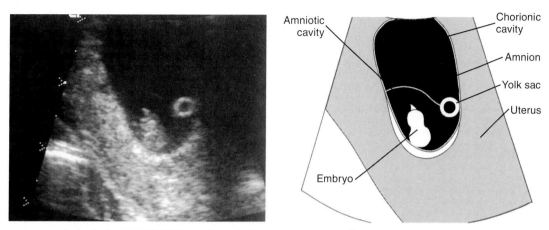

Labeled: **YOLK SAC SAG or TRV or YOLK SAC / EMBRYO SAG or TRV**

7. **LONG AXIS** image of **EMBRYO** *with length (superior to inferior) or CRL measurement.*

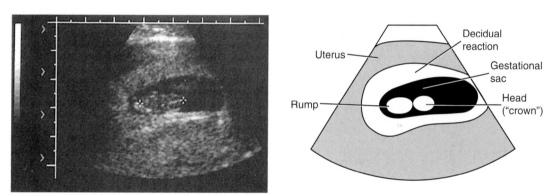

Labeled: **CRL**

8. Same image as number 7 *without calipers.*

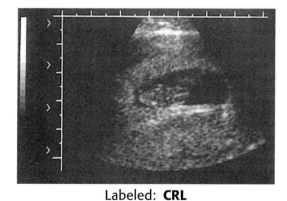

Labeled: **CRL**

9. Doppler documentation of viability.

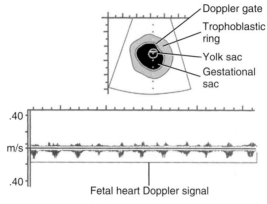

Doppler gate

Trophoblastic ring

Yolk sac

Gestational sac

Fetal heart Doppler signal

Labeled: **DOP VIAB**

Later First Trimester
Sagittal Plane • Transabdominal Approach

1. **LONG AXIS** image of the **UTERUS** showing the location of the gestational sac.

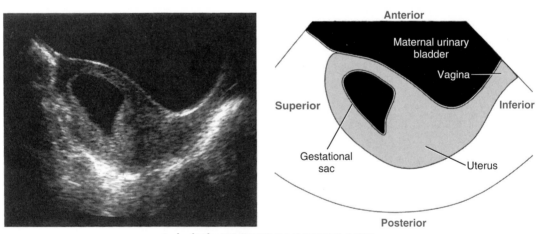

Anterior

Maternal urinary bladder

Vagina

Superior

Inferior

Gestational sac

Uterus

Posterior

Labeled: **UTERUS SAG LONG AXIS**

NOTE: Assuming an embryo is identified, the CRL measurement is taken in the scanning plane where its long axis appears.

Scanning Plane Determined by Position of Anatomy •
Transabdominal Approach

2. Longitudinal image of the **GESTATIONAL SAC** to include the embryo (if visualized) *with measurement from crown to rump* (if applicable) and placenta location (if distinguishable).

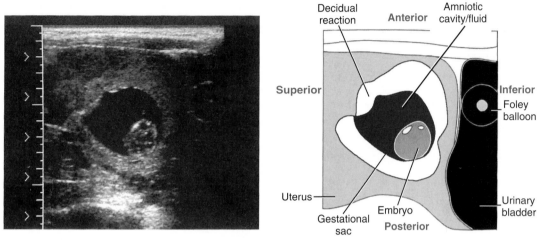

Labeled: **GS SAG or TRV**

3. Axial image of the **GESTATIONAL SAC** to include the embryo (if visualized) *with measurement from crown to rump* (if applicable) and placenta location (if distinguishable).

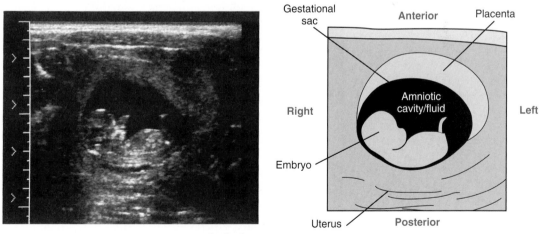

Labeled: **GS SAG or TRV**

4. Same image as number 3 *without calipers* (if applicable).

> **NOTE:** In this case, the CRL measurement was not applied to the previous image, therefore an additional image demonstrating the longest axis of the embryo with CRL measurement must be taken here.

5. **LONG AXIS** image of the **EMBRYO** *with measurement from crown to rump.*

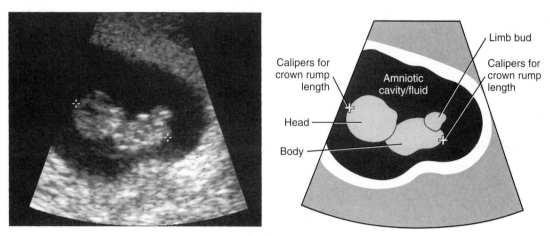

Labeled: **CRL**

6. Same image as number 5 *without calipers.*

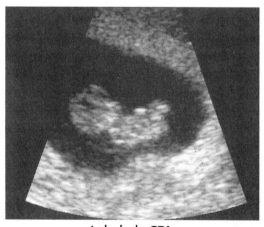

Labeled: **CRL**

NOTE: In addition to the crown rump length (CRL) measurement, some institutions require biparietal diameter, abdominal circumference, and femur length measurements of the embryo during the later part of the first trimester. However, many experts believe that these additional measurements are not necessary because they do not add any new information to the study and they are not as accurate as the CRL measurement for determining GA.

7. Optional view(s) of the embryo demonstrating **LIMBS.**

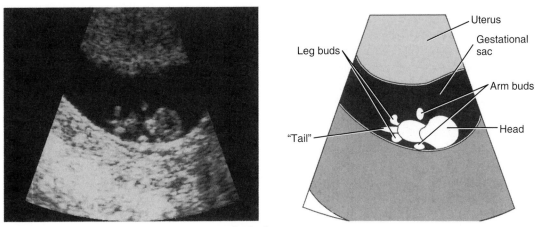

Labeled: **LIMBS**

NOTE: It may be helpful to magnify the field of view for the limb image(s).

Second and Third Trimester
Sagittal Plane • Transabdominal Approach

1. When the trimester allows, **LONG AXIS** image of the **UTERUS** and contents or best overall longitudinal representation.

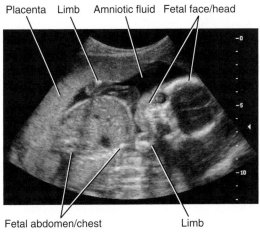

Labeled: **UTERUS SAG**

NOTE: In this case the trimester was too advanced to image the entire uterus on a single view.

Scanning Plane Determined by Position of Anatomy •
Transabdominal Approach

2. Longitudinal image of the **PLACENTA.**

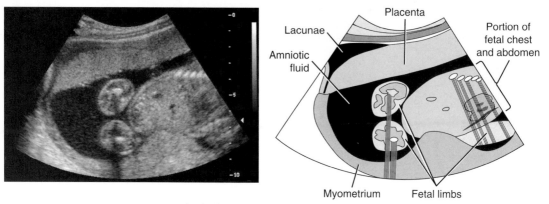

Labeled: **PLACENTA SAG or TRV**

3. Axial image of the **PLACENTA.**

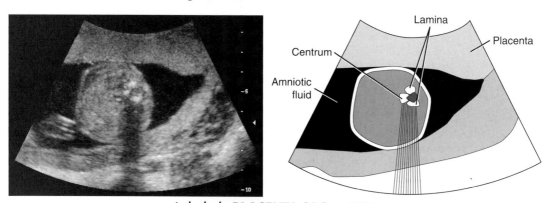

Labeled: **PLACENTA SAG or TRV**

Sagittal Plane • Transabdominal Approach

4. Longitudinal image of the **CERVIX** to include the internal os.

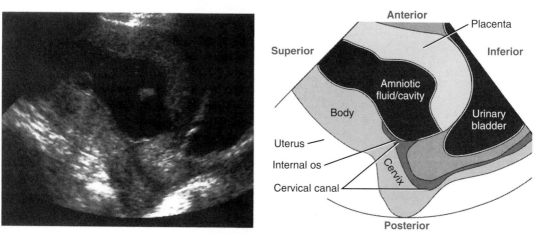

Labeled: **CERVIX SAG**

NOTE: An image of the lower uterine segment to include the internal os is required to rule out placental previa and to document the cervix. In cases where the head of the fetus or the mother's body habitus inhibit imaging of the lower uterine segment, either an endovaginal or translabial image must be obtained. The translabial image is obtained with an empty or nearly empty bladder. The transducer is covered with a sheath, condom, or glove and placed between the labia. The transducer is angled so that the cervix is nearly perpendicular to the ultrasound beam.

Longitudinal translabial image of the lower uterine segment.

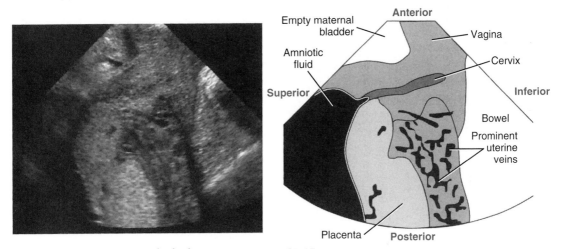

Labeled: **CERVIX TRANSLAB**

Scanning Plane Determined by Position of Anatomy • Transabdominal Approach

5. Depending on the stage of gestation, an overall longitudinal image of **AMNIOTIC FLUID** or the largest pocket *with superior to inferior measurement.*

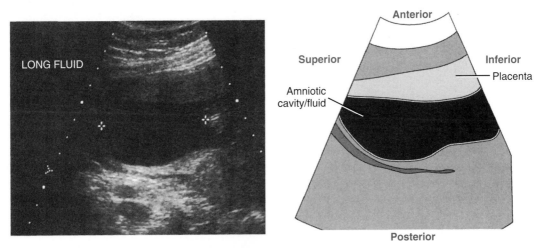

Labeled: **FLUID SAG**

NOTE: At times a quantitative measurement of amniotic fluid is required. Anteroposterior (AP) measurements are obtained for the right and left upper and lower quadrants. The sum of these AP measurements is called the amniotic fluid index (AFI). Fluid pockets that contain primarily cord or fetal parts are not included in the measurement.

6. Depending on the stage of gestation, an overall axial image of **AMNIOTIC FLUID** or the largest pocket with *anterior to posterior and right to left measurements.*

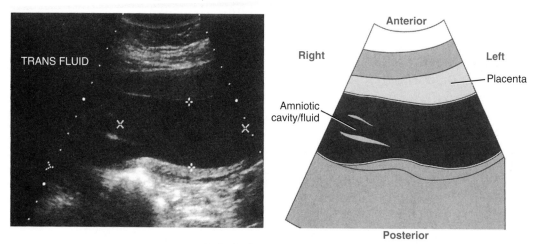

Labeled: **FLUID TRV**

NOTE: Because of the variability of fetal position and movement, the following fetal anatomy images may be taken in any sequence.

NOTE: An ultrasound examination during the second and third trimesters requires the documentation of a large number of anatomic structures, therefore 2 or more structures can be documented on a single image if they are well represented.

NOTE: Because of the variability of fetal position and movement, the scanning plane is not included as part of the film labeling for the following images.

7. Longitudinal image of the **CERVICAL SPINE.**

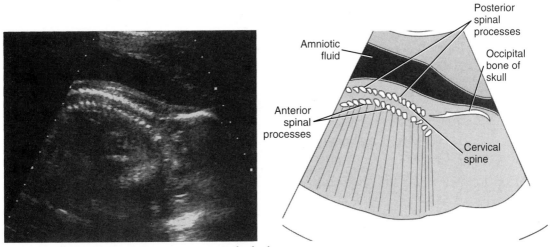

Labeled: **C SPINE**

8. Longitudinal image of the **THORACIC SPINE.**

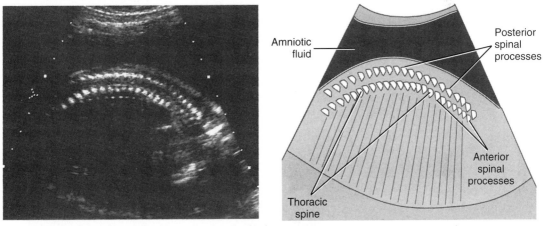

Labeled: **T SPINE**

9. Longitudinal image of the **LUMBAR SPINE.**

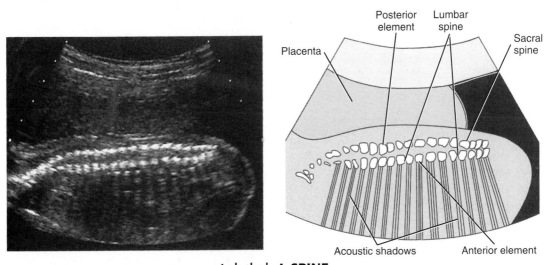

Labeled: **L SPINE**

10. Longitudinal image of the **SACRAL SPINE.**

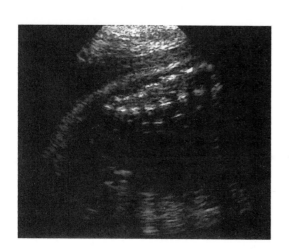
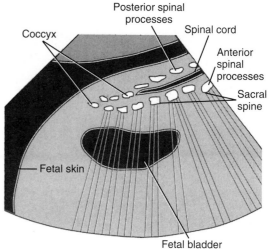

Labeled: **S SPINE**

NOTE: In some cases the long axis of the spine can be visualized on a single image. If so, take the image and label:
Labeled: **SPINE LONG AX**

11. Axial image of the **CERVICAL SPINE.**

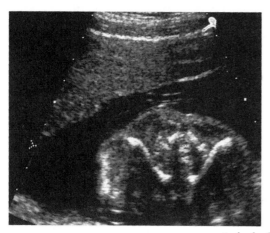
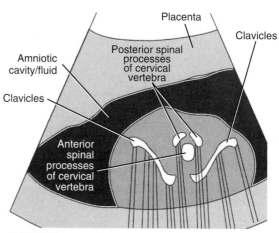

Labeled: **C SPINE**

12. Axial image of the **THORACIC SPINE.**

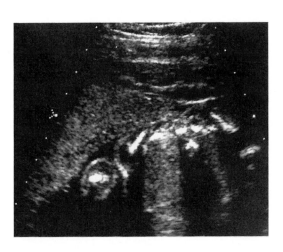 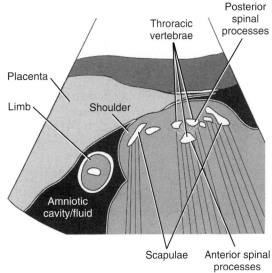

Labeled: **T SPINE**

13. Axial image of the **LUMBAR SPINE.**

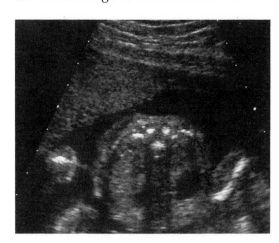 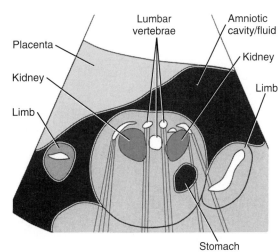

Labeled: **L SPINE**

14. **4-CHAMBER VIEW** of the fetal heart to include its location within the thorax.

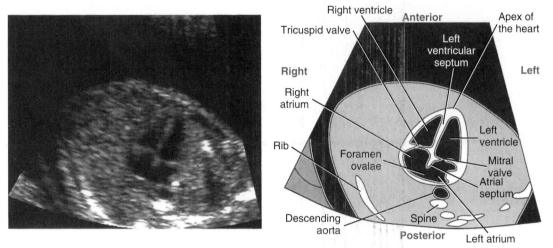

Labeled: **HEART**

15. Optional image showing the normal **RIGHT VENTRICULAR OUTFLOW TRACT.**

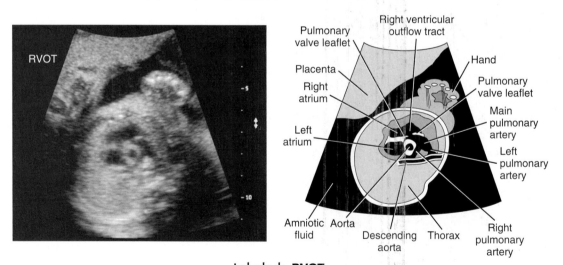

Labeled: **RVOT**

16. Optional image showing the normal **LEFT VENTRICULAR OUTFLOW TRACT.**

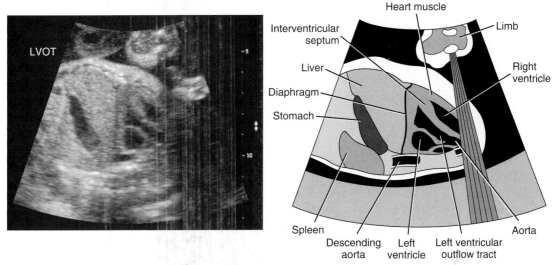

Labeled: **LVOT**

17. Axial image of **FETAL KIDNEYS** together.

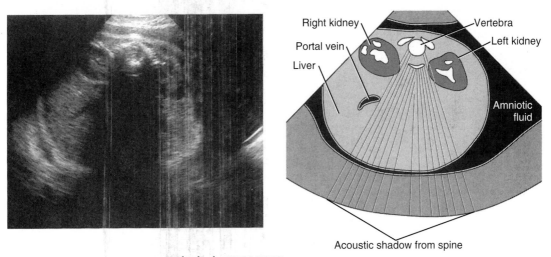

Labeled: **KIDNEYS**

NOTE: In cases where the kidneys cannot be imaged together because of fetal position or movement, take separate axial images of each kidney and label accordingly.

18. Longitudinal image of the **RIGHT KIDNEY.**

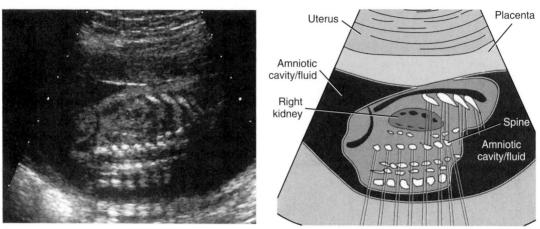

Labeled: **RT KID**

19. Longitudinal image of the **LEFT KIDNEY.**

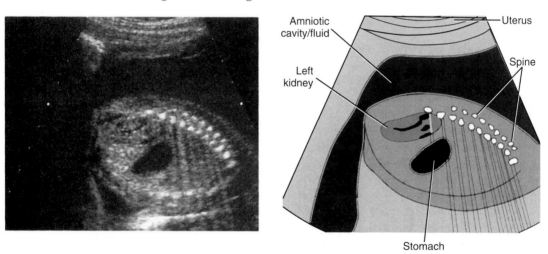

Labeled: **LT KID**

20. Image of the **URINARY BLADDER.**

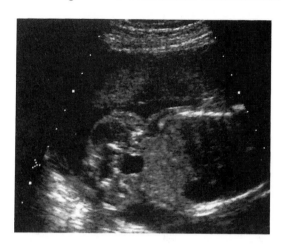
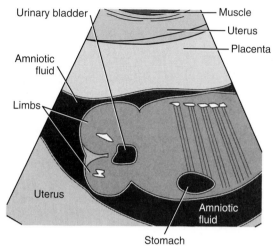

Urinary bladder
Muscle
Uterus
Placenta
Amniotic fluid
Limbs
Uterus
Amniotic fluid
Stomach

Labeled: **UR BLADDER**

21. Image of the **UMBILICAL CORD INSERTION SITE** on the anterior abdominal wall.

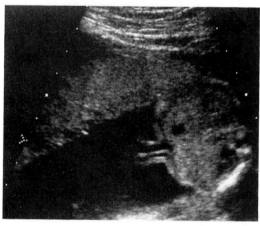
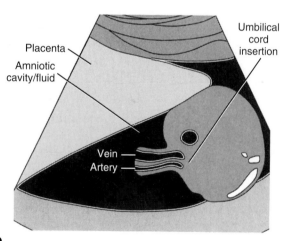

Placenta
Amniotic cavity/fluid
Umbilical cord insertion
Vein
Artery

Labeled: **CORD**

NOTE: If the insertion site image does not distinguish the 3 vessels of the cord, take an additional image of the cord to demonstrate the 3 vessels and label accordingly.

22. A magnified view of an axial section of the 3-vessel **UMBILICAL CORD.**

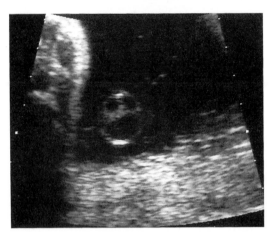 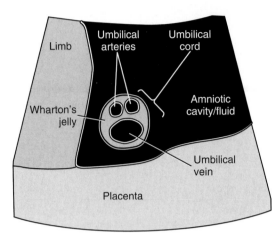

Labeled: **CORD**

23. Image of the **STOMACH** if visualized.

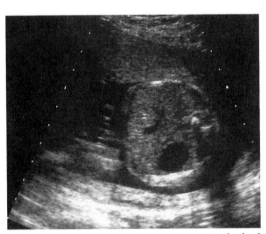 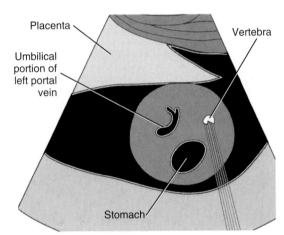

Labeled: **STOMACH**

NOTE: The image of the stomach is not necessary if the stomach was documented on any other image.

24. Image of **GENITALIA. A** and **B** provided to aid identification of the different genitalia: **(A)** Image of male genitalia. **(B)** Image of female genitalia.

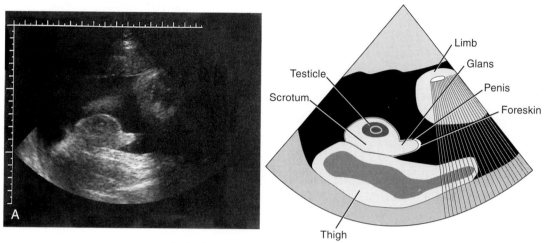

Labeled: **GENITALIA**

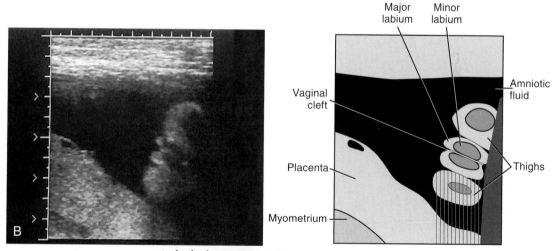

Labeled: **GENITALIA**

25. Longitudinal image of the **FETUS** to include the **DIAPHRAGM.**

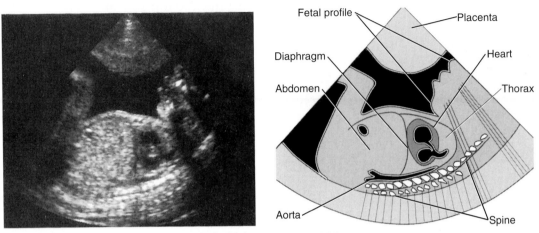

Labeled: **DIAPHRAGM**

NOTE: Because of the obvious nature of the fetal measurements, specifics are not included as part of the film labeling for the following measurement images.

26. **BIPARIETAL DIAMETER (BPD)** image at the level of the thalamus and the cavum septum pellucidi. *Measurement is from the outside of the near cranium to the inside of the far cranium (leading edge to leading edge).*

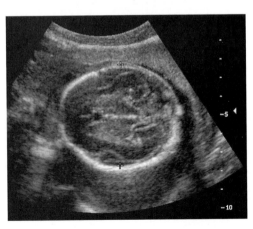
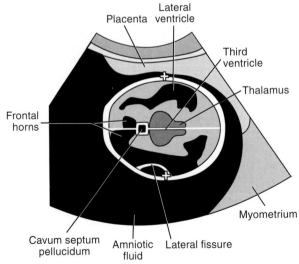

27. **CEREBELLUM** *with measurement.*

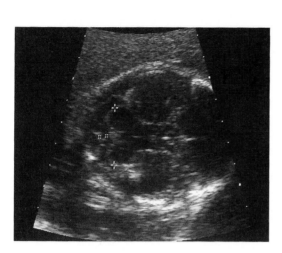

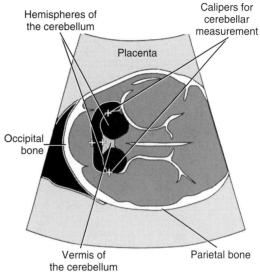

Hemispheres of the cerebellum

Calipers for cerebellar measurement

Placenta

Occipital bone

Vermis of the cerebellum

Parietal bone

28. **CISTERNA MAGNUM** *with measurement.*

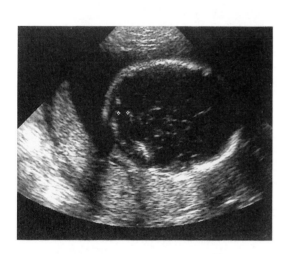

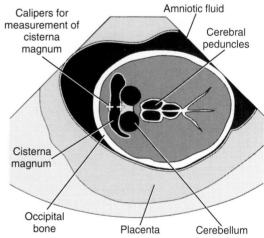

Calipers for measurement of cisterna magnum

Amniotic fluid

Cerebral peduncles

Cisterna magnum

Occipital bone

Placenta

Cerebellum

29. **NUCHAL FOLD** (done between 16 and 24 weeks) *with measurement.*

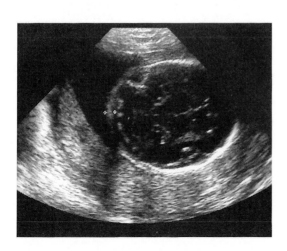

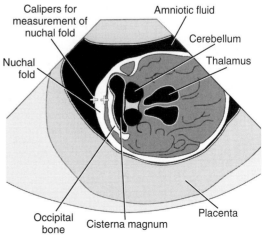

Calipers for measurement of nuchal fold

Amniotic fluid

Cerebellum

Nuchal fold

Thalamus

Occipital bone

Cisterna magnum

Placenta

NOTE: The measurement of the nuchal fold is not always routinely performed but should be considered for the fetus of patients over age 35 or when a lower-than-normal serum AFP level has been detected in the mother. The extra fold of soft tissue visualized at the back of the neck is considered a sonographic marker for the second trimester detection of Down syndrome.

30. **HEAD CIRCUMFERENCE** image at the same level as the biparietal diameter or use the BPD image. *Measurement is around the outline of the cranium.* Up-to-date ultrasound equipment provides tracking balls to trace the cranium or calipers that open to outline the cranium.

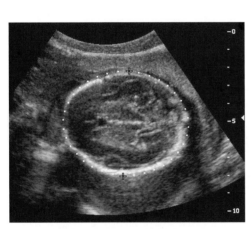
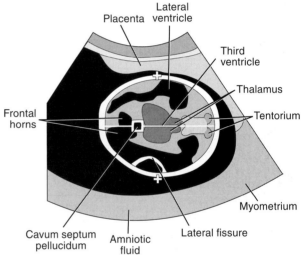

31. Image of the **CHOROID PLEXUS.**

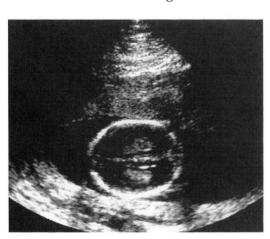
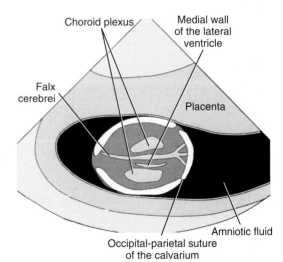

32. **LATERAL VENTRICLE** *with measurement.*

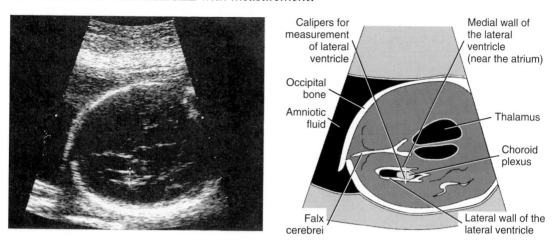

Calipers for measurement of lateral ventricle

Occipital bone

Amniotic fluid

Medial wall of the lateral ventricle (near the atrium)

Thalamus

Choroid plexus

Falx cerebrei

Lateral wall of the lateral ventricle

33. **ABDOMINAL CIRCUMFERENCE** image at the level of the junction of the umbilical vein and portal vein sinus. *Measurement is around the outline of the abdomen.* The abdomen should appear round.

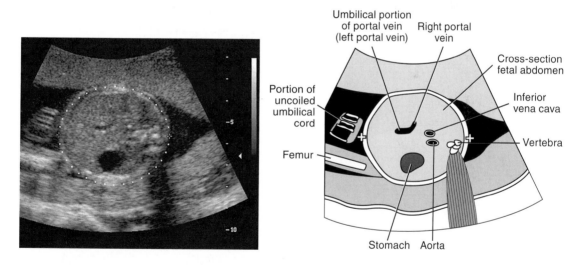

Umbilical portion of portal vein (left portal vein)

Right portal vein

Cross-section fetal abdomen

Portion of uncoiled umbilical cord

Inferior vena cava

Vertebra

Femur

Stomach   Aorta

34. **LONG AXIS** image of the femur *with measurement from one ossified end of the femur to the other ossified end.*

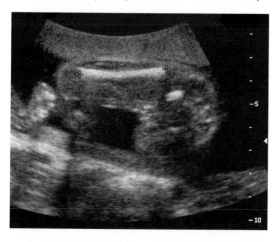

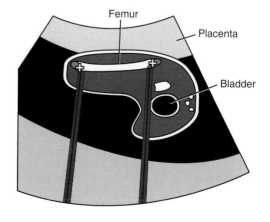

Femur

Placenta

Bladder

NOTE: For long bone measurements, cursors are placed at the bone-cartilage interface. The cartilaginous ends of the bones are not included in the measurement.

35. **LONG AXIS** image of the humerus *with measurement from one ossified end of the humerus to the other ossified end.*

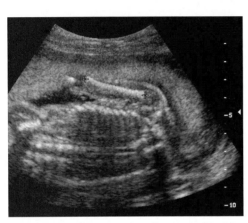
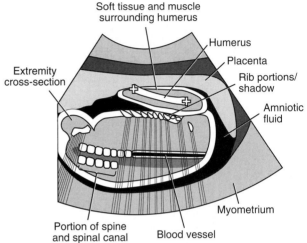

36. Image of the lower portion of the **LEG.**

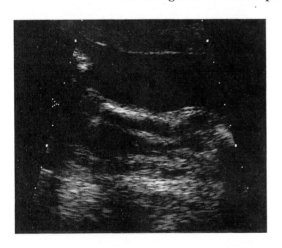
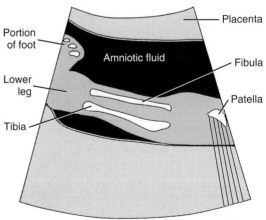

37. Image of the **RADIUS** and **ULNA**.

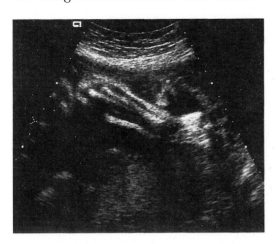 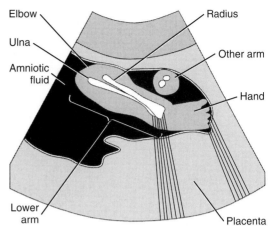

38. Image of a **HAND.**

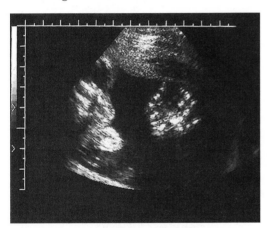 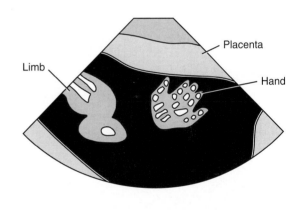

39. Another image of the **HAND.**

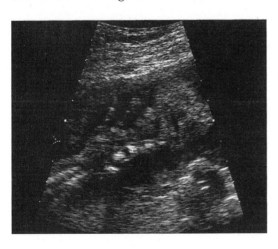 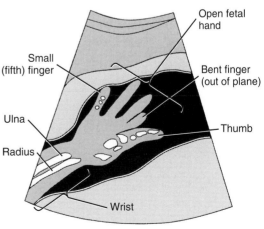

40. Image of **FACIAL PROFILE.**

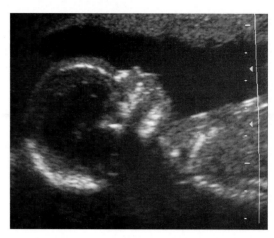

41. **CORONAL** image of the nostrils and lips.

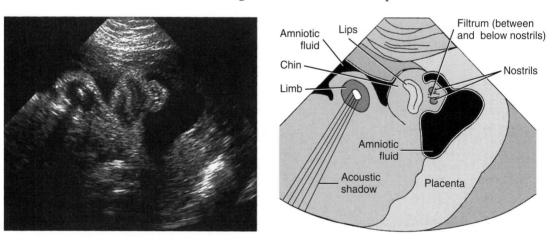

NOTE: Most physicians only require images of 1 hand, foot, arm, and leg based on the assumption that both were evaluated during the survey.

Multiple Gestations
Additional Required Images

Each fetus of a multiple gestation should be imaged as previously described for singleton pregnancies plus the following additional views as they apply:

1. Image of a twin pregnancy demonstrating separate sacs.

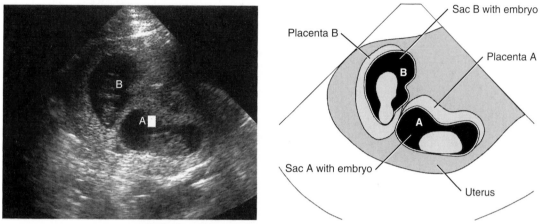

Labeled: **TWINS / SEP SACS**

2. Image of second trimester twins demonstrating the presence of a separating membrane.

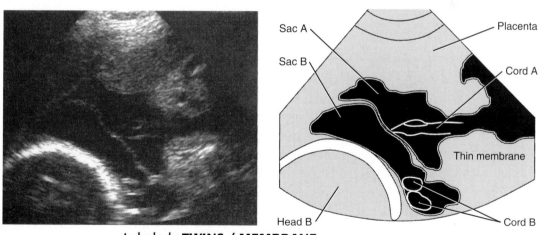

Labeled: **TWINS / MEMBRANE**

3. Image of triplets.

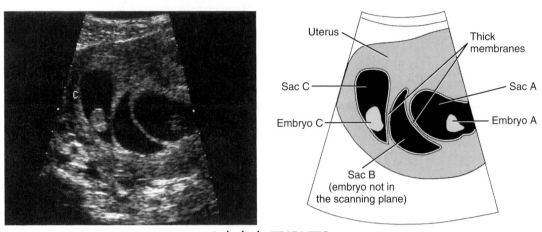

Labeled: **TRIPLETS**

NOTE: It is important to demonstrate the position of the presenting fetus. This is the fetus that is lower in the uterus, closer to the cervix, and will be delivered first. This fetus is labeled "A" and the other fetus is labeled "B." If there are more than 2 (as in Number 3) then "C," "D," etc., will be used. This labeling allows individual growth rates to be determined. If possible, determine the gender of each fetus. This information may help determine whether they are fraternal or identical.

The Biophysical Profile

An examination that is often performed during the late third trimester is the biophysical profile. This test measures fetal well-being and consists of 5 parameters. The first part of the test involves a nonstress test. This test is performed in the delivery room or in an obstetrician's office and measures spontaneous heart rate accelerations. This part of the biophysical profile (BPP) is not performed by the sonographer. The remaining 4 parameters of the BPP are measured by the sonographer. They are as follows: (1) fluid, (2) fetal respiration, (3) fetal tone, and (4) gross body motion. These parameters and scoring of this test are described in Table 13-1.

Table 13-1	Biophysical Profile Scoring	
	Criterion	**Score (points)**
Part I		
Nonstress test	2 accelerations of 15 beats/min in 30-min test	2
Part II		
Ultrasound Examination:		
Gross Movement	3 separate flexions and extensions in 30-min examination	2
Tone	1 episode of fetal opening and closing of hand or clenching of foot in 30-min examination	2
Respiration	At least 60 sec of fetal breathing in 30-min examination	2
Fluid	At least 1 pocket of amniotic fluid of at least 1 cm in 2 dimensions	2
	Unqualified Pass	8 or more
	Maximum Total	10

Data from Manning EA, Platt LD, Sipos L: Antenatal fetal evaluation: Development of a fetal biophysical profile. *Am J Obstet Gynecol.* 136:787–795, 1980.

Required Images for a Biophysical Profile

1. Demonstration of a **POCKET OF FLUID.**

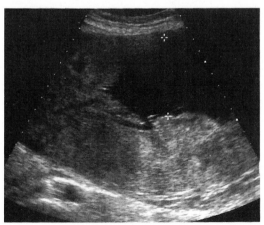

Labeled: **FLUID**

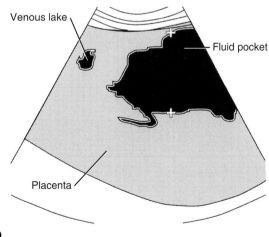

2. Demonstration of **FETAL RESPIRATION.**

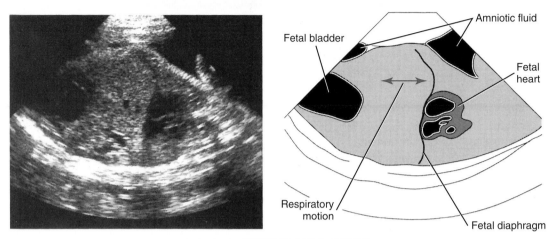

Labeled: **DIAPHRAGM / RESP**

3. Demonstration of **FETAL TONE.**

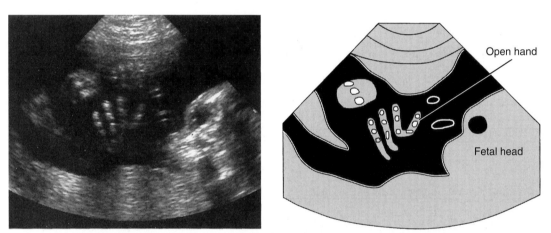

Labeled: **HAND**

4. Demonstration of **FETAL GROSS BODY MOTION.**

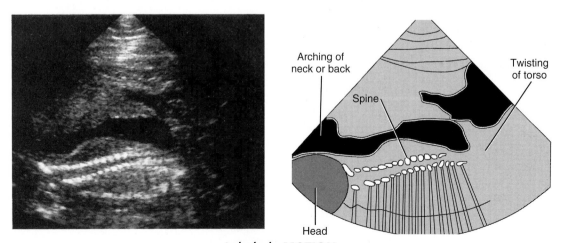

Labeled: **MOTION**

NOTE: Occasionally it is necessary to measure the resistance to blood flow within the umbilical arteries. This measurement is obtained by examining the umbilical cord artery with low-power Doppler. The ratio of the peak systolic flow to the end diastolic flow is calculated (SD ratio). This number varies with the age of the fetus and charts are available to determine if blood flow through the cord is adequate.

5. Umbilical artery Doppler measurement and determination of the SD ratio.

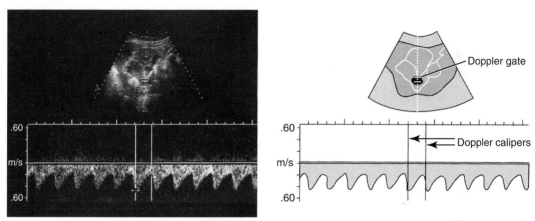

Labeled: **DOP / UMB ART**

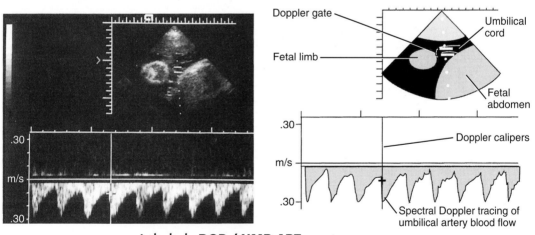

Labeled: **DOP / UMB ART**

6. Uterine artery Doppler measurement and determination of the SD ratio.

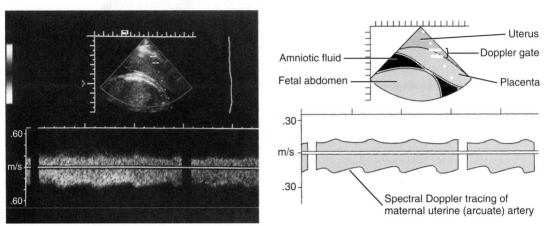

Labeled: **DOP / UT AR**

NOTE: In some cases, the physician may also want to determine if the blood flow to the placenta from the mother's circulation is adequate, so another Doppler measurement is made at the interface between the placenta and uterus or in the uterine artery if possible. The SD ratio for the Doppler wave-form is calculated and checked against a chart value for the appropriate GA.

Review Questions

Answers on page 629.

1. Using a 28-day menstrual cycle, most radiologists and obstetricians define the first trimester as the
   a) 12 weeks following the first day of the last normal menstrual period.
   b) 12 weeks beginning with the first day of the last normal menstrual period.
   c) 10 weeks beginning with the first day of the last normal menstrual period.
   d) 12 weeks following the last day of the last normal menstrual period.

2. The sonographic landmark for locating early cardiac activity is the
   a) amniotic membrane.
   b) double bleb sign.
   c) yolk sac.
   d) double sac sign.

3. When scanning the fetus, the first thing to do is
   a) determine the focal zone.
   b) take a BPD measurement.
   c) decide the plane of view.
   d) determine fetal presentation.

4. The intradecidual sign
   a) describes an abnormal early intrauterine pregnancy.
   b) describes the gestational sac's location within the endometrial cavity.
   c) describes an early intrauterine pregnancy adjacent to the endometrial cavity.
   d) occurs the eighth gestational week.

5. An intrauterine pregnancy can be confirmed before visualization of the yolk sac by identifying the
   a) fluid-filled chorionic cavity.
   b) double bleb sign.
   c) developing chorionic villi.
   d) double sac sign.

6. When the yolk sac, embryonic disk, and developing amniotic membrane are visualized together it is described as the
   a) fluid-filled chorionic cavity.
   b) double bleb sign.
   c) developing chorionic villi.
   d) double sac sign.

7. A tail-like appendage is often identified at the site of the embryo's rump. With development it
   a) becomes part of the umbilical cord.
   b) regresses.
   c) becomes part of the iliac wings of the bony pelvis.
   d) becomes the lower segment of the sacral portion of the spine.

8. Between the twelfth and sixteenth gestational weeks, the amniotic cavity has enlarged enough to
   a) obtain a mean sac diameter measurement.
   b) obliterate the yolk sac.
   c) obliterate the chorionic cavity.
   d) separate the yolk sac and the embryo.

9. When the umbilical cord enters the fetus
   a) the umbilical artery courses cephalad to join portal circulation and the umbilical veins run along each side of the urinary bladder.
   b) it joins the portal vein.
   c) the umbilical vein courses cephalad to join portal circulation and the umbilical arteries run along each side of the urinary bladder.
   d) it merges into one vessel.

10. Male gender can be established from the early second trimester by identifying the
    a) penis.
    b) urethra.
    c) scrotum.
    d) hydrocele.

11. The BPD can be measured
    a) through a single plane of section that demonstrates a symmetrical view of the third ventricle, thalami, cavum septum pellucidum, and tentorium.
    b) during the fourth gestational week.
    c) through any plane of section that demonstrates a symmetrical view of the short axes of the third ventricle and thalami.
    d) during the third gestational week.

12. The abdominal circumference (AC) is measured through a single plane of section that demonstrates where the
    a) left branch of the portal vein and both kidneys are visualized.
    b) umbilical arteries and the left and right portal veins are continuous with one another.
    c) right branch of the portal vein and the liver are visualized.
    d) umbilical vein branches and the left and right portal veins are continuous with one another.

13. Normal gut herniation should not be seen after the _____ GA week.
    a) twentieth.
    b) twelfth.
    c) tenth.
    d) sixteenth.

14. Placenta previa can be ruled out if the placenta is _____ cm from the internal os.
    a) 1.5
    b) 3
    c) 2
    d) 5

15. If an embryo is not visualized within the gestational sac, the GA in weeks can be determined by measuring the mean sac diameter and adding ____ to it.
    a) 1.5
    b) 3
    c) 2
    d) 5

16. A yolk sac is considered abnormal if it is larger than ____ mm.
    a) 3
    b) 6
    c) 2
    d) 7

17. As a trimester progresses, the crown rump length and amniotic sac diameter increase ___ mm a day.
    a) 1
    b) 3
    c) 1.5
    d) 5

18. The circular structure visualized between 4 and 10 weeks that supplies nutrition to the developing embryo is the _____.
    a) yolk sac
    b) disk
    c) amnion
    d) morula

19. For long bone measurements of the fetus, calipers are placed at the
    a) cartilage on the superior end and the bone-cartilage interface at the inferior end.
    b) bone-cartilage interface.
    c) cartilaginous ends of the bone.
    d) cartilage on the inferior end and the bone-cartilage interface at the superior end.

20. Lateral ventricle width is normal up to ____ mm.
    a) 11
    b) 7
    c) 10
    d) 5

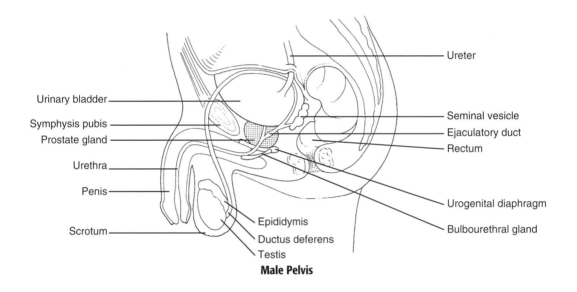

Urinary bladder

Symphysis pubis

Prostate gland

Urethra

Penis

Scrotum

Ureter

Seminal vesicle

Ejaculatory duct

Rectum

Urogenital diaphragm

Bulbourethral gland

Epididymis

Ductus deferens

Testis

Male Pelvis

CHAPTER 14

Male Pelvis Scanning Protocol for the Prostate Gland, Scrotum, and Penis

Betty Bates Tempkin

Key Words

Buck's fascia	Prostatic urethra
Central zone	Retroperitoneal
Corpora cavernosa	Scrotal sacs
Corpus spongiosum	Scrotum
Ductus epididymis	Seminal vesicles
Ejaculatory ducts	Seminiferous tubules
Epididymis	Spermatic cords
Interlobar septa	Testicles
Median raphe	Transition zone
Mediastinum testis	Tunica albuginea
Perineum	Urethra
Peripheral zone	Vas deferens ducts
Prostate gland	Verumontanum

Objectives

At the end of this chapter, you will be able to:

- Define the key words.
- Distinguish the sonographic appearance of the anatomy of the male pelvis and the terms used to describe it.
- Describe the transabdominal transducer options for scanning male pelvis anatomy.
- List the suggested patient positions (and options) when scanning male pelvis anatomy.
- Describe the patient prep for male pelvis studies.
- Name the survey steps and explain how to evaluate the entire length, width, and depth of the prostate gland, scrotum, and penis.
- Name the transducer options for endorectal scanning.
- List the scanning planes and image orientations for endorectal scanning.
- List the suggested patient position (and options) for endorectal scanning.
- Describe the patient prep for endorectal scanning.
- Explain the order and exact locations to take representative images of the prostate gland, scrotum, and penis.
- Answer the review questions at the end of the chapter.

Overview

The male pelvis contains the urinary bladder, a portion of the ureters, musculature, vasculature, and the genitourinary system, which includes the prostate gland, seminal vesicles, scrotum, testicles, and penis.

The emphasis of this scanning protocol chapter is the genitourinary system. As part of reproduction, the male genitourinary tract provides a means to perpetuate the species. The spermatozoa are manufactured in the testes; the ductal system stores and helps propel the sperm during ejaculation via the penis; the alkaline secretions from the prostate gland and seminal vesicles help the sperm survive to complete the process of reproduction.

Anatomy
Prostate Gland and Seminal Vesicles
- The *prostate gland:*
  - Is **retroperitoneal** (it lies in the portion of the abdominopelvic cavity posterior to the peritoneal sac), anterior to the rectum and inferior to the urinary bladder.
  - *Consists of* fibromuscular and glandular tissue that surrounds the neck of the urinary bladder and **prostatic urethra** (portion of male urethra surrounded by prostate gland).
  - Is about the size of a chestnut and conical in shape; approximately 3.5 cm long, 4.0 cm wide, and 2.5 cm anterior to posterior. The base, its broadest aspect, is superior to its apex.
  - The *glandular portion* of the prostate is divided into 3 zones (Figure 14-1):
    1. **Peripheral zone:** located posterior and lateral to the distal prostatic urethra. Normally, it is the *largest zone.*
    2. **Central zone:** extends from the base of the prostate to the **verumontanum** (landmark area near the center of the prostate gland) and surrounds the **ejaculatory ducts** (two ducts that transport sperm and pass through the prostate gland to empty into the prostatic urethra).
    3. **Transition zone:** located on both sides of the proximal urethra. Normally, it is the smallest zone.
- The *seminal vesicles:*
  - 2 convoluted, sac-like structures that lie superior to the prostate gland and posterior to the urinary bladder.
  - Approximately 5 cm (2 inches) in length and less than 1 cm in diameter. They join the **vas deferens ducts** (part of ductal system that transports sperm) to form the ejaculatory ducts.

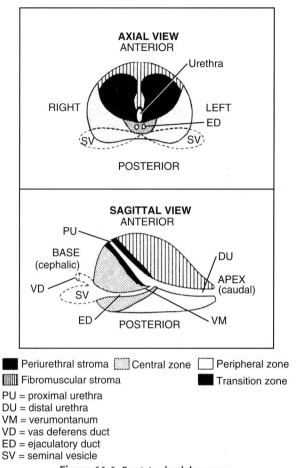

Figure 14-1 Prostate glandular zones.

Scrotum and Testicles

- The *scrotum:*
  - Is a pouch of skin that is continuous with the abdomen. It is suspended from the base of the male pelvis between the perineum (area between the anus and the scrotum) and the penis.
  - Externally, the median raphe or median ridge divides the scrotum into lateral portions.
  - Internally, the scrotum is divided into 2 sacs by a septum that is formed by the continuation of the external skin, superficial fascia, and contractile tissue. Each scrotal sac contains a *testis, epididymis,* and *proximal portion of the ductus (vas) deferens* (Figure 14-2).
  - 2 spermatic cords extend from the scrotum through the inguinal canals and internal inguinal rings into the pelvis. Each cord contains the *ductus (vas) deferens, testicular arteries, venous pampiniform plexus* (veins that drain the testes and become the spermatic veins superiorly) *lymphatics, autonomic nerves,* and *cremaster muscle fibers.*

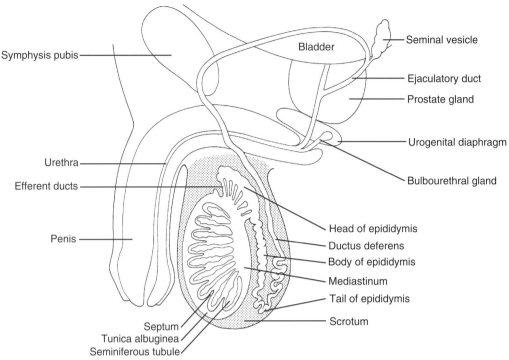

Figure 14-2 Scrotal anatomy.

- Each **testicle** is:
  - A male gonad. Male gonads are the organs that make the gametes (spermatozoa).
  - Approximately 1.5 to 2 inches (3 to 5 cm) long, 1 inch (2 to 3 cm) wide, and 1 inch (2 to 3 cm) anteroposteriorly. Before age 12, testicular volume is less than 5 mL. With maturity, the average testicular volume is approximately 25 mL. Testicular size decreases with advancing age.
  - Covered by **tunica albuginea**, a dense fibrous tissue which extends into the posterior testicle wall and forms the **mediastinum testis** and **interlobar septa**:
    - The septa of the mediastinum radiate into the testicle and separate into 200 to 300 lobules. Each lobule contains 1 to 3 convoluted **seminiferous tubules** that produce sperm then empty it into the straight tubules, which lead to a network of ducts called the rete testis. This network of ducts exits the testis through the mediastinum testis into a series of coiled epididymal efferent ducts.
    - The **epididymis** is primarily composed of the **ductus epididymis** a single convoluted, tightly wrapped, 1.5 inch, smooth muscle tube encapsulated by a serosal layer. When unwrapped, the tube measures about 20 feet (6 m) in length and 1.5 inches

(3.8 cm) in diameter. The epididymis is connected to the superior portion of the testis and runs along the posterior aspect to the base of the testis, where it drains into the ductus (vas) deferens. The ductus epididymis is subdivided into a *head, body,* and *tail:* the head (globus major) is the larger superior portion consisting mostly of the efferent ducts that empty into the ductus epididymis; the body runs along the posterior aspect of the testis and contains the ductus epididymis; the tail (globus minor) is the smaller inferior portion, where the ductus epididymis empties into the ductus (vas) deferens.

- The **ductus (vas) deferens** is a thicker, less convoluted continuation of the ductus epididymis that joins with the seminal vesicles to form the **ejaculatory ducts**, which course through the prostate and empty into the prostatic urethra.

Penis
- The *penis:*
  - Is composed of 3 cylindrical masses of smooth muscle and erectile tissue that enclose vascular cavities:
    - 2 corpora cavernosa situated dorso-laterally and
    - 1 corpus spongiosum in the midventral region, which contains the spongy urethra (longest portion of male urethra).
    - The 3 corpora are bound and separated by fibrous tissue, the *tunica albuginea.* Superficial to the tunica albuginea is a thick fibrous envelope and a loosely applied covering of skin, called Buck's fascia (Figure 14-3).
  - Along with the urethra, receives blood from the pair of *pundendal arteries,* which are branches of the internal iliac arteries. The primary veins of the penis are the superficial and *deep dorsal veins.*

Physiology
- As part of reproduction, the male genitourinary tract provides a means to perpetuate the species.
- The male gametes or spermatozoa are produced in the testes and mature in the epididymis. The function of the ductal system is to store and help propel the sperm during ejaculation via the penis. Without the alkaline secretions from the prostate gland and seminal vesicles, the sperm could not survive to complete the process of reproduction.
- The reproductive function of the penis is to eject semen into the female vagina. During ejaculation, increased pressure within the urethra causes the urinary bladder sphincter to close, which prevents urine from being expelled into the vagina and semen from entering the bladder.

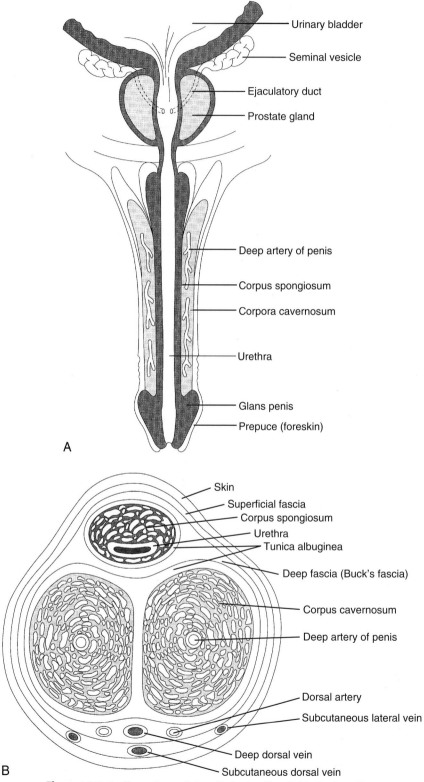

Figure 14-3 Penile anatomy. A, Longitudinal section. **B,** Short axis section.

Sonographic Appearance
Prostate Gland and Seminal Vesicles
Prostate Gland
- The majority of the parenchyma of the prostate appears homogeneous and midgray, with medium-level echoes. The periurethral glandular stroma that surrounds the urethra is slightly hypoechoic relative to surrounding prostatic parenchyma. At the midline of the gland the prostatic urethra walls appear echogenic.
- A normal prostate gland should appear symmetrical with a smooth contour and well-defined margins.
- Calcifications may be seen throughout the gland in older patients.
- The *central* and *transition zones* of the prostate are not normally distinctive. The *peripheral zone* appears homogeneous and slightly hyperechoic relative to adjacent parenchyma.

Seminal Vesicles
- These are identified as ovoid structures with low-level echoes, just superior to the prostate gland. They appear hypoechoic relative to the prostate gland.
- They should appear symmetric in size, shape, and echogenicity.
- They are horizontally oriented, therefore, they are seen in long axis on transverse plane scans.
- They are easier to visualize when the urinary bladder is partially filled.
- The *vas deferens* and *ejaculatory ducts* may be difficult to distinguish from surrounding structures. However, when seen, the vas deferens is medial to, and has an echo texture similar to, the seminal vesicles. The *ejaculatory duct* will appear as bright double lines.

Scrotum and Testicles
Scrotum
- Various layers of the scrotum are not normally differentiated on ultrasound. The combination of the scrotal wall layers typically appear as a single, bright, echogenic stripe.
- The highly echogenic *spermatic cord* may be visualized as it courses through the inguinal canal. As mentioned, the ductus deferens may be difficult to appreciate sonographically. Color flow Doppler is useful in identifying the blood vessels within the cord.

Testicles
- The parenchyma is homogeneous with medium-level echoes similar to those of the thyroid gland. Echo texture and size of each testicle should be compared to its opposite side.
- The *mediastinum testis* appears as a bright line running along the long axis of the testis.

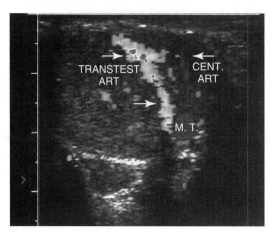

Figure 14-4 **Testicular Vascular Normal Variant.** The transtesticular artery runs in a direction opposite the centripetal arteries. See Color Plate 1.

- A few millimeters of anechoic fluid visualized between the two layers of the tunica vaginalis is a normal finding.
- The *epididymis* appears isosonic/isoechoic or slightly hyperechoic relative to the testicle. The texture of the epididymis, however, is generally more course in appearance. Echo texture and size of each epididymis should be compared to its opposite side.
- A testicular vascular normal variant identified sonographically in 10% to 20% of cases is the transtesticular artery coursing through the testis in a direction opposite the centripetal arteries (Figure 14-4).
- Color Doppler technical considerations:
  - Confirm intratesticular and epididymal flow using both color and conventional waveform analysis. Use the mediastinum testis as a point of reference when demonstrating intratesticular flow. With acute torsion less than 6 hours or chronic torsion more than 24 hours, there is absent intratesticular flow and increased peristesticular flow. Color Doppler cannot differentiate malignant hypervascularity from inflammatory hypervascularity.

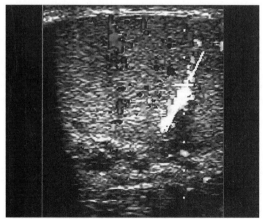

Color flow image and waveform of intratesticular arteries.
See Color Plate 2.

- Color Doppler arterial/venous flow characteristics:
  - The *testis* has low vascular resistance. Testicular, capsular, centripetal, and recurrent rami arteries have low resistance flow. Their waveforms are characterized by broad systolic peaks and high levels of diastolic flow similar to the internal carotid artery. Cremasteric and deferential arteries have high systolic peaks and lower levels of diastolic flow similar to the external carotid artery.

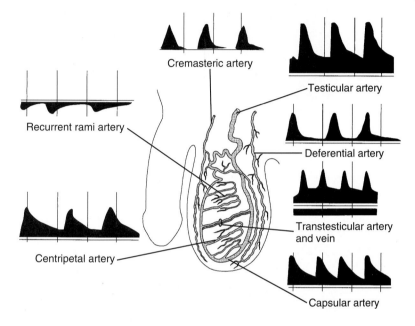

- Intratesticular veins accompany companion arteries. Their waveform is continuous or phasic.
- Spermatic cord/pampiniform plexus has minimal to moderate flow.

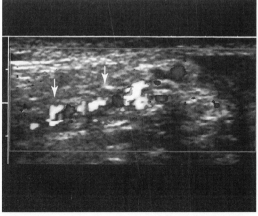

Color flow image of spermatic cord. See Color Plate 3.

- The epididymis has a very slight flicker or dashes of flow.

Color flow image of epididymis. See Color Plate 4.

- Testicular, deferential cremasteric, centripetal, and capsular arteries have moderate flow.

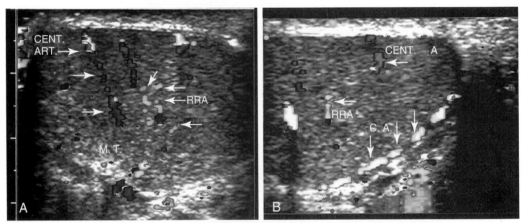

Color flow images of intratesticular arteries. **A,** See Color Plate 5. **B,** See Color Plate 6.

Penis

- *Corpus spongiosum* and *corpora cavernosa* appear homogeneous with medium-level echoes.
- The single corpus spongiosum:
  - In axial sections, is identified at the midline surrounding the urethra, which appears slightly hyperechoic compared to the corpus spongiosum.
  - Compressed by the transducer, it will appear elliptical in shape.
- The 2 corpora cavernosa:
  - Are surrounded by the *tunica albuginea,* which appears bright and distinctive.

- Are posterior to the corpus spongiosum and appear symmetrical, round or oval, with bright borders from the tunica albuginea.
- In short axis sections, the axial, anechoic lumen of the cavernosal artery is easily identified in the center of each corpus cavernosum; their pulsations can be seen in real time.
- In longitudinal sections they appear divided by the central, linear, bright appearance of the cavernosal arterial walls.

Preparation

Patient Prep
Prostate Gland
Endorectal Sonography
The prostate gland is best evaluated by endorectal (or transrectal) sonography. Transabdominal male pelvis examinations to evaluate the prostate gland are rarely performed now because the high frequency endorectal transducer can be placed closer to the area of interest and produce superior, highly detailed images.

- The patient should have a self-administered enema before the examination. If for some reason the patient cannot have the enema, the study should still be attempted.
- Explain the examination to the patient. Verbal or written consent is required and the examination should be witnessed by another health-care professional. The initials of the witness should be part of the film labeling.
- The sonographer or physician inserts the transducer.

Scrotum

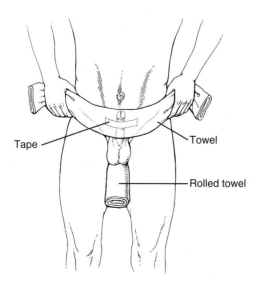

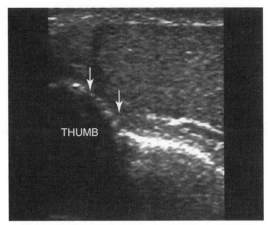

THUMB

Figure 14-5 The sonographer's thumb and fingers are easily identified when scanning the scrotum and can be used as reference points for localizing scrotal lesions.

- The scrotum should be supported on a rolled towel placed between the patient's thighs to isolate and immobilize the scrotum for scanning. Cover the penis with a towel and tape the towel to the abdominal wall.
- Explain the examination to the patient. The examination should be witnessed by another health-care professional and their initials should be part of the film labeling.
- Use warm gel as a scanning couplant.
- To scan the scrotum the sonographer's gloved fingers should be placed underneath the scrotum and the thumb over the top of the scrotum. This hand position further stabilizes the scrotum and has the advantage of allowing correlation between a palpable mass and its sonographic findings. Also, the sonographer's fingers are easily identified as they appear bright and highly reflective and are used as reference points for localizing masses (Figure 14-5).

Penis
- The penis should be supported on a rolled towel placed between the patient's thighs to isolate and immobilize the penis for scanning.
- Explain the examination to the patient. The examination should be witnessed by another health-care professional and their initials should be part of the film labeling.
- Use warm gel as a scanning couplant.

Transducer

Prostate Gland

Endorectal Sonography

- **5.0 MHz** or higher.
- Preparing the transducer includes providing a water path. Preparation includes one of the following 3 options:
  1. Some transducer manufacturers provide a finger-like sheath that slides onto the transducer head. The sheath is secured by a small rubber band, and 20 or 30 mL of nonionized water is injected into the sheath through a pathway inside the transducer handle. Tip the transducer down and tap the water-filled sheath so any air bubbles will rise to the top and can be aspirated. Fill a condom half full with sonographic gel, then insert the sheathed transducer. Apply additional lubrication to the outside of the condom before insertion. A small rubber hose can be attached to the transducer pathway to introduce or aspirate water from the sheath to adjust for any air bubbles that might occur and cause artifacts.
  2. Apply gel to the end of the transducer, then cover it with a condom. Secure the condom with a rubber band and make sure there are no air bubbles at the tip. Apply additional lubrication to the outside of the condom before insertion. Use an inner balloon filled with 30 to 50 mL of nonionized water as a water path.
  3. Cover a transducer with a disposable sheath or condom and secure it with a rubber band; lubricate the outside; then insert the transducer into the rectum. Fill the sheath or condom with 30 to 50 mL of an unionized water for a water path.
- Following the examination, any tubing or stopcocks and the disposable sheath or condom covering the endorectal probe should be disposed. The probe should be soaked in an antimicrobial solution. Follow manufacturer's instructions and infectious disease recommendations for solution type and soak time. If the sheath or condom was torn during the procedure, the probe's fluid channels must be flushed with the antimicrobial solution.

Scrotum

- **5.0 MHz or higher, real-time, linear or a curved linear transducer.**
- 7.0 MHz to 10.0 MHz is preferable for pediatric applications.
- 3.5 MHz to 7.0 MHz conventional Doppler with color flow imaging (low flow filter, scale, and optimized resolution).
- If necessary, use a gel standoff pad to improve imaging. They can be helpful when evaluating anterior lesions.

Penis
- **5.0 MHz, high resolution, real-time, linear transducer.**
- 7.5 MHz, 10.0 MHz.
- Conventional Doppler with color flow imaging (low flow filter, scale, and optimized color gain).
- In some cases, a gel standoff pad may improve imaging.

Patient Position
Prostate Gland
Endorectal Sonography
- **Left lateral decubitus with knees bent toward the chest.**
- Lithotomy position.

Scrotum
- **Supine with the legs slightly spread or in a semi frog-legged position.**
- Upright.

Penis
- **Supine with the legs slightly spread or in a semi frog-legged position.**
- Upright.

Prostate Gland Survey

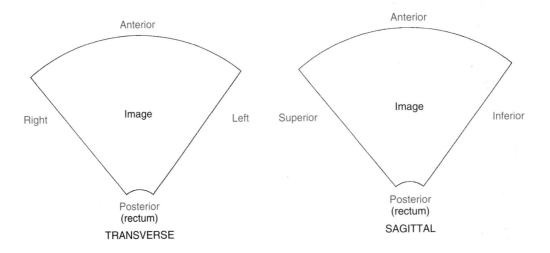

NOTE: If a male pelvis transabdominal study is ordered, the examination is systematically evaluated and documented in the same manner as the female pelvis transabdominal studies. Sagittal plane surveys extend from one side of the pelvic cavity to the other. Transverse plane surveys extend from the symphysis pubis to the umbilicus. The prostate gland is examined from an inferior transducer angle at the level of the symphysis pubis. Patient prep, patient position, and transducer choices are the same as those for the female pelvis. See Chapter 11 for specifics.

NOTE: While surveying the prostate evaluate the periprostatic fat and vessels for asymmetry and any disruption in echogenicity. Also evaluate the perirectal space, especially the area where the prostate and perirectal tissue abut. The rectal wall and lumen should be evaluated in cases where rectal pathology is clinically suspected.

Prostate • Axial Survey
Transverse Plane • Rectal Approach

NOTE: To survey the prostate in short axis, the transducer is inserted into the rectum and then withdrawn sequentially to examine the prostate superiorly (base) to inferiorly (apex).

1. With the transducer inserted, the survey begins at the level of the seminal vesicles.
2. After the seminal vesicles have been evaluated, slowly withdraw the transducer to scan through the prostate from its superior to inferior margins. The lateral margins should be well defined. Note the size, shape, and symmetry of the prostate.

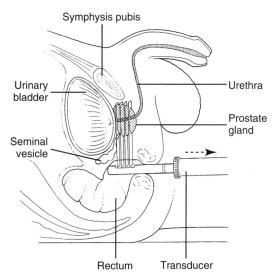

Prostate • Longitudinal Survey
Sagittal Plane • Rectal Approach

> **NOTE:** To survey the prostate longitudinally the transducer is rotated clockwise, and counterclockwise to examine the prostate from one lateral edge to the other.

1. Begin at the midline of the prostate. The superior and inferior margins should be well defined and the prostatic urethra visualized.
2. To examine the lateral aspects of the prostate and seminal vesicles slowly rotate the transducer clockwise and counterclockwise.

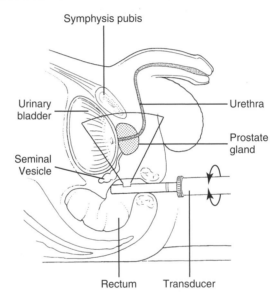

Prostate Gland Required Images*

> **NOTE:** The required images are a small representation of what a sonographer visualizes during a study. Therefore, the images should provide the interpreting physician with the most telling and technically accurate information available.

*Images in this section are by courtesy the Ultrasound Department of Methodist Hospital, Houston, Texas.

Prostate • Axial Images
Transverse Plane • Rectal Approach
1. Axial image of the **SEMINAL VESICLES.**

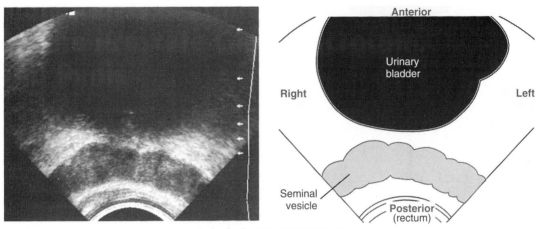

Labeled: **ER TRV SEM V**

("ER" indicates endorectal)

> **NOTE:** Because of the limited field of view, both seminal vesicles may not be entirely visible on a single view. If so, take these additional images:

2. Axial image of the **RIGHT SEMINAL VESICLE** to include its right lateral margin.

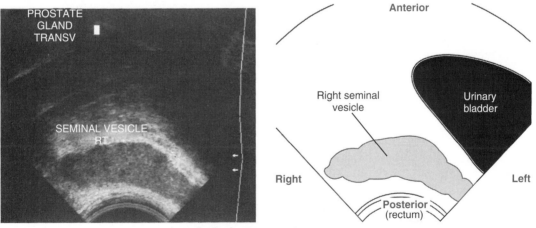

Labeled: **ER TRV SEM V RT**

3. Axial image of the **LEFT SEMINAL VESICLE** to include its left lateral margin.

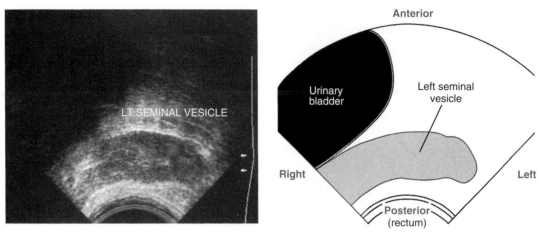

Labeled: **ER TRV SEM V LT**

4. Axial image of the **BASE** of the prostate.

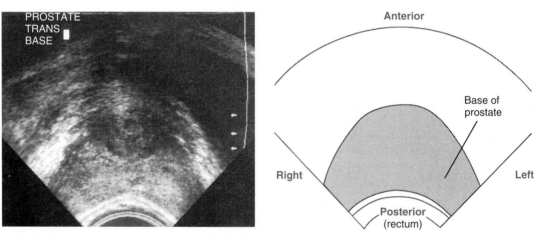

Labeled: **ER TRV BASE**

5. Axial image of the **MID** prostate.

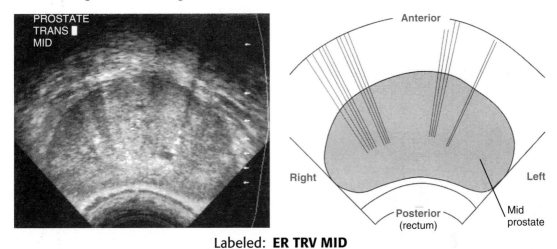

Labeled: **ER TRV MID**

6. Axial image of the **APEX** of the prostate.

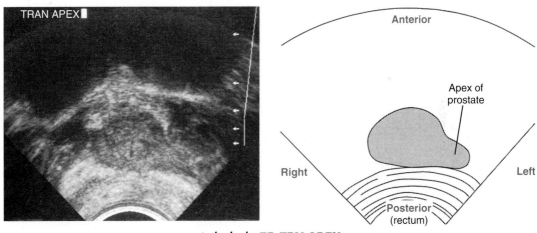

Labeled: **ER TRV APEX**

Prostate • Longitudinal Images
Sagittal Plane • Rectal Approach
7. **LONGITUDINAL MIDLINE** image of the prostate.

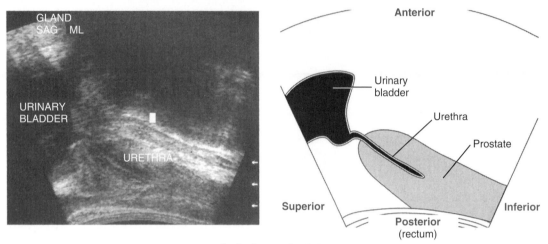

Labeled: **ER SAG ML**

8. Longitudinal image of the **RIGHT LATERAL** portion of the prostate gland including the right seminal vesicle.

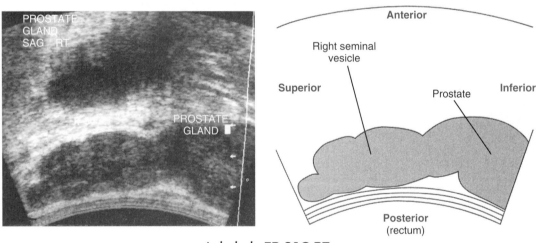

Labeled: **ER SAG RT**

9. Longitudinal image of the **LEFT LATERAL** portion of the prostate gland including the left seminal vesicle.

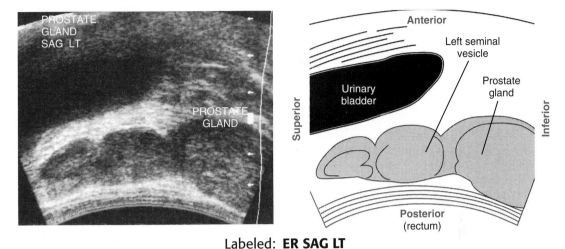

Labeled: **ER SAG LT**

Scrotum Survey

> **NOTE:** Use the following survey steps for both testes.

Scrotum • Longitudinal Survey
Sagittal Plane • Anterior Approach

> **NOTE:** Evaluation of the testis begins with a survey of the spermatic cord with the patient in normal respiration followed by having the patient perform the Valsalva maneuver to rule out varioceles.

1. Begin scanning with the transducer perpendicular at the superior midline portion of the testis at the level of the spermatic cord. The patient should be at normal respiration.

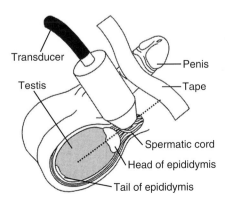

2. Keep the transducer perpendicular at the level of the spermatic cord and slowly slide the transducer medially through and beyond the cord.

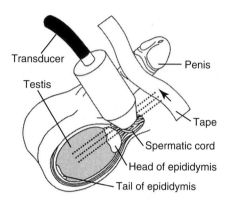

3. Scan back through the medial portion of the spermatic cord to mid testis. Keeping the transducer perpendicular, slowly slide the transducer laterally through and beyond the cord.

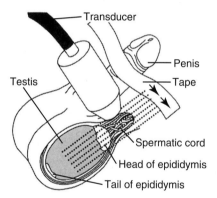

4 to 6. Repeat the above survey steps of the spermatic cord while the patient performs the Valsalva maneuver.

7. Keep the transducer perpendicular and return to the mid portion of the testis.

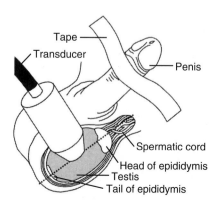

NOTE: The spermatic cord, epididymal head, and the superior and inferior margins of the testis should be visible on longitudinal sections. If not, move the transducer superior and inferior as necessary to evaluate all of the anatomy.

8. Slowly slide the transducer medially through and beyond the scrotal sac.

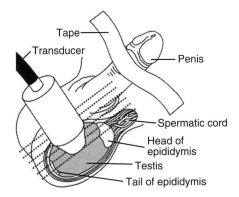

NOTE: Note scrotal skin thickness.

9. Move back to mid testis. Keep the transducer perpendicular; slowly scan laterally through and beyond the testis and scrotal sac.

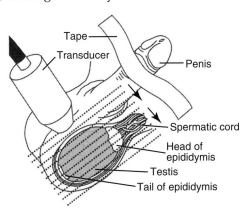

Scrotum • Axial Survey
Transverse Plane • Anterior Approach

> **NOTE:** Evaluation of the testis begins with a survey of the spermatic cord with the patient in normal respiration followed by having the patient perform the Valsalva maneuver to rule out varioceles.

1. Begin scanning with the transducer perpendicular at the superior portion of the testis at the level of the spermatic cord. The patient should be at normal respiration.

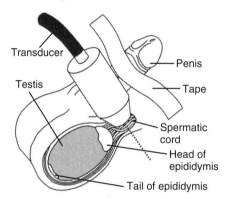

2. Keep the transducer perpendicular at the level of the spermatic cord and slowly slide the transducer superiorly, scanning through and beyond the cord.

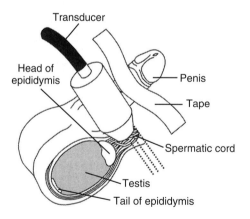

3. Scan back through the superior portion of the spermatic cord to mid cord. Keeping the transducer perpendicular, slowly scan inferiorly through and beyond the cord.

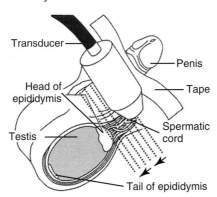

4 to 6. Repeat the above survey steps of the spermatic cord while the patient performs the Valsalva maneuver.

7. Keep the transducer perpendicular and return to the mid portion of the testis.

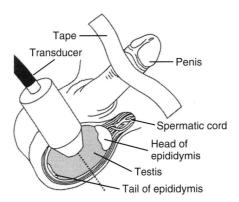

NOTE: The medial and lateral margins of the testis should be visible on axial sections. If not, move the transducer medial and lateral as necessary to evaluate all of the anatomy.

8. Slowly slide the transducer superiorly through the superior portion of the testis to the head of the epididymis.

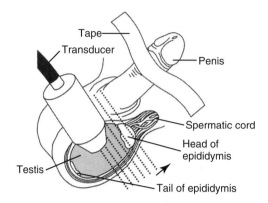

9. Keep the transducer perpendicular and continue to move the transducer superiorly through and beyond the head of the epididymis, the spermatic cord, and scrotal sac.

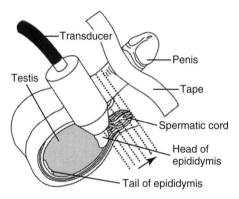

10. Move back to mid testis. Keep the transducer perpendicular; slowly scan inferiorly, through the inferior portion of the testis to the level of the tail of the epididymis.

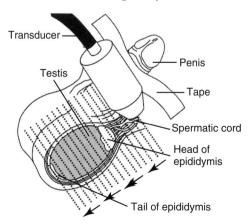

11. Continue to scan inferiorly through and beyond the scrotal sac.

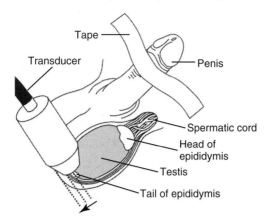

Scrotum Required Images

NOTE: The required images are a small representation of what a sonographer visualizes during a study. Therefore, the images should provide the interpreting physician with the most telling and technically accurate information available.

Scrotum • Right Hemiscrotum • Longitudinal Images
Sagittal Plane • Anterior Approach

1. **LONG AXIS** image of the **SPERMATIC CORD** at normal respiration or rest *with anterior to posterior measurement.*

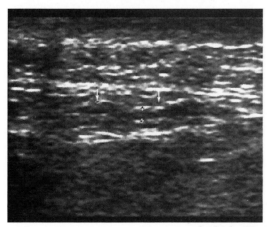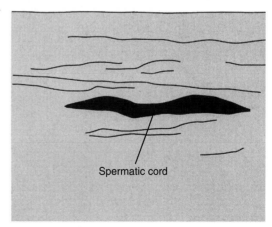

Labeled: **RT CORD SAG REST**

2. Same image as number 1 *without calipers.*

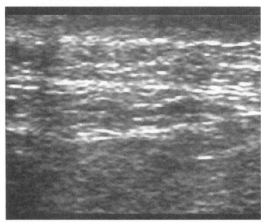

Labeled: **RT CORD SAG REST**

3. **LONG AXIS** image of the **SPERMATIC CORD** while the patient performs the Valsalva maneuver *with anterior to posterior measurement.*

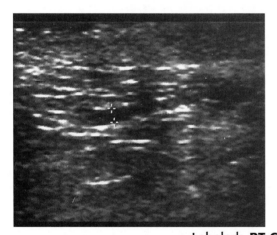 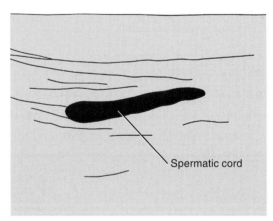

Spermatic cord

Labeled: **RT CORD SAG VAL**

4. Same image as number 3 *without calipers*.

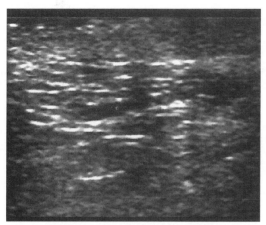

Labeled: **RT CORD SAG VAL**

5. Longitudinal image of the head of the **EPIDIDYMAL HEAD.**

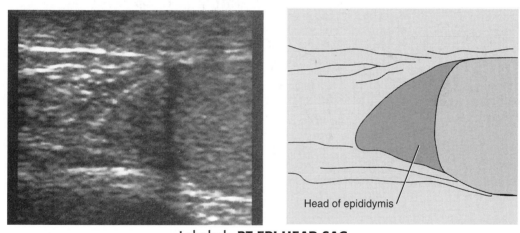

Head of epididymis

Labeled: **RT EPI HEAD SAG**

6. Longitudinal image **SUPERIOR MARGIN** of the right testis.

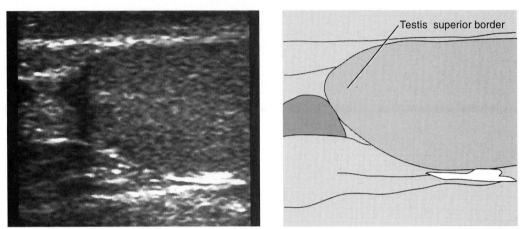

Labeled: **RT TESTIS SAG SUP**

7. Longitudinal image of the **MID PORTION** of the right testis.

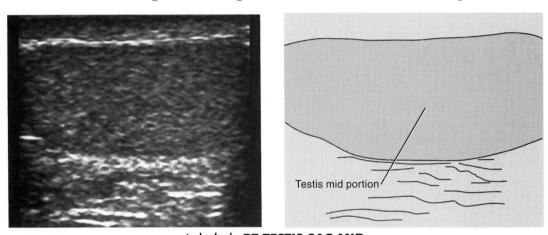

Labeled: **RT TESTIS SAG MID**

8. **LONG AXIS** image of the spermatic right testis *with superior to inferior measurement.*

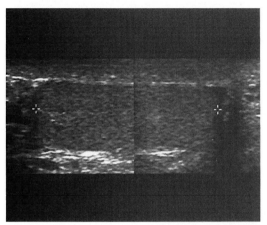 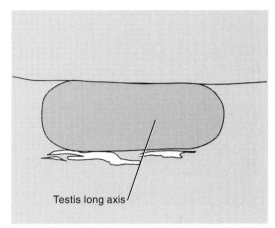

Testis long axis

Labeled: **RT TESTIS SAG LONG AXIS**

NOTE: If necessary, use dual imaging to obtain the entire long axis of the testis on the image.

9. Same image as number 8 *without calipers.*

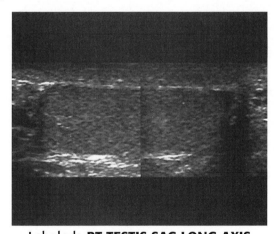

Labeled: **RT TESTIS SAG LONG AXIS**

10. Longitudinal image of the **MEDIAL PORTION** of the right testis.

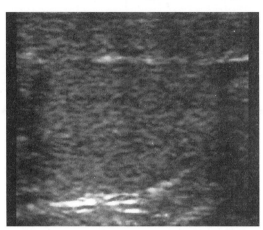   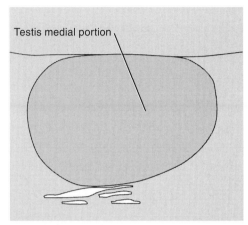

Labeled: **RT TESTIS SAG MED**

11. Longitudinal image of the **LATERAL PORTION** of the right testis.

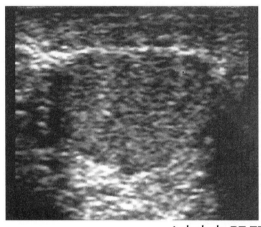   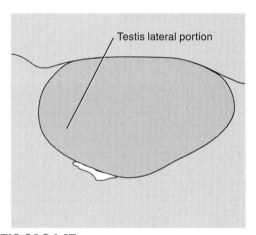

Labeled: **RT TESTIS SAG LAT**

12. Longitudinal image of the **INFERIOR MARGIN** of the right testis.

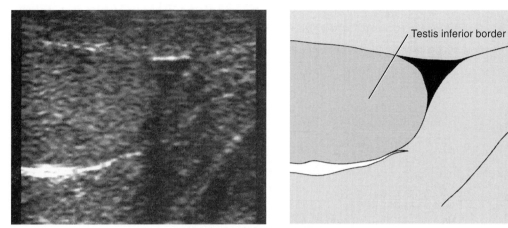

Labeled: **RT TESTIS SAG INF**

13. Longitudinal image of the **EPIDIDYMAL TAIL** (if visualized).

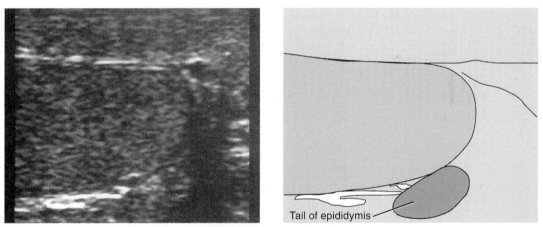

Labeled: **RT EPI TAIL SAG**

Scrotum • Right Hemiscrotum • Axial Images
Transverse Plane • Anterior Approach

14. Axial image of the **SPERMATIC CORD** at normal respiration or rest *with anterior to posterior measurement.*

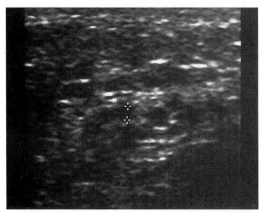 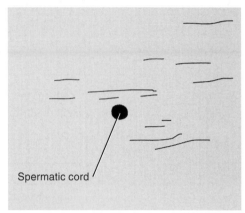

Spermatic cord

Labeled: **RT CORD TRV REST**

15. Same image as number 14 *without calipers.*

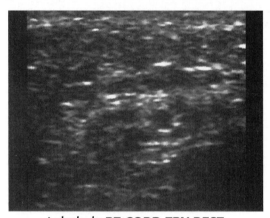

Labeled: **RT CORD TRV REST**

16. Axial image of the **SPERMATIC CORD** while the patient performs the Valsalva maneuver *with anterior to posterior measurement.*

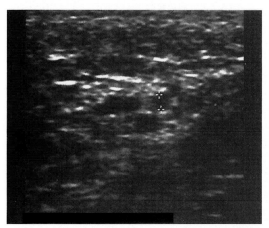 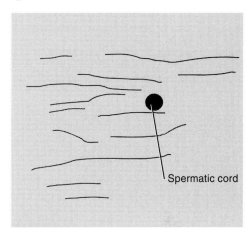

Labeled: **RT CORD TRV VAL**

17. Same image as number 16 *without calipers.*

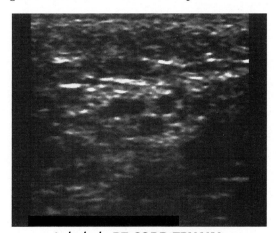

Labeled: **RT CORD TRV VAL**

18. Axial image of the **EPIDIDYMAL HEAD.**

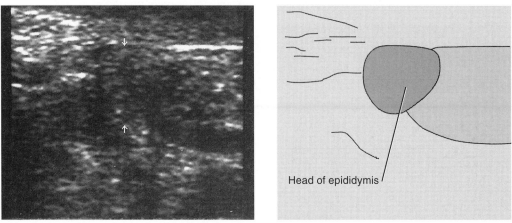

Head of epididymis

Labeled: **RT EPI HEAD TRV**

19. Axial image of the **SUPERIOR PORTION** of the right testis.

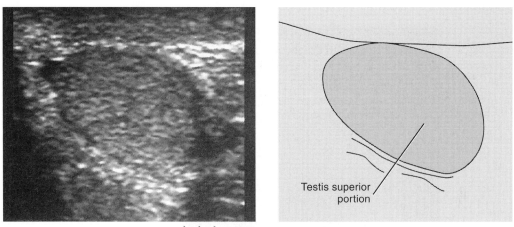

Testis superior
portion

Labeled: **RT TESTIS TRV SUP**

20. Axial image of the **MID PORTION** of the right testis *with medial to lateral measurement.*

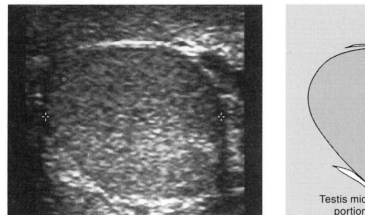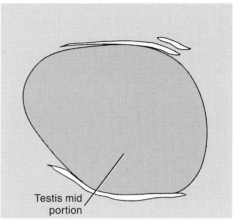

Testis mid portion

Labeled: **RT TESTIS TRV MID**

21. Same image as number 20 *without calipers.*

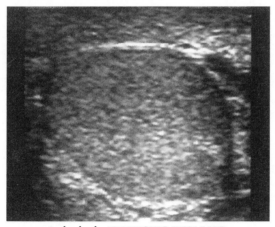

Labeled: **RT TESTIS TRV MID**

22. Axial image of the **INFERIOR PORTION** of the right testis.

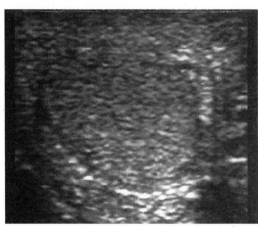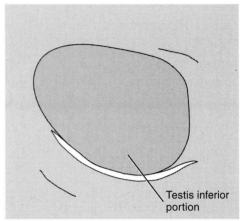

Testis inferior
portion

Labeled: **RT TESTIS TRV INF**

23. Axial image of the **EPIDIDYMAL TAIL** (if visualized).

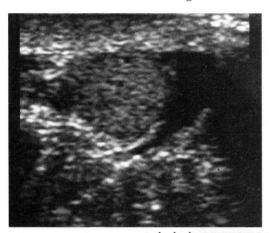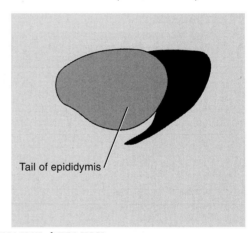

Tail of epididymis

Labeled: **RT TESTIS TRV INF / EPI TAIL**

Scrotum • Left Hemiscrotum • Longitudinal Images
Sagittal Plane • Anterior Approach
1. **LONG AXIS** image of the **SPERMATIC CORD** at normal respiration or rest *with anterior to posterior measurement.*

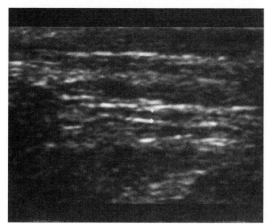 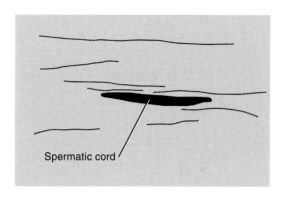

Labeled: **LT CORD SAG REST**

2. Same image as number 1 *without calipers.*

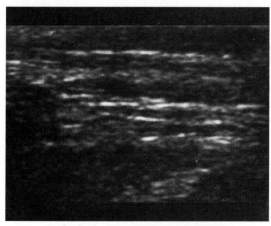

Labeled: **LT CORD SAG REST**

3. **LONG AXIS** image of the **SPERMATIC CORD** while the patient performs the Valsalva maneuver *with anterior to posterior measurement.*

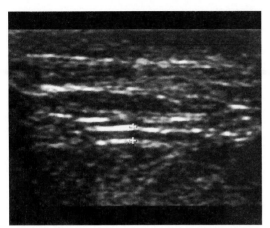 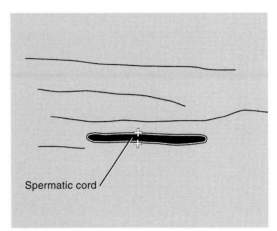

Spermatic cord

Labeled: **LT CORD SAG VAL**

4. Same image as number 3 *without calipers.*

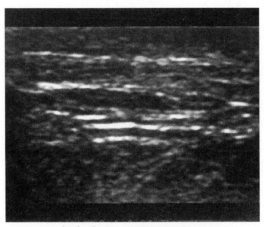

Labeled: **LT CORD SAG VAL**

5. Longitudinal image of the **EPIDIDYMAL HEAD.**

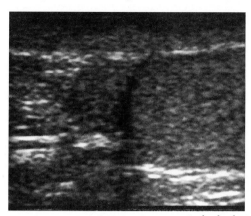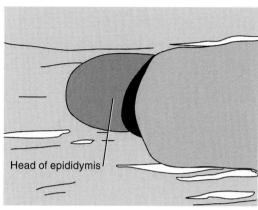

Head of epididymis

Labeled: **LT EPI HEAD SAG**

6. Longitudinal image of the **SUPERIOR MARGIN** of the left testis.

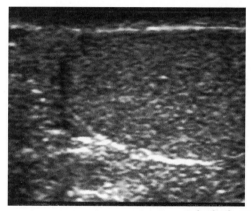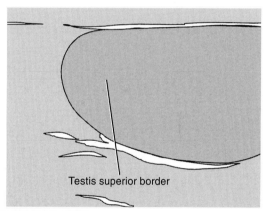

Testis superior border

Labeled: **LT TESTIS SAG SUP**

7. Longitudinal image of the **MID PORTION** of the left testis.

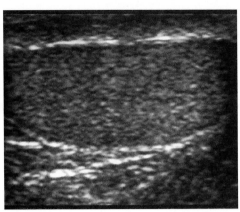

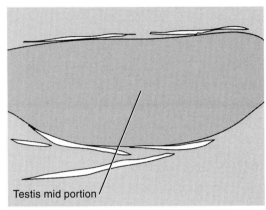

Testis mid portion

Labeled: **LT TESTIS SAG MID**

8. **LONG AXIS** image of the left testis *with superior to inferior measurement.*

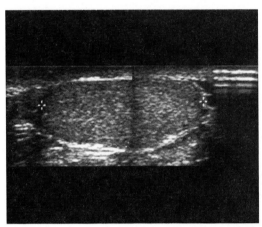

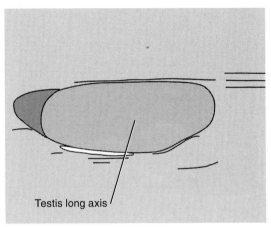

Testis long axis

Labeled: **LT TESTIS SAG LONG AXIS**

NOTE: If necessary, use dual imaging to obtain the entire long axis of the testis on the image.

9. Same image as number 8 *without calipers*.

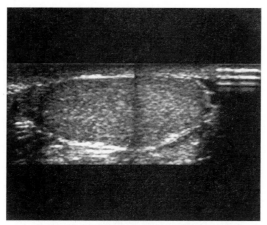

Labeled: **LT TESTIS SAG LONG AXIS**

10. Longitudinal image of the **MEDIAL PORTION** of the left testis.

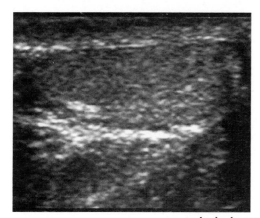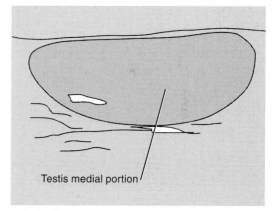

Testis medial portion

Labeled: **LT TESTIS SAG MED**

11. Longitudinal image of the **LATERAL PORTION** of the left testis.

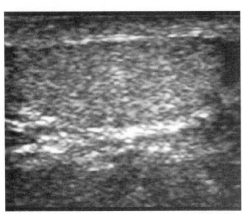 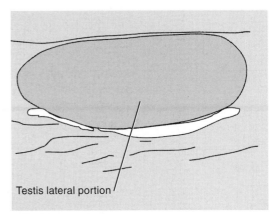

Labeled: **LT TESTIS SAG LAT**

12. Longitudinal image of the **INFERIOR MARGIN** of the left testis.

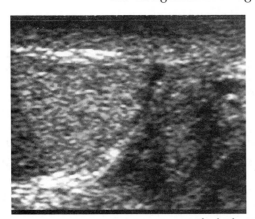 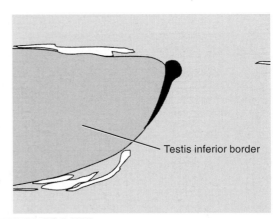

Labeled: **LT TESTIS SAG INF**

13. Longitudinal image of the **EPIDIDYMAL TAIL** (if visualized).

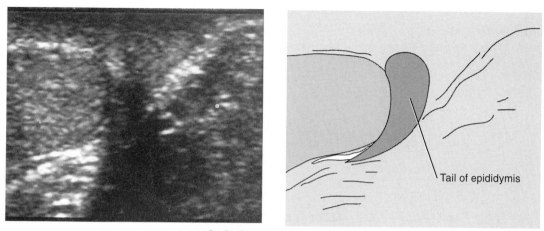

Labeled: **LT EPI TAIL SAG**

Scrotum • Left Hemiscrotum • Axial Images
Transverse Plane • Anterior Approach

14. Axial image of the **SPERMATIC CORD** at normal respiration or rest *with anterior to posterior measurement.*

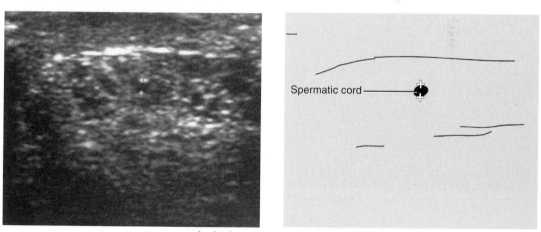

Labeled: **LT CORD TRV REST**

15. Same image as number 14 *without calipers*.

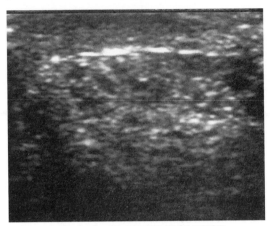

Labeled: **LT CORD TRV REST**

16. Axial image of the **SPERMATIC CORD** while the patient performs the Valsalva maneuver *with anterior to posterior measurement*.

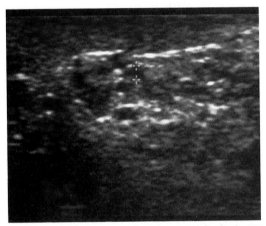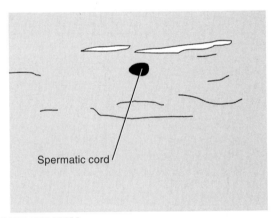

Spermatic cord

Labeled: **LT CORD TRV VAL**

17. Same image as number 16 *without calipers*.

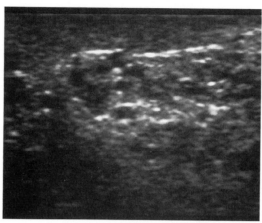

Labeled: **LT CORD TRV VAL**

18. Axial image of the **EPIDIDYMAL HEAD.**

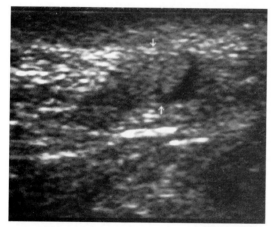 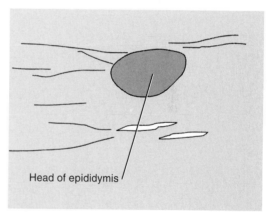

Head of epididymis

Labeled: **LT EPI HEAD TRV**

19. Axial image of the **SUPERIOR PORTION** of the left testis.

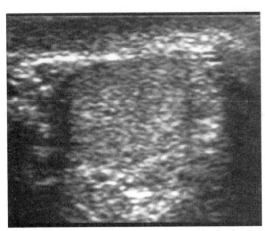
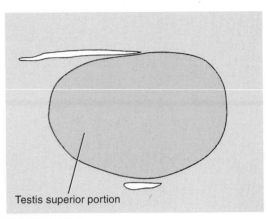

Labeled: **LT TESTIS TRV SUP**

20. Axial image of the **MID PORTION** of the left testis *with medial to lateral measurement.*

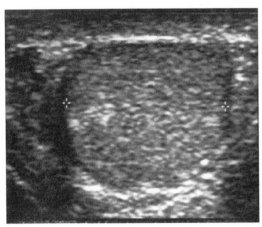
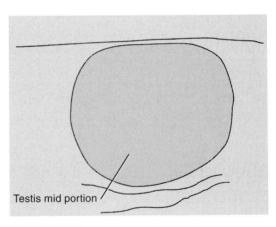

Labeled: **LT TESTIS TRV MID**

21. Same image as number 20 *without calipers*.

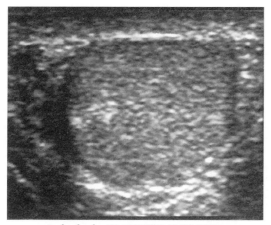

Labeled: **LT TESTIS TRV MID**

22. Axial image of the **INFERIOR PORTION** of the left testis.

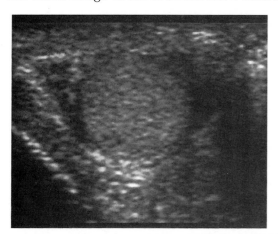
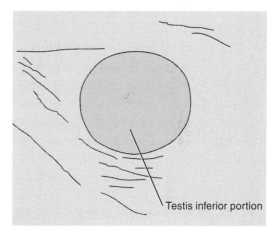

Testis inferior portion

Labeled: **LT TESTIS TRV INF**

23. Axial image of the **EPIDIDYMAL TAIL** (if visualized).

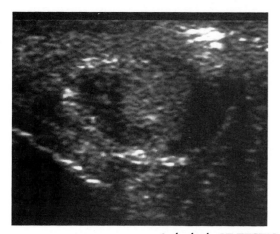
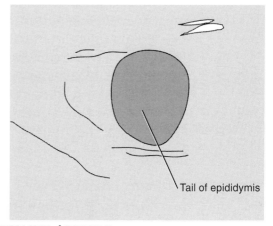

Tail of epididymis

Labeled: **LT TESTIS TRV INF / EPI TAIL**

24. Axial image of the **MID PORTION BOTH TESTES.**

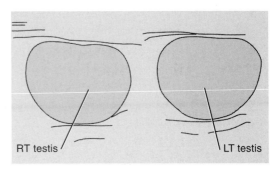

RT testis   LT testis

RT   LT

Labeled: **BILAT TESTES TRV**

Penis Survey

Penis • Longitudinal Survey
Sagittal Plane • Anterior Approach

1. Begin scanning with the transducer perpendicular at the midline of the most superior portion of the penis. Very slowly slide the transducer inferiorly, scanning along the length of the penis until you are beyond it. Notice how the corpora cavernosum stops at the area of the glans penis. Anteriorly, the homogeneous long section represents the corpus spongiosum. Note the highly echogenic appearance of the anterior and posterior margins formed by the tunica albuginea and Buck's fascia.

2. Return to the superior, midline position then move the transducer toward the patient's left side to include the left margin of the penis. Very slowly slide the transducer inferiorly, scanning along the length of the penis until you are beyond it. Notice the centrally located, bright, thin, parallel lines, representing a longitudinal section of the cavernosal arterial walls.

3. Return to the superior, midline position then move the transducer toward the patient's right to include the right margin of the penis. Very slowly slide the transducer inferiorly, scanning along the length of the penis until you are beyond it. Notice the centrally located, bright, thin, parallel lines, representing a longitudinal section of the cavernosal arterial walls.

Penis • Axial Survey
Transverse Plane • Anterior Approach

1. Remain in the sagittal scanning plane and return to the superior, midline position of the penis. Rotate the transducer 90 degrees into the transverse scanning plane. The short axis view of the penis

will include the anteroposterior and right and left lateral margins. Note the smaller corpus spongiosum just anterior to the pair of corpora cavernosa. Notice how the centrally located, bright walls, and anechoic, short axis lumen of the cavernosal arteries disrupts the otherwise homogeneous echo texture of each corpus cavernosum.

2. Keep the transducer perpendicular and very slowly slide the transducer inferiorly, scanning through and beyond the penis. Notice how the corpora cavernosum stops at the area of the glans penis.

Penis Required Images

NOTE: The required images are a small representation of what a sonographer visualizes during a study. Therefore, the images should provide the interpreting physician with the most telling and technically accurate information available.

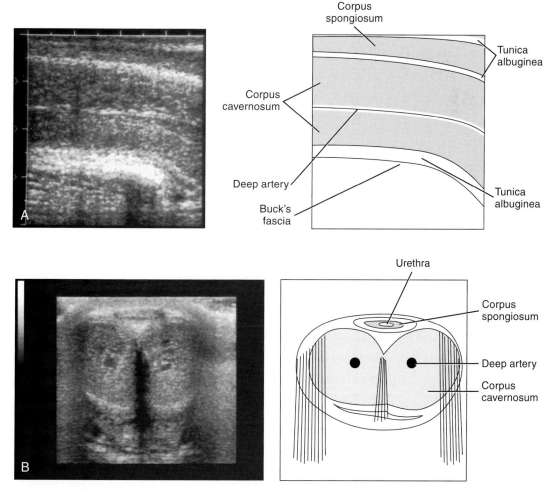

Representative longitudinal **(A)** and short axis **(B)** image sections of the penis.

Penis • Longitudinal Images
Sagittal Plane • Anterior Approach

1. Longitudinal image of the left lateral, superior portion of the penis to include the corpus spongiosum, corpus cavernosum, and cavernosal artery.
   Labeled: **SAG PENIS LT SUP**

2. Longitudinal image of the left lateral, mid portion of the penis to include the corpus spongiosum, corpus cavernosum, and cavernosal artery.
   Labeled: **SAG PENIS LT MID**

3. Longitudinal image of the left lateral, inferior portion of the penis to include the corpus spongiosum, corpus cavernosum, and cavernosal artery.
   Labeled: **SAG PENIS LT INF**

4. Longitudinal image of the left lateral glans penis.
   Labeled: **SAG PENIS LT GLANS**

5. Longitudinal image of the right lateral, superior portion of the penis to include the corpus spongiosum, corpus cavernosum, and cavernosal artery.
   Labeled: **SAG PENIS RT SUP**

6. Longitudinal image of the right lateral, mid portion of the penis to include the corpus spongiosum, corpus cavernosum, and cavernosal artery.
   Labeled: **SAG PENIS RT MID**

7. Longitudinal image of the right lateral, inferior portion of the penis to include the corpus spongiosum, corpus cavernosum, and cavernosal artery.
   Labeled: **SAG PENIS RT INF**

8. Longitudinal image of the right lateral glans penis.
   Labeled: **SAG PENIS RT GLANS**

Penis • Axial Images
Transverse Plane • Anterior Approach

9. Axial image of the superior portion of the penis to include the corpus spongiosum, corpus cavernosum, and cavernosal arteries.
   Labeled: **TRV PENIS SUP**

10. Axial image of the mid portion of the penis to include the corpus spongiosum, corpus cavernosum, and cavernosal arteries.
    Labeled: **TRV PENIS MID**

11. Axial image of the inferior portion of the penis to include the corpus spongiosum, corpus cavernosum, and cavernosal arteries.
    Labeled: **TRV PENIS INF**

12. Axial image of the glans penis.
    Labeled: **TRV PENIS GLANS**

Review Questions

Answers on page 630.

1. The male genitourinary system includes the
   a) prostate gland, seminal vesicles, scrotum, testicles, and penis.
   b) urinary bladder, prostate gland, scrotum.
   c) kidneys, a portion of the ureters, musculature, urinary bladder.
   d) kidneys, a portion of the ureters, urinary bladder, prostate gland.

2. The prostate gland is located
   a) intraperitoneal, anterior to the rectum; inferior to urinary bladder.
   b) retroperitoneal, posterior to the rectum; inferior to urinary bladder.
   c) retroperitoneal, anterior to the rectum; inferior to urinary bladder.
   d) intraperitoneal, around the base of the urethra.

3. The peripheral zone is
   a) located on both sides of the proximal urethra.
   b) the smallest zone.
   c) located posterolateral to the distal prostatic urethra.
   d) the extension of the base of the prostate gland to the verumontanum.

4. The two convoluted sac-like structures that lie superior to the prostate and posterior to the urinary bladder are the
   a) testes.
   b) vas deferens ducts.
   c) verumontanum.
   d) seminal vesicles.

5. Each scrotal sac contains a
   a) testis, epididymis, portion of vas deferens duct.
   b) testis, seminal vesicle, portion of vas deferens duct.
   c) testis, epididymis, seminal vesicles.
   d) testis, epididymis, portion of ejaculatory duct.

6. _____and_____ join to form the ejaculatory ducts.
   a) Seminal vesicles, vas deferens ducts.
   b) Epididymis, seminal vesicles.
   c) Epididymis, vas deferens ducts.
   d) Vas deferens ducts, proximal prostatic urethra.

7. Which zone(s) of the prostate gland is normally sonographically distinguishable?
   a) All zones
   b) Peripheral zone only
   c) Central and peripheral zones
   d) Transition zone only

8. The ovoid structures with low-level echoes, just superior to the prostate gland are the
   a) vas deferens ducts.
   b) seminal vesicles.
   c) ejaculatory ducts.
   d) epididymis.

9. Compared to the testicle, the echo texture of the epididymis is
   a) hypoechoic.
   b) slightly hyperechoic and smoother.
   c) slightly hyperechoic and more coarse.
   d) extremely hyperechoic.

10. The bright line seen running along the long axis of the testis is the
    a) epididymis.
    b) verumontanum.
    c) mediastinum testis.
    d) efferent duct.

11. In short axis sections, the corpus spongiosum is identified
    a) posterior to the copora cavernosa.
    b) at the midline surrounding the urethra.
    c) by the centrally located cavernosal artery.
    c) posterolateral to the urethra.

12. The prostate gland is about the size of a
    a) chestnut.
    b) pea.
    c) plum.
    d) the collapsed urinary bladder.

13. The bright covering of the testes is the
    a) spermatic cord.
    b) inguinal rings.
    c) cremaster muscle.
    d) tunica albuginea.

14. What ducts enter the base of the prostate gland and pass through to the urethra?
    a) Ejaculatory
    b) Vas deferens
    c) Epididymal
    d) Inguinal

15. The normal corpus spongiosum and corpora cavernosa will appear _____ with _____ echoes.
    a) homogeneous, low-level echoes
    b) heterogeneous, bright
    c) homogeneous, inguinal ring
    d) homogeneous, medium-level echoes

16. The corpora cavernosa are surrounded by the tunica albuginea, which appears _____.
    a) hypoechoic in comparison
    b) homogeneous
    c) bright
    c) heterogeneous

17. The epididymis appears _____ or slightly _____ compared to the testicle.
    a) darker, hypoechoic
    b) isosonic, hypoechoic.
    c) isosonic, hyperechoic
    d) bright, hyperechoic

18. The periurethral glandular stroma that surrounds the urethra is _____ compared to surrounding prostatic parenchyma.
    a) slightly hyperechoic
    b) slightly hypoechoic.
    c) bright
    d) hyperechoic

19. In short axis sections of the corpus cavernosum, _____ are easily identified in the center.
    a) axial sections of the capsular artery
    b) axial sections of the corpus spongiosum
    c) axial sections of the cavernosal artery
    d) long sections of the urethra

20. Superficial to the tunica albuginea is a thick fibrous envelope and a loosely applied covering of skin, called
    a) Buck's fascia.
    b) median raphe.
    c) interlobar septa.
    d) perineum.

PART V

SMALL PARTS SCANNING PROTOCOLS

Musculoskeletal Scanning Protocol for Rotator Cuff, Carpal Tunnel, and Achilles Tendon

Amy T. Dela Cruz

Key Words

Achilles tendon	Plantaris tendon
Aponeurosis	Retrocalcaneal bursa
Biceps tendon	Rotator cuff
Bicipital groove	Subacromial bursa
Bouffard position	Subcutaneous calcaneus bursa
Bursae	Subdeltoid bursa
Carpal tunnel	Subscapularis muscle/tendon
Guyon's canal	Supraspinatus muscle/tendon
Infraspinatus muscle/tendon	Synovial sheath
Krager's fat pad	Teres minor muscle/tendon
Median nerve	Transverse ligament
Neutral position	

Objectives

At the end of this chapter, you will be able to:

- Define the key words.
- Distinguish the sonographic appearance of the musculoskeletal system and the terms used to describe it.
- Describe the transducer options for scanning the musculoskeletal system.
- List the suggested patient position (and options) when scanning structures in the musculoskeletal system.
- Name the survey steps and explain how to evaluate the structures in the musculoskeletal system.
- Explain the order and exact locations to take representative images of the structures in the musculoskeletal system.
- Answer the review questions at the end of the chapter.

Rotator Cuff Scanning Protocol Overview

Location

The rotator cuff is located at the humeral head sitting in the shallow glenoid fossa at the proximal humerus. It surrounds the shoulder joint, providing stability.

Anatomy

- The rotator cuff consists of 4 muscles and the corresponding tendons
  1. Subscapularis muscle/tendon: largest muscle in the rotator cuff complex. The subscapularis originates from the scapula and drapes along the anterior surface of the scapula, inserting by way of subscapularis tendon to the lesser tuberosity of the humeral head.The transverse ligament is a lateral extension of the subscapularis tendon that covers the anterior aspect of the biceps tendon (a landmark for locating rotator cuff anatomy).
  2. Supraspinatus muscle/tendon: originates and courses along the anterior and superior scapula, inserting by way of the supraspinatus tendon to the greater tuberosity.
  3. Infraspinatous muscle/tendon: originates and courses along the posterior scapular inferior to the supraspinatus, attaching by way of the infraspinatous tendon to the greater tuberosity.
  4. Teres minor muscle/tendon: courses inferior to infraspinatus muscle along the posterior scapula, attaching by way of teres minor tendon to the greater tuberosity.
- The shoulder complex contains 2 bursae, which are fluid-filled sacs aiding in the movement of the shoulder joint and protection from the bone causing friction with the soft tissue:
  1. Subdeltoid bursa (largest in the shoulder complex)
  2. Subacromial bursa

Physiology

- The rotator cuff surrounds the shoulder joint, providing stability to the head of the humerus sitting in the shallow glenoid fossa. The tendons provide the attachment for the muscles to the bones.
- The muscles and tendons creating the cuff aid in movement:
  1. **Subscapularis muscle** and **tendon** aid in *internal rotation* of the shoulder.
  2. **Supraspinatous muscle** and **tendon** aid in *abduction* of the shoulder.
  3. **Infraspinatous muscle** and **tendon** aid in *external rotation* of the shoulder.
  4. **Teres minor muscle** and **tendon** aid in *external rotation* of the shoulder.

Sonographic Appearance

- Most *muscles* appear very low-gray and hypoechoic relative to adjacent structures, often having a compartment type feature caused by the connective tissue that surrounds the bundles of muscle fibers. Axially, the muscles can appear speckled as a result of the perimysium separating the muscle fibers into small bundles. Longitudinally, the muscle will appear more fibrillar. The technique of rotating the transducer to confirm the change from speckled to striated appearance is helpful in distinguishing muscle from other structures. The aponeurosis is the tissue that binds the muscle fibers together and aids in the connection to the bone. Sonographically it will appear as a bright reflecting linear structure.
- *Tendons* such as the biceps tendon appear midgray (and often have bright reflectors throughout) with medium to high level echoes that are hyperechoic to adjacent muscles. Some tendons, like the biceps tendon, are surrounded by a synovial sheath, a membrane or bursa that contains a small amount of fluid or mucinoid material, aiding in movement. The fluid will appear hypoechoic around the tendon. Excess fluid may accumulate during some pathological processes.
- *Ligaments* are thin structures coursing in many different directions, making their sonographic identification challenging. When visualized, ligaments will typically appear highly echogenic.

Preparation

Patient Prep
- No prep needed.

Transducer
- Linear 7 MHz to 18 MHz.

Patient Position
- Sitting.
- Arm in neutral, external rotation, or Bouffard position (hand in back pocket; elbow extending posteriorly).

Breathing Technique
- None.

Rotator Cuff Survey and Required Images

Biceps Tendon
1. Patient position should be sitting with the arm in a neutral position resting on the thigh with the hand facing upward.

As illustrated below, begin with the transducer in transverse orientation just inferior to the humeral head. The image demonstrates how the biceps tendon sits within the **bicipital groove** *(arrows)* of the humerus between the greater and lesser humeral tuberosities (GT, LT). The tendon appears as a midgray, ovoid structure with medium- to high-level echoes that are hyperechoic compared to the deltoid muscle. It is normal to see a very small amount of anechoic fluid surrounding the tendon. Notice how the transverse ligament appears as a bright band sandwiched between the deltoid muscle (anteriorly) and biceps tendon (posteriorly).

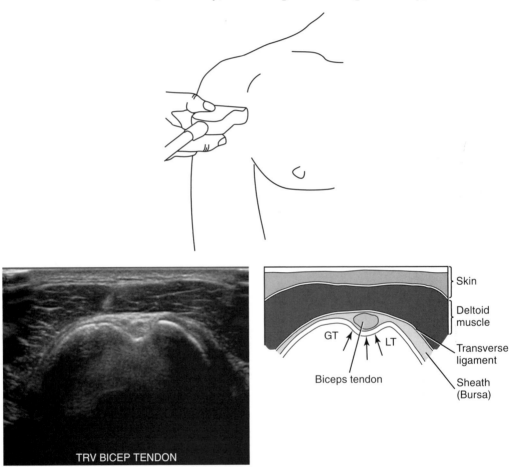

2. As illustrated on the facing page, rotate the transducer 90 degrees into the longitudinal plane to image the full length of the biceps tendon. The image demonstrates the tendon anterior to the

*Images in this chapter courtesy of the University of Virginia Imaging Center, Charlottesville, Virginia.

humeral shaft and posterior to the deltoid muscle. Note the consistent architecture of the biceps tendon; any disruption is indicative of an abnormality.

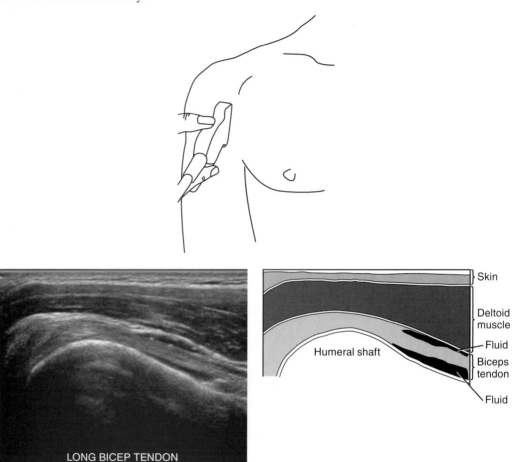

LONG BICEP TENDON

Subscapularis

1. The patient should begin with the arm in a neutral position. As illustrated on the following page, return the transducer to the transverse orientation and image the axial biceps tendon, then move the transducer slightly superior and medial (toward the humeral head) to image the long axis of the subscapularis tendon. The image demonstrates how the long axis of the subscapularis tendon appears as a fibrillar band of medium level echoes posterior to the deltoid muscle. Dynamic imaging during internal and external rotation will provide full evaluation of the tendon. (*S*, Subscapularis tendon; *BT*, biceps tendon; *D*, deltoid muscle; *C*, coracoid process.)

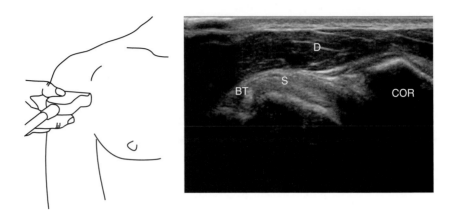

2. With the patient still in the neutral position, rotate the transducer 90 degrees into the longitudinal plane, as illustrated below. The image demonstrates how the subscapularis tendon *(S)* will be seen in short axis just anterior to the humeral head *(H)*. *(D, Deltoid muscle.)*

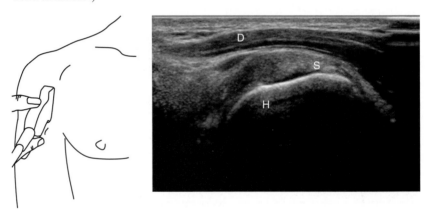

Supraspinatus

1. The patient should be placed into the Bouffard position with hand in back pocket and elbow extended posteriorly. In a slightly oblique transverse scanning orientation move the transducer laterally, superiorly and slightly posteriorly. The medial edge of the transducer will be pointing in the direction of the patient's ear. The following image shows that in this plane the long axis of the supraspinatus tendon *(SS)* can be evaluated just anterior to the echogenic line of the humeral head *(H)*. *(D, Deltoid muscle.)*

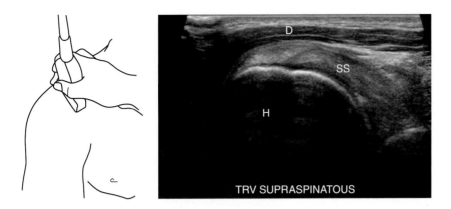

TRV SUPRASPINATOUS

2. Maintaining the Bouffard position, the supraspinatus tendon should be evaluated in a longitudinal plane by rotating the transducer 90 degrees from the previous oblique transverse position. The critical zone of the rotator cuff is located here, about 1 cm lateral and posterior to the biceps tendon. (*D*, Deltoid muscle; *H*, humeral head; *SS*, supraspinatus tendon.)

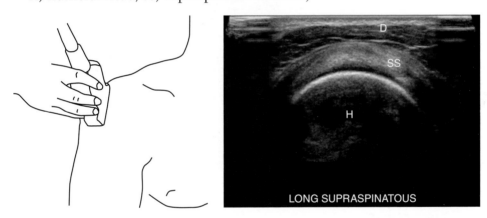

LONG SUPRASPINATOUS

Infraspinatus

1. Return patient to neutral position. Turn the transducer to an oblique transverse orientation to align with the infraspinatus tendon. Move the transducer posteriorly and laterally just inferior to the spine of the scapula. The following image shows the deltoid muscle *(solid arrow)* anterior to the echogenic appearing infraspinatus tendon *(dashed arrow)*. The echogenic line of the humeral head *(dotted arrow)* and scapula are posterior. Internal and external rotation or movement from neutral to hand reaching to opposite shoulder can be used for identification and evaluation.

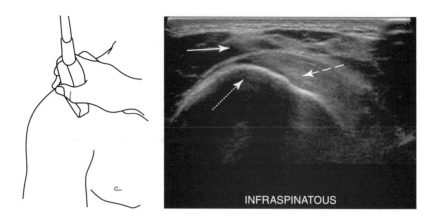

2. Turn the transducer to an oblique longitudinal orientation. The following image shows the infraspinatus tendon *(IT)* between the medially placed glenoid *(G)* and the laterally placed humeral head *(HH).* (*D*, Deltoid muscle.)

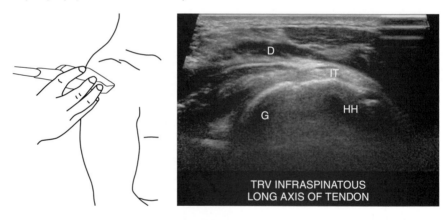

Teres Minor

1. The patient should be in the neutral position. Return transducer to transverse position and move slightly inferior to image the trapezoidal shaped tendon in the long axis. The humeral head *(HH)* will be lateral and the deltoid muscle *(solid arrow)* anterior to the teres minor tendon *(dashed arrow).*

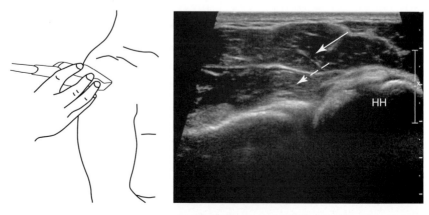

2. Turn the transducer to the longitudinal position to evaluate the tendon in the transverse axis.

Carpal Tunnel Scanning Protocol Overview

Location

Carpal tunnel region is located along the midwrist proximal to the crease toward the forearm and distal to the wrist crease toward the fingers.

Anatomy

- The carpal tunnel houses bones, tendons, nerves, ligaments, muscles and vessels, all providing the hand with the ability to function properly.
- The carpal tunnel consists of a bundle of tendons coursing from the flexor muscles in the forearm through the wrist and into the hand. At the level of the midwrist the superficial border to the tunnel is the transverse carpal tunnel ligament or flexor retinaculum. The tendons coursing through the tunnel are divided into 2 groups:
  1. The more posteriorly situated tendons originate from the flexor digitorum profundus muscle in the forearm and travel through the tunnel to the fingers as the flexor profundus tendons.
  2. The anteriorly placed tendons originate from the flexor digitorum superficialis muscle in the forearm and travel through the tunnel also to the fingers as the flexor superficialis tendons. The muscle and tendon aiding the first digit, or the thumb, originate from the flexor pollicis longus muscle on the radial side of the forearm. The tendons are all covered by a synovial sheath.
- The median nerve runs just anteriorly to the bundle of tendons and slightly toward the radial edge. The transverse carpal tunnel ligament or flexor retinaculum covers the tunnel transversely just anterior to the median nerve. The nerve is naturally elliptical in shape and will flatten slightly as it courses distally into the hand.
- The *proximal carpal tunnel* is located just before the crease in the wrist on the side of the forearm. Here, with the hand supinated, at the proximal region the *pisiform* stands as the bony landmark on the medial edge, *scaphoid* on the lateral edge, and *lunate* posteriorly. The profundus and superficialis tendons and median nerve are midline as described above. The flexor pollicis tendon courses laterally along the border of the scaphoid. Also at this level, the ulnar nerve and artery course along

the medial edge adjacent and slightly anterior to the pisiform border. This anatomical area is known as Guyon's canal. The carpal tunnel anatomy is draped anteriorly by the flexor retinaculum.

- The *distal tunnel* is located just past the crease in the wrist and is distinguished by the bony landmarks of the hamate medially, trapezium laterally and posteriorly by the capitate. The profundus and superficialis tendons continue along the middle of the tunnel with the flexor pollicis tendon far laterally along the border of the trapezium. The median nerve continues its course anteriorly and slightly laterally. All of these structures continue to be draped anteriorly by the flexor retinaculum.

Physiology

- The carpal tunnel houses the tendons that connect the muscles in the forearm to each of the digits in the hand. These tendons aid in movement of the fingers. Nerves coursing through the carpal tunnel, including the most prominent median nerve, provide sensation and muscle function to the fingers. These structures are surrounded by a tunnel of bones that provide stability, not only for the structures inside the carpal tunnel but to the entire wrist and hand.

Sonographic Appearance

- The tendons running midline through the carpal tunnel will appear hypoechoic compared to adjacent structures and will move with flexion of the fingers.
- The radial and ulnar arteries on the lateral and medial edges respectively, will appear anechoic and can prove to be a valuable landmark when color is used for identification.
- The median nerve coursing anterior to the tendons will also be hypoechoic relative to adjacent structures but the shape may be slightly elliptical and a thin hyperechoic ring can be seen around the periphery.
- Proximally, the echogenic curve of the bony surface of the pisiform on medial edge and scaphoid on the lateral edge is visualized. Moving distally, the bony surface of the hamate and trapezium, medially and laterally, respectively, can be located.

Preparation

Patient Prep
- No patient prep.

Transducer
- Linear 10 to 18 MHz.

Patient Position
- The patient should be sitting with the arm at 90 degrees and palm facing up in a resting position on a stable surface.
- A towel rolled and placed under the wrist can add stability and aid with neutral positioning of the anatomy.

Breathing Technique
- No breathing technique required.

Carpal Tunnel Survey

Transverse Plane
1. Toward the forearm side of the wrist place the transducer adjacent to the wrist crease to visualize the proximal carpal tunnel.
2. Identify the flexor superficialis and flexor profundus tendons midline and the flexor pollicis along the radial edge by having the patient flex the fingers. Identify the more hypoechoic median nerve (MN) anterior to the group of tendons.

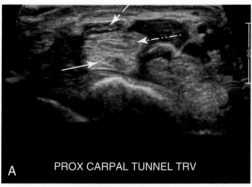 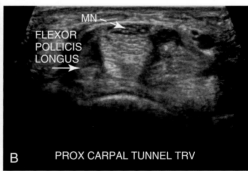

A, *Dashed arrow:* Median nerve; *dash-dotted arrow:* flexor superficialis tendon; *solid arrow:* flexor profundus tendon. **B,** *Dashed arrow:* Median nerve.

3. This gray-scale version of color Doppler shows how it can be used to identify Guyon's canal with the ulnar artery and nerve along the medial edge. (*Dashed arrow: MN,* Median nerve.)

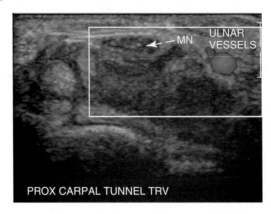

4. Locate the midline posterior bony edge of the lunate. (*Dashed arrow: MN,* Median nerve.)

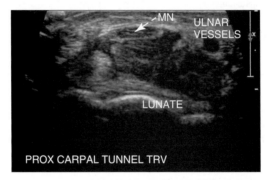

5. Move the transducer distally toward the fingers, staying adjacent to the crease of the wrist and angling slightly toward the proximal region.
6. Identify the central bundle of tendons and the anteriorly placed median nerve as described in the proximal carpal tunnel.
7. Locate the midline posterior boney edge of the capitate. (*Dashed arrow:* Median nerve.)

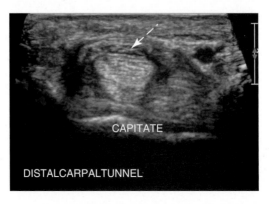

Sagittal Plane

1. Place the transducer along the midline wrist 90 degrees from transverse image of median nerve.
2. Move the transducer toward the forearm to image the proximal carpal tunnel.
3. Identify the hypoechoic median nerve most anteriorly.
4. Identify the bundle of superficialis and profundus tendons just posterior to median nerve *(dashed arrow)*. With flexion of the fingers the tendons will move in a sliding motion. In the proximal carpal tunnel the boney landmark seen posterior to the midline will be the lunate. *(Dashed arrow:* Median nerve; *dash-dotted arrow:* flexor superficialis tendon; *solid arrow:* flexor profundus tendon.)

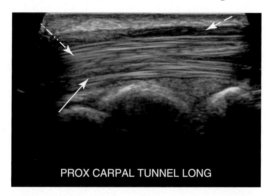

PROX CARPAL TUNNEL LONG

5. Move the transducer toward the fingers into the distal carpal tunnel region, staying in the midline of the wrist. Identify the median nerve and tendons in the same placement as the proximal carpal tunnel.

Carpal Tunnel Required Images

Transverse Images

1. Transverse image of the proximal carpal tunnel. *(Dashed arrow:* Median nerve; *dash-dotted arrow:* flexor superficialis tendon; *solid arrow:* flexor profundus tendon.)

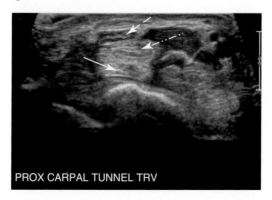

PROX CARPAL TUNNEL TRV

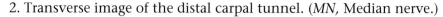

2. Transverse image of the distal carpal tunnel. (*MN*, Median nerve.)

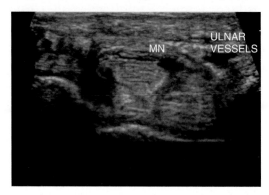

Sagittal Images

3. Sagittal image of the proximal carpal tunnel. (*Dashed arrow:* Median nerve; *dash-dotted arrow:* flexor superficialis tendon; *solid arrow:* flexor profundus tendon.)

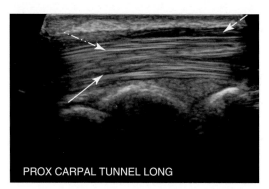

4. Sagittal image of the distal carpal tunnel. (*Dashed arrow:* Median nerve; *solid arrow:* flexor superficialis tendon; *dotted arrow:* flexor profundus tendon.)

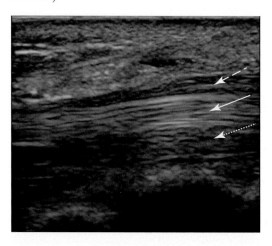

Achilles Tendon Scanning Protocol Overview

Location

- The insertion of the *Achilles tendon* is positioned along the posterior calcaneus bone. The Achilles tendon continues to course along the posterior lower leg until it forms with the gastrocnemius and soleus calf muscles located in the mid to upper posterior lower leg.

Anatomy

- The **Achilles tendon** connects the lateral and medial gastrocnemius calf muscles and the soleus calf muscle to the calcaneus or heel bone. The **plantaris tendon**, also originating from the gastrocnemius muscle will insert along the medial and posterior edge of the calcaneus bone.
- 2 bursae are located just superior to or at the insertion of the Achilles tendon.
  1. The **subcutaneous calcaneus bursa** sits along the posterior heel superficial to the tendon and is sometimes referred to as the *retro-Achilles bursa* and does not always contain fluid.
  2. The **retrocalcaneal bursa** is located between the posterior and superior aspect of the calcaneus bone and the Achilles. This bursa should normally contain fluid which can make for easier identification.
- **Krager's fat pad** is an area of fatty tissue located just posterior to the Achilles tendon. The posterior and superior edge of the calcaneus bone forms the inferior border, whereas the retrocalcaneal bursa will be located along the most inferior and posterior edge.

Physiology

- The Achilles tendon is the strongest tendon in the body. The tendon aids in the movement of the foot downward and the ability to put weight and balance on the toes, which are necessary for walking and running motion.

Sonographic Appearance

- In the longitudinal plane the Achilles tendon appears as a fibrillar pattern of thin echogenic lines having uniform thickness throughout the midsection. Distally at the muscle interface and proximally at the insertion the tendon will become narrower. A thin echogenic border surrounds the tendon.
- At the insertion point the echogenic border of the calcaneus bone will be seen posteriorly.
- As the tendon continues superiorly up the leg and gets closer to the muscle interface it will begin to appear less prominent and blend in with the surrounding muscular structure.

- With dorsiflexion and plantar flexion of the foot the tendon will move in a sliding motion, which can be helpful for identification.
- At the midsection the tendon should measure between 5 and 6 mm in the anterior posterior dimension.
- Transversely the tendon will appear elliptical and possibly slightly concave in shape with the same fibrillar pattern and thin echogenic rim.
- The retrocalcaneal bursa can be identified along the deep edge of the calcaneus bone by the small pocket of hypoechoic fluid surrounding it. Krager's fat pad adjacent to this bursa and just posterior to the Achilles tendon is more echogenic than the surrounding tissue and has an irregular shape on ultrasound.

Preparation

Patient Prep
- None required.

Transducer
- 5 MHz to 12 MHz.

Breathing Technique
- None required.

Patient Position
- When possible the patient should be lying prone with feet hanging off the end of the stretcher.

Achilles Tendon Survey

Longitudinal Survey
1. Begin scanning with transducer placed along the posterior calcaneus bone.
2. Identify the insertion point of the Achilles tendon with slight movements of the transducer to avoid anisotropy
3. Slowly move the transducer superiorly following the tendon until it blends into the muscles at the distal end, approximately at the mid to upper calf.

Transverse Survey
1. Begin scanning with the transducer placed along the posterior calcaneus bone.
2. Identify the insertion point of the Achilles tendon.
3. Slowly move the transducer superiorly following the tendon until it blends into the muscles at the distal end approximately at the mid to upper calf.

Achilles Tendon Required Images

Longitudinal Images

1. **LONG AXIS** of the Achilles tendon at the insertion point. (*Arrow: Achilles tendon*)

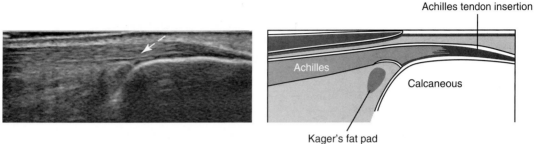

Labeled: **SAG AT INS PT**

2. **LONG AXIS** of **PROXIMAL** Achilles tendon just superior to the point of insertion.

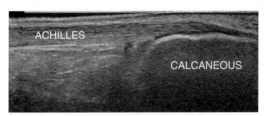

Labeled: **SAG AT PROX**

3. **LONG AXIS** of the **MID** Achilles tendon.

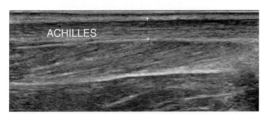

Labeled: **SAG AT MID**

4. **LONG AXIS** of the **DISTAL** Achilles tendon. (*Arrow: Achilles tendon*)

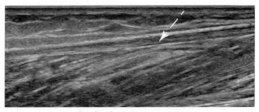

Labeled: **SAG AT DIS**

5. **PANORAMIC VIEW** of entire length of Achilles tendon.

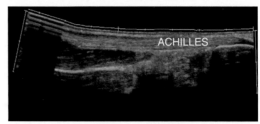

Labeled: **SAG AT**

Transverse Images

6. Achilles tendon at **INSERTION POINT.**

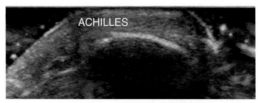

Labeled: **TRV AT INS PT**

7. **PROXIMAL** Achilles tendon proximally just superior to insertion point.

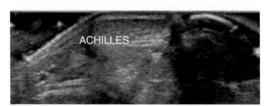

Labeled: **TRV AT PROX**

8. **MID** Achilles tendon.

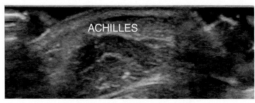

Labeled: **TRV AT MID**

9. **DISTAL** Achilles tendon.

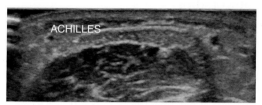

ACHILLES

Labeled: **TRV AT DIS**

Review Questions

Answers on page 630.

1. Sonographically, muscles appear _____ compared to most adjacent structures.
   a) echogenic.
   b) hypoechoic.
   c) hyperechoic.
   d) cystic.

2. How many muscles make up the rotator cuff complex?
   a) 1
   b) 2
   c) 3
   d) 4

3. What is a function of the bursa?
   a) Stabilize the joint
   b) House the nerves supplying the muscle
   c) Aid in movement
   d) Help to attach the bone to the muscle

4. Which is the largest muscle in the rotator cuff?
   a) Supraspinatus
   b) Subscapularis
   c) Teres minor
   d) Infraspinatus

5. Tendons attach muscles to
   a) bones.
   b) other muscles.
   c) ligaments.
   d) organs.

6. Which is the largest bursa in the rotator cuff?
   a) Subhumeral bursa
   b) Acromial bursa
   c) Subacromial bursa
   d) Subdeltoid bursa

7. What is the Bouffard position?
   a) Hand resting on thigh
   b) Hand across body touching opposite shoulder
   c) Hand in back pocket of affected side
   d) Hand reaching for opposite back pocket

8. Which of the rotator cuff muscles may have a trapezoidal shape in the long axis?
   a) Subscapularis
   b) Supraspinatus
   c) Infraspinatus
   d) Teres minor

9. To image the rotator cuff muscles in the long axis how must the transducer be oriented?
   a) Longitudinally
   b) Transversely

10. Which rotator cuff muscle contains the critical zone for rotator cuff tears?
    a) Subscapularis
    b) Supraspinatus
    c) Infraspinatus
    d) Teres minor

11. What is the name of the ligament that stretches across the carpal tunnel and forms the most anterior border?
    a) Flexor digitorum ligament
    b) Median nerve ligament
    c) Flexor pollicis ligament
    c) Flexor retinaculum ligament

12. The ulnar nerve and artery make up what anatomical area in the wrist?
    a) Carpal tunnel
    b) Guyon's canal
    c) Synovial sheath
    d) Anterior compartment

13. What are the most posteriorly located tendons in the carpal tunnel?
    a) Flexor superficialis tendons
    b) Flexor profundus tendons
    c) Flexor pollicis longus tendons
    d) Flexor retinaculum tendons

14. What are the more anteriorly placed tendons in the carpal tunnel?
    a) Flexor superficialis tendons
    b) Flexor profundus tendons
    c) Flexor pollicis longus tendons
    d) Flexor retinaculum tendons

15. What bones form the medial and lateral borders in the proximal carpal tunnel?
    a) Ulnar and radius
    b) Metacarpals
    c) Hamate and trapezium
    d) Pisiform and the scaphoid

16. What bones form the medial and lateral borders in the distal carpal tunnel?
    a) Ulnar and radius
    b) Metacarpals
    c) Hamate and trapezium
    d) Pisiform and scaphoid

17. What is the sonographic appearance of the median nerve?
    a) Hypoechoic with echogenic border
    b) Hyperechoic with echogenic border
    c) Hypoechoic with thick striations
    d) Hyperechoic with hypoechoic ring

18. What tendon connects to the first digit?
    a) Flexor superficialis tendon
    b) Flexor profundus tendon
    c) Flexor pollicis longus tendon
    d) Flexor retinaculum tendon

19. In the sagittal plane of the carpal tunnel the median nerve will appear in what position?
    a) Anteriorly
    b) Posteriorly
    c) Medially
    d) Laterally

20. When scanning the carpal tunnel in what position should the hand be placed?
    a) Medial edge down
    b) Lateral edge down
    c) Palm facing up
    d) Palm facing down

21. At the midsection of the Achilles tendon what is the normal anteroposterior measurement?
    a) 1 to 2 mm
    b) 3 to 4 mm
    c) 5 to 6 mm
    d) 7 to 8 mm

22. What two calf muscles does the Achilles tendon attach to in the lower posterior leg?
    a) Calcaneus muscle
    b) Gastrocnemius muscle
    c) Soleus muscle
    d) a and b
    e) b and c

23. Where is the insertion point of the Achilles tendon?
    a) At the gastrocnemius muscle
    b) At the soleus muscle
    c) At the lateral malleolus bone
    d) At the posterior calcaneus bone

24. The Achilles tendon is necessary for walking.
    a) True
    b) False

25. What is another name for the subcutaneous calcaneus bursa?
    a) Retro–Achilles bursa
    b) Retrocalcaneal bursa
    c) Posterior heel bursa
    d) Krager's bursa

26. Which is true about the outer border of the Achilles tendon?
    a) The border is hypoechoic.
    b) The border has a fibrillar pattern.
    c) The border is indistinguishable from the surrounding muscle tissue.
    d) The border is echogenic.

27. Which bursa near the insertion of the Achilles tendon can be identified by a small amount of hypoechoic fluid?
    a) Subcutaneous calcaneus bursa
    b) Retrocalcaneal bursa
    c) Posterior heel bursa
    d) Krager's bursa

28. In what region of the Achilles tendon is it the thickest?
    a) The proximal region
    b) The midregion
    c) The distal region
    d) The normal Achilles tendon should be the same thickness throughout

29. Which of the following correctly describes the shape of the Achilles tendon in the transverse plane?
    a) Irregular shape with fibrillar pattern
    b) Circular shape and hypoechoic
    c) Elliptical shape with fibrillar pattern
    d) Elliptical shape with echogenic center

30. What is the best patient position for imaging the Achilles tendon?
    a) Patient lying prone with feet hanging off the end of the stretcher
    b) Patient lying supine with feet hanging off the end of the stretcher
    c) Patient standing with even weight on both feet
    d) Patient standing with all weight on affected leg

31. At what region of the Achilles tendon will the tendon begin to blend in with the muscle?
    a) The insertion
    b) The proximal region
    c) The midregion
    d) The distal region.

32. What is the name of the fatty tissue located just posterior to the Achilles tendon?
    a) Subcutaneous fat pad
    b) Achilles fat pad
    c) Krager's fat pad
    d) Retrocalcaneal fat pad

33. Which tendon is considered to be the strongest in the body?
    a) Biceps tendon
    b) Achilles tendon
    c) Patellar tendon
    d) Hamstring tendon

34. What technology can the sonographer use to show the entire length of the Achilles tendon?
    a) Panoramic imaging
    b) Harmonic imaging
    c) 3D technology
    d) Widescreen imaging

35. Which of the following correctly describes how the Achilles tendon will move with dorsiflexion of the foot?
    a) The tendon will move in a sliding motion.
    b) The tendon will move anterior to posterior.
    c) The tendon will become smaller and larger with movement.
    d) The tendon does not move with dorsiflexion movement.

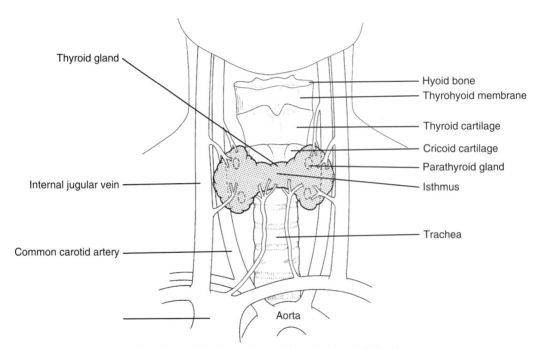

Thyroid gland

Internal jugular vein

Common carotid artery

Hyoid bone
Thyrohyoid membrane

Thyroid cartilage

Cricoid cartilage

Parathyroid gland

Isthmus

Trachea

Aorta

Location and Anatomy of Thyroid and Parathyroid Glands

CHAPTER 16

Thyroid and Parathyroid Glands Scanning Protocol

Wayne C. Leonhardt

Key Words

Adenomas	Parathormone (PTH)
Anterior strap muscles	Posterior longus colli muscle
Calcitonin	Pyramidal lobe
Dilated follicles	Recurrent laryngeal nerve
Ectopic parathyroid glands	Thyroxine (T4)
Ectopic thyroid	Trachea
Endocrine gland	Triiodothyronine (T3)
Esophagus	Vagus nerve
Isthmus	Variant parathyroid gland
Minor neurovascular bundle	shapes

Objectives

At the end of this chapter, you will be able to:

- Define the key words.
- Distinguish the sonographic appearance of the thyroid and parathyroid glands and the terms used to describe them.
- List the transducer options for scanning the thyroid and parathyroid glands.
- Name the suggested breathing techniques for patients when scanning the thyroid and parathyroid glands.
- List the suggested patient position (and options) when scanning the thyroid and parathyroid glands.
- Explain the patient prep for a thyroid and parathyroid glands study.
- Distinguish the thyroid and parathyroid glands normal variants.
- Name the survey steps and explain how to evaluate the entire length, width, and depth of the thyroid and parathyroid glands.
- Explain the order and exact locations to take representative images of the thyroid and parathyroid glands.
- Answer the review questions at the end of the chapter.

Overview

Location

Thyroid Gland

- Located in the lower, anterior portion of the neck, anterior to the trachea and inferior to the larynx.

- Has bilateral lobes that lie on each side of the trachea. They are bordered laterally by the common carotid artery and internal jugular vein.
- The **isthmus** of the thyroid gland unites the lobes at the level of the second, third, and fourth tracheal rings.
- Lies between the **anterior strap muscles:** (*sternocleidomastoid, sternothyroid,* and *sternohyoid* muscles) and the **posterior longus colli muscle** and **minor neurovascular bundle** (consisting of the *inferior thyroid artery* and *recurrent laryngeal nerve*).

Parathyroid Glands
- The 4 glands lie between the posterior aspect of the thyroid gland and the longus colli muscle.
- The 2 superior parathyroid glands are situated slightly more medial than the 2 inferior parathyroid glands.
- Typically, the parathyroid glands are symmetric in position.
- Lie deep to the cricoid cartilage, midway between the Adam's apple (apex of thyroid cartilage) and the suprasternal notch.

Anatomy
Thyroid Gland
- A superficial, butterfly-shaped gland that is variable in size but weighs approximately 25 to 35 g.
- The size and shape of the thyroid gland is greatly influenced by body habitus and gender, therefore, normal thyroid gland measurements have a wide range of variability:
  - Tall, thin individuals have elongated lateral lobes that can measure up to 8 cm long.
  - Short, obese people's lateral lobes are 5 cm or less.
  - The thyroid gland is normally larger in women and becomes enlarged during pregnancy.
- The average, normal adult thyroid gland is approximately 4-6 cm long, 1.3 to 1.8 cm anteroposteriorly, and 3 cm at its greatest width. The anteroposterior measurement of the isthmus is approximately 2 to 6 cm.
- In newborns and children, the gland is approximately 2 to 3 cm long, 0.2 to 1.2 cm anteroposteriorly, and 1.5 cm at its greatest width.
- The thyroid is highly vascular; its blood supply consists of paired superior and inferior arteries and veins, and often, middle thyroid veins.

Parathyroid Glands
- The oval or bean shaped parathyroid glands are approximately 5 to 7 mm long, 1 to 2 mm thick, and 3 to 4 mm wide.
- Parathyroid glands are supplied blood by separate small branches of the inferior and superior thyroid arteries. Venous drainage is via the superior, inferior, and middle thyroid veins.

Physiology

Thyroid Gland

- An endocrine gland (ductless gland that secretes hormones directly into the bloodstream) that is responsible for secreting the *hormones* thyroxine (T4) (regulates metabolism), triiodothyronine (T3) (regulates metabolism), and calcitonin (decreases blood calcium levels, preventing hypercalcemia) that assist in regulating the metabolic rate and the metabolism of lipids, proteins, and carbohydrates and in the absorption of calcium from the blood for storage in the bones.

Parathyroid Glands

- Endocrine glands that secrete the *hormone* parathormone (PTH) which acts as the antagonist for calcitonin and controls the calcium level in the bloodstream.

Sonographic Appearance

Thyroid Gland

- Appears homogeneous and moderately echogenic. It is similar in appearance to normal liver and testes parenchyma and hyperechoic compared to adjacent musculature.
- For appearance's sake, the long axis of the thyroid gland is situated horizontally in the neck. Therefore, longitudinal and long axis views of the entire gland would be visualized in transverse scanning planes. However, for diagnostic purposes the thyroid's right and left lobes and the isthmus that connects them are examined separately.
  - Each *lobe* is oriented vertically in the neck; therefore, the long axes are visualized in sagittal scanning planes. The long sections of the lobes appear sandwiched between the hypoechoic strap muscles anteriorly and longus colli muscles posteriorly (Figure 16-1).
  - Axial sections of the right and left lobes are seen extending laterally from each side of the isthmus to axial sections of the common carotid arteries and internal jugular veins, which appear as anechoic round or oval structures with bright walls. In transverse scanning plane images showing axial sections of the thyroid lobes, adjacent neck structures such as the *vagus nerve, recurrent laryngeal nerve*, the *esophagus*, and various *muscles* are routinely identified (Figure 16-2).
    - The vagus nerve (part of the major neurovascular bundle) is visualized as a hypoechoic dot posterolateral to the thyroid lobe, usually between the carotid artery and jugular vein.
    - The recurrent laryngeal nerve (part of the minor neurovascular bundle) is best identified as an echogenic rim located between the trachea, esophagus, and left posterior thyroid lobe.

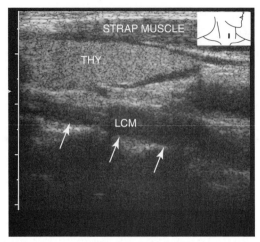

FIGURE 16-1 Sagittal scanning plane image of the left lobe of the thyroid gland and adjacent vasculature. *THY,* Thyroid gland; *LCM,* longus colli muscle *(arrows).*

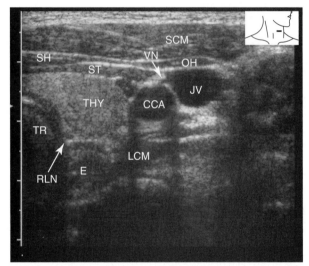

FIGURE 16-2 Transverse scanning plane section of the thyroid gland's left lobe and relevant adjacent anatomic structures. *THY,* Thyroid; *CCA,* common carotid artery; *JV,* jugular vein; *E,* esophagus; *TR,* trachea; *LCM,* longus colli muscle; *RLN,* recurrent laryngeal nerve; *VN,* vagus nerve; *SH,* sternohyoid muscle; *ST,* sternothyroid muscle; *SCM,* sternocleidomastoid muscle; *OH,* omohyoid muscle.

- The **esophagus** (part of the alimentary canal that connects the throat to the stomach) is seen just to the left of the midline of the neck, posterior to the left thyroid lobe, between the **trachea** (large membranous tube reinforced by rings of cartilage, extending from the larynx to the bronchial tubes and conveying air to and from the lungs) and longus colli muscle. Its axial section appears round to oval; the outer wall is hypoechoic relative to the bright appearance of the inner lumen wall. The lumen can, however, appear anechoic or with a centrally located, moderately echogenic line or dot representing mucosa. The longus colli muscle extends laterally to lie posterior to the common carotid artery.

■ Neck muscles appear distinctively hypoechoic compared to the thyroid gland. Anteriorly, the strap muscles (sternohyoid, sternothyroid, omohyoid, and sternocleidomastoid) are easily distinguished as is the longus colli muscle posteriorly.

- The long axis of the *isthmus* is situated horizontally and viewed from a transverse scanning plane at the midline of the neck, just anterior to the bright cartilaginous rings of the trachea.
- Branches of the inferior and superior thyroid arteries and veins appear as 1 to 2 mm anechoic structures with thin, bright walls. Color Doppler can be helpful in differentiating intra- and extrathyroidal vessels.

Parathyroid Glands

- By using newer high frequency transducers, normal parathyroid glands are occasionally visualized sonographically, especially in young children. When identified, they appear as a flat, hypoechoic structure lying between the thyroid gland anteriorly and longus colli muscle posteriorly.

Color Flow Doppler Characteristics

- Utilize color Doppler to differentiate vascular from nonvascular structures.
- Adjust color Doppler parameters to detect normal or increased flow in the thyroid gland.
- Color Doppler shows increased vascularity within and in the periphery of autonomous functioning **adenomas** (a benign tumor formed from glands) and thyroid cancer.
- Utilize color Doppler to follow the superior or inferior thyroid arteries to locate parathyroid adenomas.

Normal Variants
Thyroid Gland

- **Pyramidal lobe:** Triangular-shaped, superior extension of the isthmus. Present in 15% to 30% of thyroid glands. Variable in size and extends more often to the left side. Parenchyma appears the same as the normal thyroid.
- **Dilated follicles:** Interspersed throughout the thyroid, they appear as 1- to 3-mm cystic areas.
- **Ectopic thyroid:** Lingual thyroids account for 90% of ectopic thyroids.

Parathyroid Glands

- Ectopic parathyroid glands: Represent approximately 15% to 20% of the total.
- Variant parathyroid gland shapes: Elongated (11%), bi-lobed (5%), or multi-lobed (1%).

Preparation

Patient Prep

- None.

Transducer

- "Small Parts" indicates a structure that is superficial or close to the surface of the skin. In most cases, it requires a real-time, high-frequency transducer.
- **7.5 MHz** to **10 MHz** high resolution, real-time, linear transducer.
- According to the transducer and machine used, a water path or standoff pad may be necessary.
- Doppler color flow imaging (low-flow filter, scale, and optimized color gain).

Breathing Technique

- Normal respiration.

Patient Position

- The patient should be **supine with the neck mildly hyperextended and the head turned slightly away from the side of interest**.
- Place a sponge, pillow, or rolled towel under the patient's shoulders to maintain hyperextension of the neck.

Thyroid Gland Survey Steps

NOTE: Patient comfort and the amount of transducer pressure on the skin surface is always an important consideration when scanning any structure, but the significance is more acute with small part structures. Generally, a lighter approach is recommended.

NOTE: The thyroid gland is small and can be seen in its entirety by some transducers, but it is still evaluated by viewing the lobes individually.

Lobes: Axial Survey Isthmus • Longitudinal Survey
Transverse Plane • Anterior Approach

1. Begin with the transducer perpendicular at the sternal notch. Move the transducer slightly superior and toward the patient's right, lateral enough to view the right lobe from its medial to lateral margins.

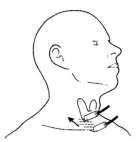

2. Keep the transducer perpendicular and scan superiorly through and beyond the right lobe to the level of the mandible. Note the isthmus medially.

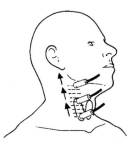

3. Move the transducer inferiorly from the mandible back through and beyond the inferior margin of the right lobe to the level of the sternal notch.

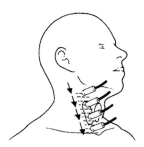

4. Move the transducer slightly superior and toward the patient's left, lateral enough to view the left lobe from its medial to lateral margins.

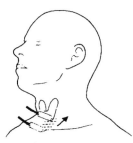

5. Keep the transducer perpendicular and scan superiorly through and beyond the right lobe to the level of the mandible. Note the isthmus medially.

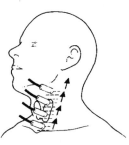

6. Move the transducer inferiorly from the mandible back through and beyond the inferior margin of the left lobe to the level of the sternal notch.

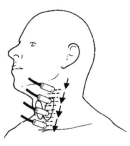

7. Move to the midline of the sternal notch and scan superiorly until you scan through and beyond the isthmus.

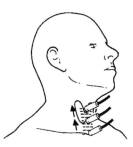

Lobes • Longitudinal Survey
Sagittal Plane • Anterior Approach

> **NOTE:** Imaging the inferior portion of the lobes can be improved by having the patient swallow. This raises the gland superiorly.

8. Begin with the transducer perpendicular at the midline of the sternal notch. Move the transducer slightly superior and toward the patient's right, enough to view the right lobe from its superior to inferior margins.

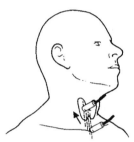

9. Keep the transducer perpendicular and move toward the patient's right, scanning laterally through and beyond the right lobe.

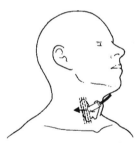

10. Move back onto the right lobe and scan through and beyond the lobe to the midline.

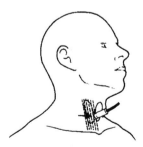

11. From the midline move the transducer slightly toward the patient's left, enough to view the left lobe from its superior to inferior margins.

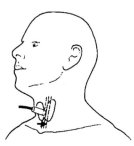

12. Keep the transducer perpendicular and move toward the patient's left, scanning laterally through and beyond the left lobe.

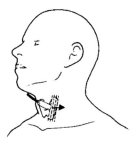

13. Move back onto the left lobe and scan through and beyond to the midline.

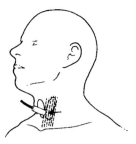

Thyroid Gland Required Images

Thyroid • Right Lobe • Axial Images
Transverse Plane • Anterior Approach
1. Axial image of the **INFERIOR** right lobe.

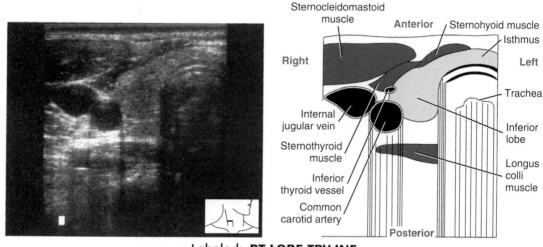

Labeled: **RT LOBE TRV INF**

2. Axial image of the **MID** right lobe.

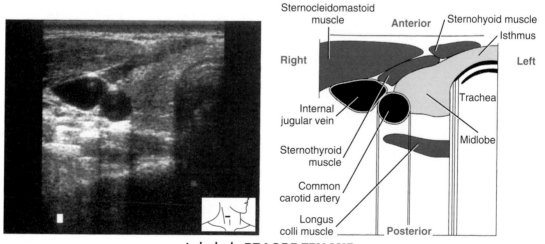

Labeled: **RT LOBE TRV MID**

3. Axial image of the **SUPERIOR** right lobe.

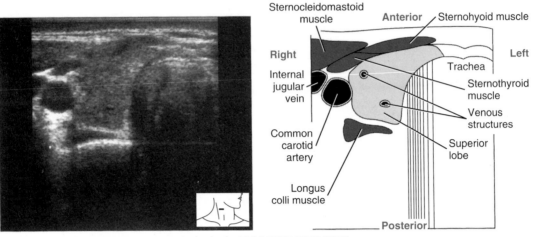

Labeled: **RT LOBE TRV SUP**

4. Longitudinal image of the **ISTHMUS** to include both the right and left lobe attachments.

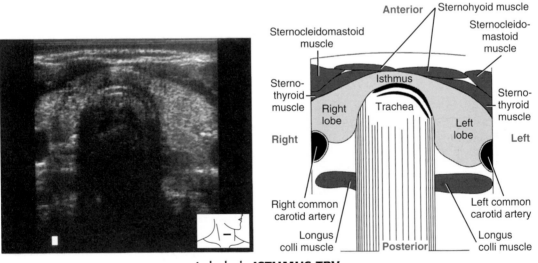

Labeled: **ISTHMUS TRV**

Thyroid • Right Lobe • Longitudinal Images
Sagittal Plane • Anterior Approach
5. Longitudinal image of the **MEDIAL** right lobe.

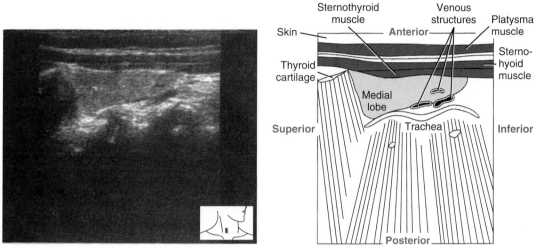

Labeled: **RT LOBE SAG MED**

6. Longitudinal image of the **LATERAL** right lobe.

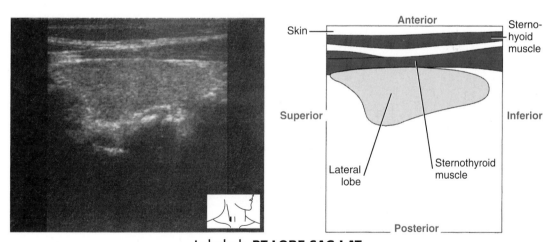

Labeled: **RT LOBE SAG LAT**

Thyroid • Left Lobe • Axial Images
Transverse Plane • Anterior Approach
7. Axial image of the **INFERIOR** left lobe.

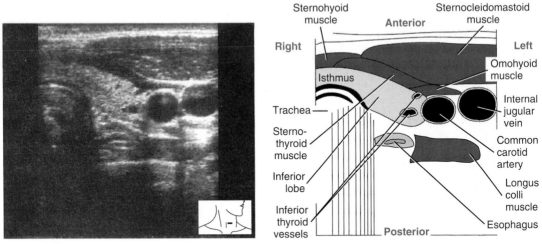

Labeled: **LT LOBE TRV INF**

8. Axial image of the **MID** left lobe.

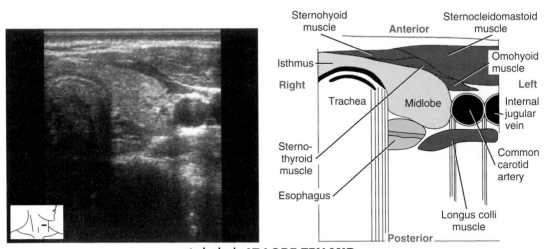

Labeled: **LT LOBE TRV MID**

9. Axial image of the **SUPERIOR** left lobe.

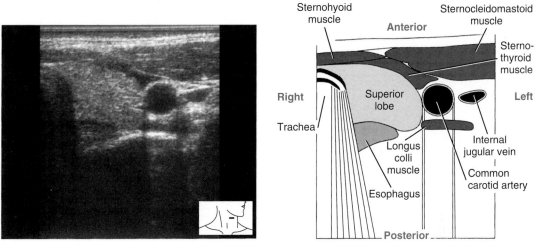

Labeled: **LT LOBE TRV SUP**

Thyroid • Left Lobe • Longitudinal Images
Sagittal Plane • Anterior Approach

10. Longitudinal image of the **MEDIAL** left lobe.

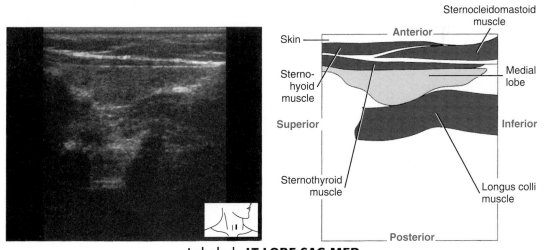

Labeled: **LT LOBE SAG MED**

11. Longitudinal image of the **LATERAL** left lobe.

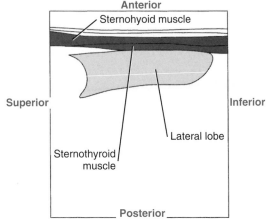

Labeled: **LT LOBE SAG LAT**

Review Questions

Answers on page 630.

1. The thyroid gland is located
   a. between the trachea and longus colli muscle.
   b. lateral to the trachea and superior to the larynx.
   c. in the lower, anterior portion of the neck, anterior to the trachea and inferior to the larynx.
   d. in the lower, anterior portion of the neck, posterior to the trachea and superior to the larynx.

2. The normal thyroid gland generally appears as
   a. medium to low-level echoes.
   b. uniform echoes, hypoechoic relative to testes parenchyma.
   c. uniform echoes, isosonic to liver parenchyma.
   d. high-level echoes with coarse echo texture.

3. Normal parathyroid glands
   a. are occasionally identified in young children.
   b. appear isosonic to the thyroid gland.
   c. are not sonographically appreciated.
   d. appear as a bright rim posterior to the thyroid and anterior to the longus colli muscle.

4. The best way to image the inferior portion of the thyroid lobes is to
   a. use a stand-off pad.
   b. have the patient swallow.
   c. use a water path.
   d. have the patient hold their breath.

5. The thyroid gland is connected in the middle by the
   a. pyramidal lobe.
   b. isthmus.
   c. parathyroid glands.
   d. recurrent laryngeal nerve.

6. The longus colli muscle is located
   a. posterior to each thyroid lobe.
   b. anterior to the thyroid gland.
   c. between the trachea, esophagus, and sternothyroid muscle.
   d. lateral to the internal jugular vein.

7. The best approach when scanning the thyroid gland is
   a. lateral and coronal.
   b. to compress the thyroid with the transducer to improve imaging.
   c. to use a light touch with the transducer.
   d. to use a stand-off pad.

8. The size of the thyroid gland is
   a. influenced by body habitus.
   b. larger in men.
   c. the same size in men and women.
   d. constant.

9. The best patient position to scan the thyroid gland is
   a. sitting upright; chin relaxed.
   b. supine; head to the side.
   c. standing; head extremely hyperextended.
   d. supine; neck mildly hyperextended.

10. The thyroid gland is
    a. the master gland.
    b. an exocrine gland.
    c. a gastrointestinal accessory gland.
    d. an endocrine gland.

11. The lobes of the thyroid gland are bordered laterally by the _____ and _____.
    a. longus colli muscle, common carotid artery.
    b. common carotid artery, internal jugular vein.
    c. longus colli muscle, internal jugular vein.
    d. common carotid artery, sternohyoid muscle.

12. The average, normal adult thyroid gland is approximately _____cm long, _____cm anteroposteriorly, and _____ cm at its greatest width.
    a. 5; 3; 3
    b. 4 to 6; 3; 3
    c. 4 to 6; 1.3 to 1.8; 3
    d. 7; 1.3 to 1.8; 3

13. The thyroid gland has two lateral _____ connected by the _____.
    a. lobes; strap muscles.
    b. lobes; isthmus.
    c. lobes; longus colli muscle.
    d. parathyroid glands; isthmus.

14. The thyroid gland is located on the _____ side of the trachea.
    a. posterior.
    b. anterior.
    c. right lateral.
    d. left lateral.

15. The main function of thyroid hormones is to _____.
    a. increase metabolism.
    b. regulate iodine levels.
    c. stimulate the pituitary gland.
    d. stimulate the hypothalamus.

16. The parathyroid glands lie between the ____aspect of the thyroid gland and the ____.
    a. posterior; longus colli muscle
    b. anterior; longus colli muscle
    c. posterior; trachea
    d. anterior; trachea

17. The long axis of the isthmus is situated _____ and viewed from a _____ scanning plane at the midline of the neck,
    a. horizontally, coronal.
    b. horizontally, transverse.
    c. horizontal oblique, transverse oblique.
    d. horizontally, sagittal.

18. The long sections of the lobes appear sandwiched between the _____ anteriorly and _____ posteriorly.
    a. strap muscles, trachea.
    b. strap muscles, longus colli muscles.
    c. strap muscles, common carotid artery.
    d. longus colli muscles, strap muscles.

19. Each lobe is oriented vertically in the neck; therefore, the long axes are visualized in sagittal scanning planes.
    a. horizontally, coronal.
    b. vertically, transverse.
    c. horizontally, coronal.
    d. vertically, sagittal.

20. The thyroid gland is _____ relative to the strap muscles.
    a. hypoechoic.
    b. isosonic.
    c. anechoic.
    d. hyperechoic.

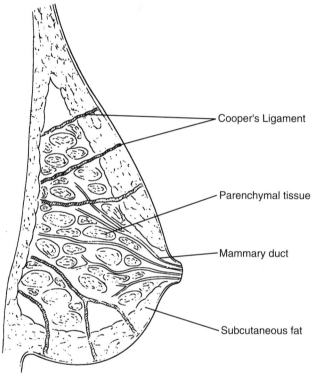

Cooper's Ligament

Parenchymal tissue

Mammary duct

Subcutaneous fat

Breast Anatomy

CHAPTER 17

Breast Scanning Protocol

Betty Bates Tempkin

Key Words

Breast parenchyma	Mammary layer
Breasts	Parenchymal elements
Cooper's ligaments	Pectoralis major muscle
Exocrine glands	Retromammary layer
Lactation	Stromal elements
Lactiferous ducts	Subcutaneous layer

Objectives

At the end of this chapter, you will be able to:

- Define the key words.
- Distinguish the sonographic appearance of the breast and the terms used to describe it.
- List the transducer options for scanning the breast.
- List the suggested patient position (and options) when scanning the breast.
- Explain the patient prep for a breast study.
- Name the survey steps and how to evaluate the entire breast.
- Distinguish the normal variants of the breast.
- Explain the order and exact locations to take representative images of the breast/lesion.
- Answer the review questions at the end of the chapter.

Clinical Reasoning

- In most cases—for women under 30 and for lactating and pregnant women—breast sonography has become the first phase of imaging for evaluating palpable masses. Breast sonography, however, is not recognized as a screening study for microcalcifications.
- Breast sonography is generally performed to determine the composition or characterization of a localized lesion(s) (that may or may not be palpable) and to further evaluate mammographic and clinical findings.
- Additional indications for breast sonography include ultrasound-guided biopsies, treatment plans for radiation therapy, and evaluating complications associated with breast implants.
- In some cases, whole-breast scanning may be recommended for diffuse diseases, such as fibrocystic disease.

Overview

Anatomy

- Each breast lies anterior to the sixth rib, pectoralis major, serratus, and external oblique muscles. The second and third ribs form the superior border of each breast and the seventh costal cartilage is the inferior border. The medial border of each breast is the sternum and laterally the breasts are bound by the margin of the axilla. The most anterior aspect of the breast is attached to the skin.
- Breast tissue is supported by Cooper's ligaments, suspensory ligaments that extend posteriorly from the deep muscle fascia, through the breast, to the skin.
- The breast is comprised of:
  - Parenchymal elements (lobes, ducts, and alveoli).
  - Stromal elements (connective tissue and fat).
- The breast is described in terms of 3 layers:
  1. Subcutaneous layer: Skin and subcutaneous fat lobules.
  2. Mammary layer: 15 to 20 lobes that contain alveoli (multiple glandular tissue lobules), and ducts that drain to the nipple; fat lobules, and connective tissue.
  3. Retromammary layer: Fat lobules and connective tissue.

Physiology

- The breasts or mammary glands are exocrine glands (release secretions through ducts) whose primary function is lactation (the secretion of milk) through lactiferous ducts (ducts in breast parenchyma) following pregnancy.

Sonographic Appearance

- As shown in the image on the facing page, the 3 layers of the breast are sonographically distinguishable; their normal appearance is described as follows:
  1. The *subcutaneous layer* is the most anterior layer bordered anteriorly by the bright skin line and posteriorly by the mammary layer. In between, the subcutaneous fat lobules appear as low-level echoes with bright margins.
  2. The *mammary layer* is the middle layer of the breast that contains glandular tissue or breast parenchyma. Typically it appears hyperechoic compared to the subcutaneous and retromammary layers due to its mixed parenchymal appearance depending on the amount of fat that is present:
     - The appearance with the presence of little fat is highly echogenic due to the reflective appearance of the existing connective tissue (collagen and fibrotic tissue).

- When fat is present, the appearance is of areas of low-level echoes (fat) mixed with areas of high echogenicity (connective tissue). When visualized, the ducts appear as small anechoic branches running throughout the layer.
3. The *retromammary layer* is generally hypoechoic relative to the mammary layer and hyperechoic compared to the posterior border, the **pectoralis major muscle** (large chest muscle), which has a low- to very low–level echo texture.

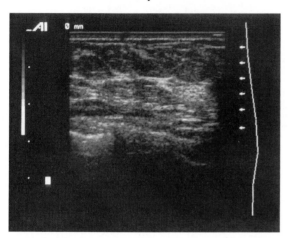
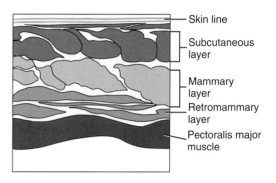

- Although all the breast layers are influenced by the age of the woman and the functional state of the breast, the mammary layer shows the greatest changes sonographically.
- The sonographic appearance of the breast changes with age.
  - The breasts of young women contain a high percentage of parenchymal elements and little fat. This causes the breast to be dense and appear highly echogenic.
  - Conversely, as seen in the following image, in older women the subcutaneous and retromammary layers become more prominent when the mammary layer in the breast decreases in size as parenchymal tissues atrophy and are replaced by fat tissue.

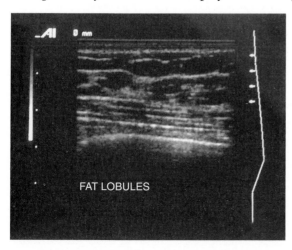
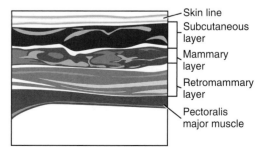

- The next image demonstrates the thin, linear, bright appearance of Cooper's ligament. Notice how the ligament appears hyperechoic relative to adjacent structures.

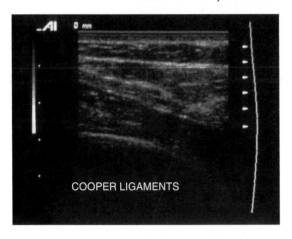

COOPER LIGAMENTS

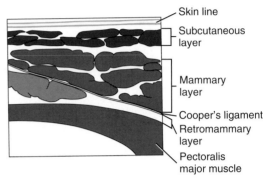

Skin line
Subcutaneous layer
Mammary layer
Cooper's ligament
Retromammary layer
Pectoralis major muscle

Normal Variants

- **Fatty breast:** Increased fatty components throughout the breast resulting from age, parity, and menopause. When fat is present, the sonographic appearance is areas of low level echoes (fat) mixed with areas of high echogenicity (connective tissue surrounding mammary ducts).
- **Fibrocystic breast:** Commonly found in women of childbearing age. Fibrous tissues and cystic areas occur throughout the breast, as well as an increase in the amount of dense connective tissue, which will cause the breast to appear highly echogenic.

Preparation

Patient Prep

- None.

Transducer

- 10 to 18 MHz linear.
- Use compression sonography when assessing fibrocystic breasts.

Patient Position

Patient Position for Breast Lesion Scanning

- Position the patient to minimize the thickness of the portion of the breast being evaluated.

Patient Position for Whole Breast Scanning

- Supine.
- Sitting erect.

NOTE: When positioning patients it may be helpful to use wedges, sponges, or rolled towels.

Breast Lesion Survey Steps

NOTE: A localized lesion or any area of interest of the breast must be evaluated in at least two scanning planes.
NOTE: A stand-off device may be helpful for the evaluation of superficial lesions.

Longitudinal Survey
Scanning Plane Determined by Lesion Shape and Lie •
Approach Determined by Lesion Location
1. Begin scanning with the transducer perpendicular at the midpoint of the most superior aspect of the lesion or area of interest.
2. Keeping the transducer perpendicular, slowly scan through and beyond all of the margins of the lesion.

Axial Survey
Scanning Plane Determined by Lesion Shape and Lie •
Approach Determined by Lesion Location
1. Begin scanning with the transducer perpendicular at the midpoint of the lesion or area of interest.
2. Keeping the transducer perpendicular, slowly scan through and beyond all of the margins of the lesion

Required Images for Breast Lesion

NOTE: The location of the lesion must be recorded to accompany the required images. The location of the lesion can be indicated by one of the following methods:
- Shown on a diagram of the breast
- Specifying the quadrant
- Using clock notation and distance from the nipple

NOTE: Image labeling should include right or left breast, location of the lesion, and transducer orientation with regard to the breast (axial or longitudinal, radial or anti-radial).

Breast Lesion • Right Breast or Left Breast • Longitudinal Images

Scanning Plane Determined by Lesion Shape and Lie • Approach Determined by Location

1. Longitudinal image of the **LESION** *with measurement from the most superior to the most inferior margin.*
   Labeled: **SITE LOCATION AND SCANNING PLANE**
2. Same image as number 1 *without measurement calipers.*
   Labeled: **SITE LOCATION AND SCANNING PLANE**

Breast Lesion • Right Breast or Left Breast • Axial Images

Scanning Plane Determined by Lesion Shape and Lie • Approach Determined by Location

3. Axial image of the **LESION** *with measurements from the most anterior to the most posterior margin and from the most lateral to lateral or lateral to medial margin.*
   Labeled: **SITE LOCATION AND SCANNING PLANE**
4. Same image as number 3 *without measurement calipers.*
   Labeled: **SITE LOCATION AND SCANNING PLANE**

Breast Lesion • Right Breast or Left Breast • Longitudinal and Axial High and Low Gain Images

Scanning Plane Determined by Lesion Shape and Lie • Approach Determined by Location

5. Longitudinal image of the **LESION** with high gain technique.
   Labeled: **SITE LOCATION, SCANNING PLANE, HIGH GAIN**
6. Axial image of the **LESION** with high gain technique.
   Labeled: **SITE LOCATION, SCANNING PLANE, HIGH GAIN**
7. Longitudinal image of the **LESION** with low gain technique.
   Labeled: **SITE LOCATION, SCANNING PLANE, LOW GAIN**
8. Axial image of the **LESION** with low gain technique.
   Labeled: **SITE LOCATION, SCANNING PLANE, LOW GAIN**

NOTE: Depending on the size and complexity of the lesion, additional images (in at least two scanning planes) may be necessary to document the extent of the lesion.

Whole Breast Survey

Whole Breast Survey • Right Breast or Left Breast

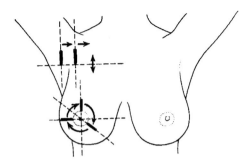

1. Begin scanning the breast in question at the 12 o'clock position.
2. Transducer orientation is set up so that the breast is viewed in sections from the nipple outward, where the orientation notch is located.
3. Scan around the breast in a clockwise manner, covering all anatomy, including the axillary regions.

NOTE: For diffuse disease, both breasts must be scanned.

Whole Breast Required Images

Whole Breast Images • Right Breast or Left Breast

1. **12 O'CLOCK IMAGE OF BREAST TISSUE** with the base of the transducer toward the nipple and the end of the transducer facing outward so that the nipple area is closest to the top of the imaging screen.
   Labeled: **12 O'CLOCK RT LT**
2. **3 O'CLOCK** image (same orientation as number 1).
   Labeled: **3 O'CLOCK RT LT**
3. **6 O'CLOCK** image.
   Labeled: **6 O'CLOCK RT LT**
4. **9 O'CLOCK** image.
   Labeled: **9 O'CLOCK RT LT**
5. Axial image through the **NIPPLE.**
   Labeled: **NIP TRV RT LT**
6. Longitudinal image through the **NIPPLE.**
   Labeled: **NIP SAG RT LT**
7. Longitudinal image of the **AXILLARY** region.
   Labeled: **AXILLARY SAG RT LT**

8. Axial image of the **AXILLARY** region.
   Labeled: **AXILLARY TRV RT LT**
9. The same corresponding images of the **OTHER BREAST.**

> **NOTE:** In some cases, whole breast scanning includes images from 12 o'clock, 1 o'clock, 2 o'clock, 3 o'clock, etc. If so, label accordingly and include nipple and axillary images.

Review Questions

Answers on page 630.

1. Breast sonography is used primarily
   a) for breast microcalcification screening.
   b) to assess breast ducts during lactation.
   c) to characterize breast lesions.
   d) for breast cyst aspirations.

2. The layers of the breast are
   a) subcutaneous, mammary, retromammary.
   b) mammary, retromammary.
   c) fat, glandular, boney.
   d) skin, parenchymal, stromal.

3. Sonographic appearance of the breast is influenced by
   a) patient parity.
   b) menopause.
   c) patient age.
   d) all of the above.

4. Sonographic findings of the breast are described by
   a) clock notations.
   b) quadrants.
   c) a diagram of the breast.
   d) any of the above.

5. Breast tissue is bordered by the
   a) skin anteriorly; Cooper's ligament posteriorly and laterally; sternum medially.
   b) skin anteriorly; pectoralis muscle posteriorly; axilla laterally; sternum medially.
   c) nipple anteriorly; pectoralis muscle posteriorly; Cooper's ligament laterally; sternum medially.
   d) nipple anteriorly; Cooper's ligament posteriorly; axilla laterally; sternum medially.

6. Whole breast scanning is recommended for evaluating
    a) complications associated with breast implants.
    b) diffuse diseases.
    c) impalpable breast lesions.
    d) palpable masses.

7. Breast lesions are characterized
    a) by their composition.
    b) as benign or malignant.
    c) by size, shape, and echogenicity.
    d) by size, shape, attenuation, and echogenicity.

8. Compression sonography is recommended when
    a) scanning fibrocystic breasts.
    b) assessing fatty breasts.
    c) taking lesion measurements within dense breast tissue.
    d) cystic lesions are evaluated.

9. The breast layer(s) that exhibits the most changes sonographically is (are) the
    a) mammary and retromammary layers.
    b) mammary layer.
    c) subcutaneous layer.
    d) stromal layer.

10. The normal sonographic appearance of the breast
    a) is heterogeneous.
    b) is primarily low- to very low–level echo textures.
    c) is homogeneous.
    d) is primarily medium-level echo textures.

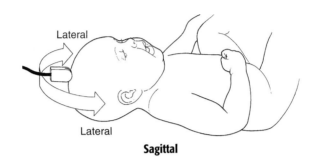

Lateral

Lateral

Sagittal

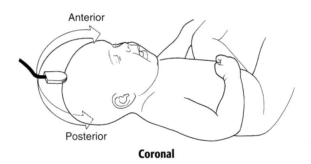

Anterior

Posterior

Coronal

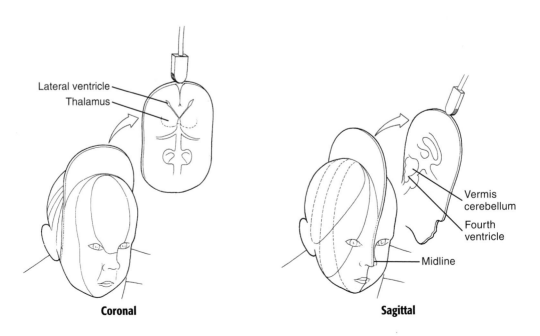

Lateral ventricle

Thalamus

Coronal

Vermis cerebellum

Fourth ventricle

Midline

Sagittal

CHAPTER 18

Neonatal Brain Scanning Protocol

Kristin Dykstra Downey; Betty Bates Tempkin

Key Words

Anterior fontanelle
Aqueduct of Sylvius
Brain stem
Caudate nucleus
Cavum septum pellucidum and cavum vergae
Cerebellum
Cerebral peduncle
Cerebrospinal fluid (CSF)
Cerebrum
Choroid plexus
Cisterna magna
Corpus callosum
Falx cerebri
Foramen of Magendie

Foramen of Monro
Foramina of Lushka
Germinal matrix
Hippocampal gyrus (choroidal fissure)
Interhemispheric fissure
Lateral ventricles
Massa intermedia
Quadrigeminal plate
Sulci
Sylvian fissure
Tentorium
Thalamus
Vermis

Objectives

At the end of this chapter, you will be able to:

- Define the key words.
- Distinguish the sonographic appearance of the neonatal brain and the terms used to describe it.
- Describe the transducer options for scanning the neonatal brain.
- List the suggested patient positions (and options) when scanning the neonatal brain.
- Explain the patient prep for a neonatal brain study.
- Distinguish neonatal brain normal variants.
- Name the survey steps and explain how to evaluate the entire length, width, and depth of the neonatal brain.
- Explain the order and exact locations to take representative images of the neonatal brain.
- Answer the review questions at the end of the chapter.

Overview

Cranial Vault Anatomy and Sonographic Appearance

- **Four ventricles**
  - **Two** lateral ventricles
    - *Anatomy:* Cerebrospinal fluid-filled cavities within each cerebral hemisphere. Cerebrospinal fluid (CSF) is a clear liquid produced continuously in the ventricles that continually circulates through the ventricles and subarachnoid space to distribute nutrients and to serve as a shock absorber against injury for the brain and spinal cord. Each ventricle is divided segmentally into a *frontal horn, body, occipital horn,* and *temporal horn.* The atrium or trigone is the junction of the body and occipital and temporal horns.
    - *Sonographic appearance:* The ventricle walls appear echogenic and curvilinear. These slit-like structures lie the same distance from the interhemispheric fissure. The ventricle cavities contain CSF and appear anechoic.
  - **Third ventricle**
    - *Anatomy:* The third ventricle is a small, teardrop-shaped, midline cavity that lies between the thalami and is connected to the lateral ventricles via the foramen of Monro (midline channels that mark the communication between the lateral ventricles and third ventricle).
    - *Sonographic appearance:* Walls appear echogenic. The cavity contains CSF and appears anechoic.
  - **Fourth ventricle**
    - *Anatomy:* A small, thin, arrowhead-shaped, midline cavity that appears to project into the cerebellum. It is vaguely seen except with massive ventricular dilatation. It is located below and connected to the third ventricle by a small channel, the aqueduct of Sylvius, a narrow opening for the passage of CSF. It directs CSF into the subarachnoid space through the foramen of Magendie and foramina of Lushka, three small holes in the floor of the fourth ventricle.
    - *Sonographic appearance:* Walls appear echogenic. The cavity contains CSF and appears anechoic when seen.
- Corpus callosum
  - *Anatomy:* Flat, broad nerve fibers between the right and left cerebral hemispheres that form the roof of the lateral ventricles.
  - *Sonographic appearance:* The parenchyma appears midgray or as medium-level echoes.
- Cerebrum
  - *Anatomy:* The largest part of the brain that is divided into two identical, symmetrical right and left hemispheres that communicate through the corpus callosum and are separated from each

other at the midline by a deep groove, the interhemispheric fissure. Each cerebral hemisphere is divided into four lobes, named after the overlying cranial bones:

- Frontal lobe
- Parietal lobe
- Temporal lobe
- Occipital lobe

- *Sonographic appearance:* Midgray with medium-level echoes.
- Cavum septum pellucidum (anterior portion) and cavum vergae (posterior portion)
  - *Anatomy:* Small cavities filled with CSF that filters from the ventricles through the septal laminae. They have no connection with the ventricles. They separate the frontal horns of the lateral ventricles, forming their medial margins at the midline of the brain. They close before birth.
  - *Sonographic appearance:* Appear moderately gray and comma-shaped sagittally or triangular coronally.
- Thalamus
  - *Anatomy:* Two large, egg-shaped thalami lie on each side of the third ventricle, forming most of its lateral walls.
  - *Sonographic appearance:* Homogeneous and midgray with medium-level echoes.
- Cerebellum
  - *Anatomy:* Constitutes the second-largest portion of the brain, it lies immediately posterior to the fourth ventricle and occupies the majority of the posterior fossae of the skull. Composed of symmetrical, bilateral hemispheres connected by the vermis, its medial portion.
  - *Sonographic appearance:* parenchyma appears midgray or as medium-level echoes. The central echogenic portion of the cerebellum is the vermis.
- Cisterna magna
  - *Anatomy:* Largest expanded subarachnoid space in the brain. Located at the base of the cerebellum in the posterior portion of the brain.
  - *Sonographic appearance:* The cavity contains CSF and appears anechoic.
- Choroid plexus
  - *Anatomy:* Special blood vessels located in the ventricles that produce CSF.
  - *Sonographic appearance:* Consists of two curvilinear, highly echogenic structures that arch around the thalami anteriorly from the floor of the body of the lateral ventricle and posteriorly to the tip of the temporal horn. Note that the choroid plexus does not extend into the frontal or occipital horns.

- Aqueduct of Sylvius
  - *Anatomy:* Midline channel that connects the third and fourth ventricles.
  - *Sonographic appearance:* Rarely seen sonographically unless dilated.
- Foramen of Monro
  - *Anatomy:* Narrow, midline channels that connect the third ventricle with each lateral ventricle for the passage of CSF.
  - *Sonographic appearance:* Anechoic area just posterior to the level of the frontal horn of each lateral ventricle.
- Brain stem
  - *Anatomy:* Columnar-appearing structure that connects the forebrain and the spinal cord. Consists of the midbrain, pons, and the medulla oblongata.
  - *Sonographic appearance:* Midgray with medium- to low-level echoes.
- Interhemispheric fissure
  - *Anatomy:* Deep groove or indentation separating the right and left cerebral hemispheres. Contains the **falx cerebri** (fold of the dura mater).
  - *Sonographic appearance:* Thin, linear, echogenic, midline structure.
- Massa intermedia
  - *Anatomy:* Pea-shaped, soft tissue structure that is suspended within the third ventricle with no known function.
  - *Sonographic appearance:* Midgray with medium-level echoes and is best seen with ventricular dilatation.
- Hippocampal gyrus (choroidal fissure)
  - *Anatomy:* Convolution on the inner surface of the temporal lobe of the cerebrum.
  - *Sonographic appearance:* Echogenic, spiral-like fold embodying each temporal horn.
- Cerebral peduncle
  - *Anatomy:* Y-shaped structure inferior to the thalami and fused at the level of the pons.
  - *Sonographic appearance:* Midgray with low-level echoes.
- Sulci
  - *Anatomy:* Grooves separating the gyri on the surface of the brain.
  - *Sonographic appearance:* Echogenic, spider-like fissures separating the gyri or folds of the brain. The premature neonate usually has fewer sulci than a full-term infant.
- Tentorium
  - *Anatomy:* Dura mater flap that separates the cerebral hemispheres from the other structures in the brain.
  - *Sonographic appearance:* Echogenic structure (tent-shaped coronally).

- Sylvian fissure
  - *Anatomy:* Groove separating the frontal and temporal lobes of the brain.
  - *Sonographic appearance:* Resembles an echogenic "Y" turned on its side. The middle cerebral artery can be seen pulsating here.
- Caudate nucleus
  - *Anatomy:* Located within the concavity of the lateral angles of each lateral ventricle.
  - *Sonographic appearance:* Midgray with medium-level echoes.
- Germinal matrix/caudothalamic groove
  - *Anatomy:* Vascular network located in the region of the caudate nucleus and thalamus called the caudothalamic groove.
  - *Sonographic appearance:* When visualized, it appears small and echogenic. Note that this is the most common site for a subependymal hemorrhage.
- Quadrigeminal plate
  - *Anatomy:* Posterior to the third ventricle.
  - *Sonographic appearance:* Echogenic structure immediately superior to the apex of the tentorium resembling the top of a pine tree.

Preparation

Patient Prep
- Keeping the baby warm is of utmost importance.
- The baby should be disturbed as little as possible, preferably left in the isolette.
- If the baby is in a high-oxygen environment, this should be maintained as much as possible, even though the baby must be scanned there.
- Gowns and gloves are recommended.
- The portable ultrasound system should be wiped down with a cleaning agent.
- Coupling gel should be at body temperature.

Transducer
- 7.5 MHz for premature infants less than 32 weeks' gestation or less than 1500 g.
- 5.0 to 3.0 MHz for term and older infants with open anterior fontanelle.

Patient Position
- **Supine with the head face up.**
- Prone with the head lying on either side.
- It can be helpful to place a small cloth or towel under and/or beside the baby's head to help immobilize it during the scan.

Neonatal Brain Survey

NOTE: Use the **anterior fontanelle** (soft, unossified membrane-covered space between the sutures of the skull) at the top of the head as a window through which to angle or pivot the transducer. The diameter of the fontanelle may restrict the amount of angulation and anatomy seen. The posterior fontanelle may also be used.

NOTE: Use an ample amount of gel to help avoid too much transducer pressure.

NOTE: While surveying the brain, close attention should be paid to all intracranial anatomy and its symmetry.

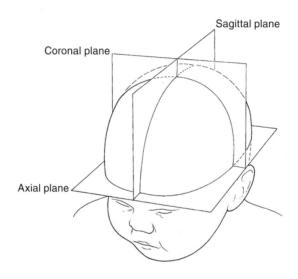

Coronal Survey
Coronal Plane • Anterior Fontanelle Approach

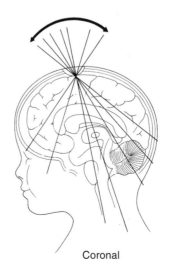

Coronal

1. Begin with the transducer perpendicular at the anterior fontanelle.
2. Slowly angle the transducer toward the face. Scan through the frontal horns into the frontal lobes of the brain.
3. Slowly angle the transducer back to perpendicular.
4. Slowly angle the transducer posteriorly. Scan through the occipital horns into the occipital lobes of the brain.
5. Slowly angle the transducer back to perpendicular.

Sagittal Survey
Sagittal Plane • Anterior Fontanelle Approach

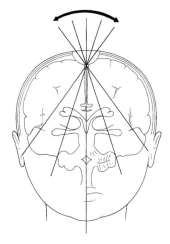

1. Begin with the transducer perpendicular at the anterior fontanelle.
2. Slowly angle the transducer laterally toward the right lateral ventricle. Scan through the temporal lobe of the brain to the level of the Sylvian fissure.
3. Slowly angle the transducer back to perpendicular.
4. Repeat the first, second, and third steps, but angle the transducer through the left hemisphere.

Neonatal Brain Required Images

Coronal Images
Coronal Plane • Anterior Fontanelle Approach

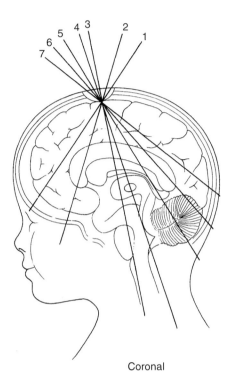

Coronal

1. Coronal image of the **FRONTAL LOBES** of the brain with the interhemispheric fissure. Include the orbital cones and ethmoid sinus.

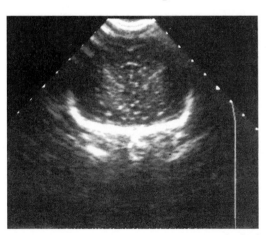
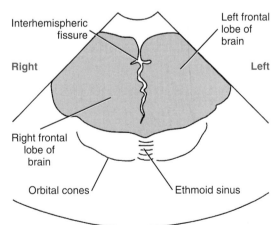

Labeled: **CORONAL**

2. Coronal image of the **FRONTAL HORNS** of the ventricles encompassing the caudate nucleus. Include the germinal matrix adjacent to the ventricles and corpus callosum.

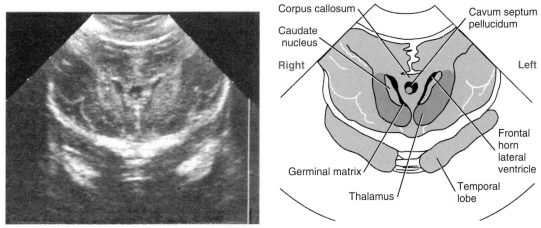

Labeled: **CORONAL**

3. Coronal image of the **FRONTAL HORNS** and **THALAMI.** Include the Sylvian fissures, septum pellucidum, third ventricle, and foramen of Monro.

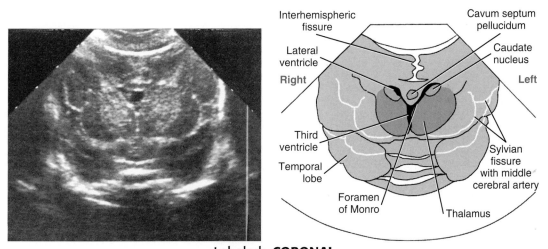

Labeled: **CORONAL**

4. Coronal image of the bodies of the **LATERAL VENTRICLES, THALAMI, SYLVIAN FISSURES, CHOROIDAL FISSURES,** and **TEMPORAL HORNS.**

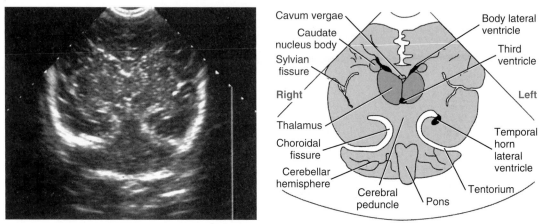

Labeled: **CORONAL**

5. Coronal image of the **TENTORIUM CEREBELLI.** Include the Sylvian fissures and the cisterna magna.

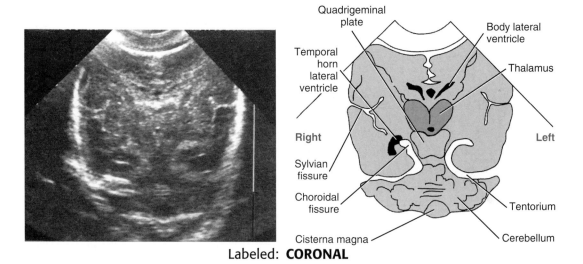

Labeled: **CORONAL**

6. Coronal image of the **CHOROID PLEXUS** in the atrium or trigone region.

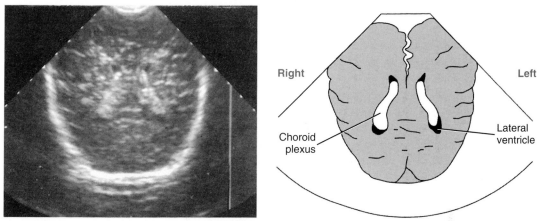

Labeled: **CORONAL**

7. Coronal image of the **OCCIPITAL LOBES** of the brain.

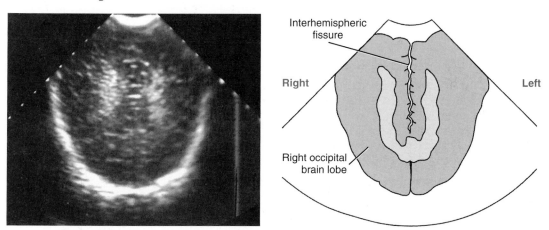

Labeled: **CORONAL**

Sagittal Images
Sagittal Plane • Anterior Fontanelle Approach

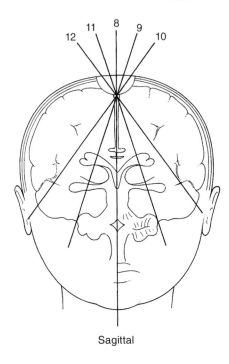

Sagittal

Midline Image

8. Sagittal midline image of the **CAVUM SEPTUM PELLUCIDUM, CORPUS CALLOSUM, THIRD VENTRICLE, FOURTH VEN-TRICLE,** and **CEREBELLUM,** including the massa intermedia (seen in two thirds of infants).

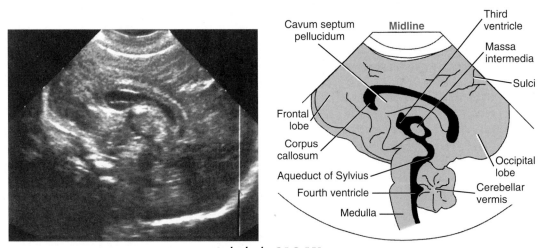

Labeled: **SAG ML**

NOTE: This image should be perpendicular at the midline.

Right Hemisphere Images

9. Sagittal image of the **RIGHT VENTRICLE, GERMINAL MATRIX, CAUDATE NUCLEUS, THALAMUS,** and **CHOROID PLEXUS.**

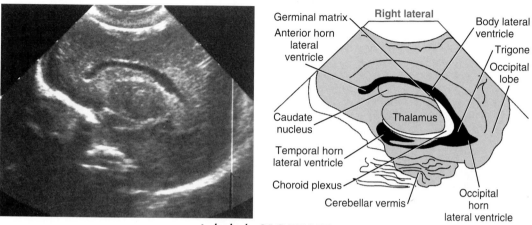

Labeled: **SAG RT LAT**

> **NOTE:** In some cases the frontal horn, body, temporal horn, and occipital horn cannot be imaged in the same plane. Therefore an additional image(s) may be necessary.

10. Sagittal image of the **RIGHT TEMPORAL LOBE** of the brain at the level of the Sylvian fissure.

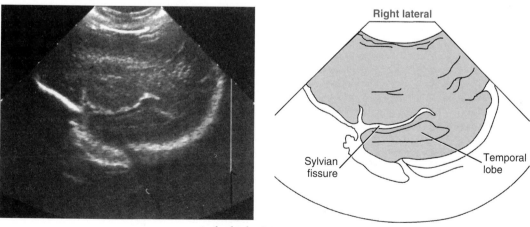

Labeled: **SAG RT LAT**

Left Hemisphere Images

11. Sagittal image of the **LEFT VENTRICLE, GERMINAL MATRIX, CAUDATE NUCLEUS, THALAMUS,** and **CHOROID PLEXUS.**

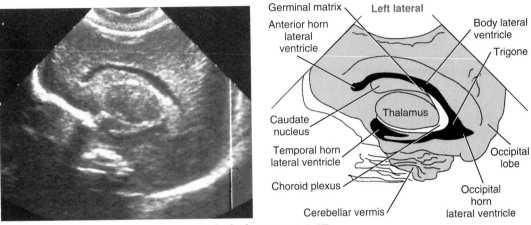

Labeled: **SAG LT LAT**

> **NOTE:** In some cases the frontal horn, body, temporal horn, and occipital horn cannot be imaged in the same plane. Therefore an additional image(s) may be necessary.

12. Sagittal image of the **LEFT TEMPORAL LOBE** of the brain at the level of the Sylvian fissure.

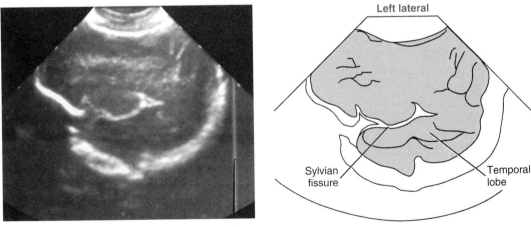

Labeled: **SAG LT LAT**

> **NOTE:** Alternative axial views through the temporal recess or posterior fontanelle are options to further evaluate the lateral ventricular walls and/or the occipital horns, respectively.

Review Questions

Answers on page 630.

1. The structures in the brain that appear anechoic on a sonogram are the
   a) four ventricles; cavum septum pellucidum and cavum vergae; cisterna magnum; tentorium.
   b) four ventricles; cavum septum pellucidum and cavum vergae; tentorium; foramen of Monro.
   c) four ventricles; cavum septum pellucidum and cavum vergae; cisterna magnum; corpus callosum.
   d) four ventricles; cavum septum pellucidum and cavum vergae; cisterna magnum; foramen of Monro.

2. The two curvilinear, bright structures that arch around the thalami anteriorly from the floor of the body of the lateral ventricle and posteriorly to the tip of the temporal horn are the
   a) corpus callosum.
   b) caudate nucleus.
   c) choroid plexus.
   d) thalamus.

3. The midline falx is
   a) a fold of dura mater that lies in the interhemispheric fissure.
   b) the interhemispheric fissure.
   c) the channel that connects the third and fourth ventricles.
   d) the echogenic portion of the cerebellum.

4. The brain stem consists of
   a) pons, medulla oblongata, cerebellum.
   b) midbrain, pons, medulla oblongata.
   c) midbrain, pons, cerebellum, medulla oblongata.
   d) aqueduct of Sylvius, cerebellum, medulla oblongata, caudate nucleus.

5. The linear, echogenic structure seen at the midline of the cerebrum is the
   a) quadrigeminal plate.
   b) caudothalamic groove.
   c) Sylvian fissure.
   d) interhemispheric fissure.

6. The midgray, homogeneous, egg-shaped structures that lie on either side of the third ventricle are the
   a) lateral ventricles.
   b) thalami.
   c) cerebral hemispheres.
   d) vermis.

7. The central echogenic portion of the otherwise midgray cerebellum is the
   a) hippocampal gyrus.
   b) thalamus.
   c) tentorium.
   d) vermis.

8. The echogenic, spider-like fissures separating the gyri of the brain are the
   a) massa intermedia.
   b) choroid plexi.
   c) sulci.
   d) choroidal fissures.

9. The four ventricles are
   a) frontal, lateral, occipital, and third.
   b) frontal, body, occipital, and temporal.
   c) two lateral, third and fourth.
   d) two frontal, lateral, and third.

10. The small, thin, anechoic, arrowhead-shaped midline structure that appears to project into the cerebellum is the
    a) fourth ventricle.
    b) temporal horn.
    c) quadrigeminal plate.
    d) tentorium.

11. In the cerebellum, the _____ connects the two hemispheres.
    a) vermis
    b) tentorium
    c) massa intermedia
    d) corpus callosum

12. The _____ is a midline channel that connects the third and fourth ventricles.
    a) vermis
    b) aqueduct of Sylvius
    c) massa intermedia
    d) foramen of Monro

13. The _____ is a midline channel that marks the communication between the lateral ventricles and third ventricle.
    a) vermis
    b) aqueduct of Sylvius
    c) massa intermedia
    d) foramen of Monro

14. The _____directs CSF into the subarachnoid space through the foramen of Magendie and foramina of Lushka.
    a) fourth ventricle
    b) temporal horn
    c) quadrigeminal plate
    d) tentorium

15. The _____ is a Y-shaped structure inferior to the thalami and fused at the level of the pons.
    a) fourth ventricle
    b) temporal horn
    c) cerebral peduncle
    d) tentorium

PART VI

VASCULAR SCANNING
PROTOCOLS

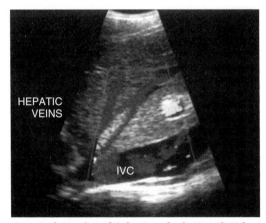

**Gray-Scale Version of Color Doppler in Hepatic Veins.
See Color Plate 7.**

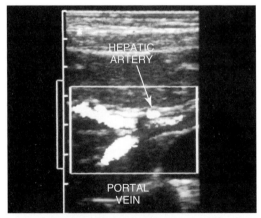

**Gray-Scale Version of Color Doppler Image of Flow in the
Portal Vein. See Color Plate 8.**

CHAPTER 19

Abdominal Doppler and Color Flow Imaging

Marsha M. Neumyer

Key Words

Angle control	Phasicity
Color Doppler	Power Doppler
Color priority	Pulsed-wave (PW) Doppler
Continuous-wave (CW) Doppler	Pulsatility index
	Renal–aortic velocity ratio
Diagnostic frequency range	Resistive index
Diastolic-to-systolic ratio	Saturation
Doppler gain	Vascular resistance
Doppler shift	Velocity scale
Gray-scale	Wall filter
Hue	Zero baseline
Luminosity	

Objectives

At the end of this chapter, you will be able to:

- Define the key words.
- Describe the anatomy of the abdominal vascular system.
- Differentiate low-resistance and high-resistance blood flow patterns.
- Describe techniques used to assess patency of vessels, rule out arterial stenosis and venous thrombosis, and determine flow direction.
- Describe the duplex scanning protocols used for evaluation of the mesenteric and renal vascular systems.
- Define methods for quantitating vascular resistance using resistive index (RI), pulsatility index (PI), and diastolic-to-systolic ratio (DSR).
- Differentiate vascular from avascular abdominal masses.
- Describe blood flow patterns commonly found in gynecologic, obstetric, and scrotal sonographic studies.
- Answer the review questions at the end of the chapter.

Basic Principles

The Doppler Equation

$$fd = \frac{2\, fo\, V\, \text{Cos}\, \theta}{C}$$

fd = Doppler shifted frequency
fo = Carrier (operating) Doppler frequency
C = Speed of sound in soft tissue
Cos ignore θ = Doppler beam angle relevant to the path of blood
V = Velocity (speed) of blood

- As the sound beam is sent into the body, any motion detected in the path of the beam is depicted as a change or shift in frequency.
  - This is referred to as the **Doppler shift** frequency (fd).
  - fd increases as the operating *frequency (fo) increases*. They are directly proportional as seen in the Doppler equation.
  - The fd usually falls within the audible frequency range.

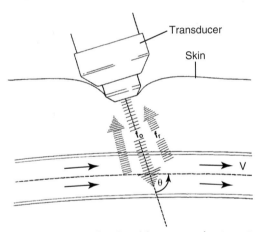

Obtaining a Doppler signal from a moving target.

General Information

Frequency Range
- The **diagnostic frequency range** for ultrasound is 1 MHz to 20 MHz.
- The frequency chosen depends on the depth of penetration required and the resolution necessary to achieve diagnostic information.

Images in this section courtesy Penn State Hershey Vascular Noninvasive Diagnostic Laboratory, Hershey, Pa., unless otherwise noted.

- As the frequency increases, resolution and blood flow detection also increase, but the depth of penetration decreases.
- If quantitative information is needed, the angle of the Doppler beam relevant to the path of blood flow must be known.
- The Doppler shift decreases as the Doppler angle increases. The angle of insonation is usually controlled by the operator.
- It must be remembered that if Doppler-shifted signals are collected at an angle of 0 degrees, the cosine of 0 is 1.0; therefore, a very accurate estimation of velocity is possible.
- An angle of insonation between 45 and 60 degrees usually ensures maximum signal return. It is important to ensure that the angle cursor is aligned parallel to the vessel wall or to the path of blood flow.

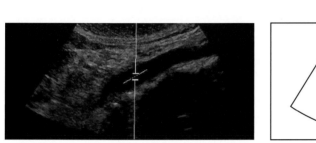
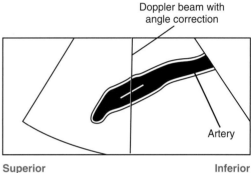

Frequency Range. B-Mode image of abdominal aorta demonstrating appropriate angle of Doppler insonation with cursor aligned parallel to the vessel wall.

- If the angle of insonation is 90 degrees (i.e., perpendicular to flow), the ultrasound system's computer will not be able to differentiate forward from reverse flow.
- When examining abdominal vessels with very small diameters, sample volume size may be initially enlarged to ensure that all returning Doppler-shifted signals are detected.
- When examining vessels with larger diameters, the sample volume size should be kept smaller.
- Sampling should be complete throughout the entire vessel lumen because peak velocities and regions of disordered flow may be encountered not only at midvessel but also adjacent to the vessel wall, depending on the amount and surface contour of lesions.

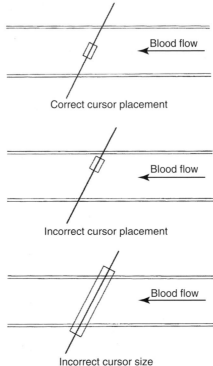

Illustrated examples of cursor size and placement.

Doppler Gain

- Doppler spectral gain should be optimized to ensure display of the full range of velocity information without introduction of an inappropriate signal-to-noise ratio.
- An appropriate gain level can be achieved by increasing the Doppler gain until "noise" is apparent and the Doppler spectral envelope is disturbed. Decrease the gain level just to the point where the spectral envelope is clear.

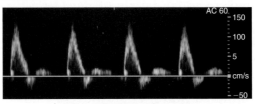

Appropriate Doppler gain.

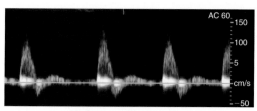
Slight Doppler overgain.

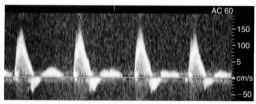
Doppler overgained. Inappropriate signal-to-noise ratio.

Most Frequently Used Doppler Controls

- Doppler gain: will increase or decrease the total gain applied to the Doppler spectral information.
- Wall filter: high-pass filters. The wall filter eliminates signals based on their frequency. Signals with a frequency higher than the filter setting will pass, whereas lower frequency signals are filtered out. Care must be taken not to set the wall filter too high or useful information will be deleted.
- Angle control: as discussed previously.
- Zero baseline: may be adjusted to allow display of the full range of velocities in a spectral waveform.
- Velocity scale: same as pulse repetition frequency (PRF). Used with pulse Doppler to help eliminate aliasing and to optimize Doppler spectral display. Remember that the Nyquist limit is half the PRF, and aliasing occurs when the Nyquist limit is exceeded.

Doppler Instrumentation

- Continuous-wave (CW) Doppler
  - Cheaper.
  - Generally a small pencil probe.
  - Employs two crystals. One continuously sends signals, one continuously receives returning echoes.
  - Lacks axial resolution.
    - Cannot determine vessel depth.
    - Filters may be used to help decrease interference from noise.

- An area of overlap between the outgoing and incoming signals is used as a basis for comparison to determine the Doppler shift frequency.
  - A demodulator (often a quadrature phase detector) is used to determine the Doppler shift frequency.

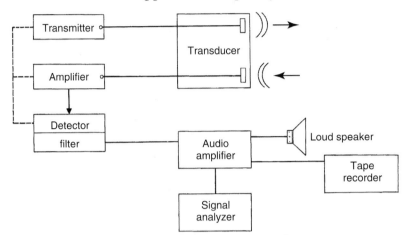

Block diagram of a continuous-wave Doppler system.

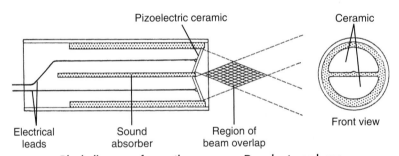

Block diagram of a continuous-wave Doppler transducer.

- **Pulsed-wave (PW) Doppler**
  - Often duplex instrumentation. A combination of real-time Doppler velocity spectral display and B-Mode image instrumentation.
    - The Doppler velocity information may be collected from discrete sample sites within the gray-scale image.
    - The Doppler crystals are located within the imaging transducer.
  - Allows Doppler velocity spectral analysis (temporal display) from a small, specific operator-controllable region (sample volume).
  - Capable of examining only a limited frequency range.
    - Will alias because the Doppler shift frequencies are determined by sampling multiple times along the same pulse line. Because of time and depth limitations (i.e., PRF), the internal computer may not be able to sample often enough within a given time frame to allow display of the full range of frequencies.

- Has poor signal-to-noise ratios; therefore, it may be difficult to detect very low flow signals due to noise interference.
  - Hard to remove noise without removing real information.
- May use high levels of power.
  - Spatial peak temporal average (SPTA) levels may reach 1 W/cm^2.
- The use of an operator-set Doppler angle correction allows easy calculation of flow velocity by the internal computer, which uses the Doppler equation.

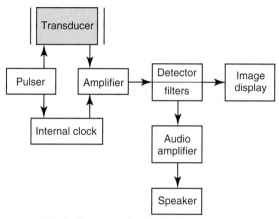

Block diagram of a duplex instrument.

- Color Doppler
  - Color encodement is dependent on Doppler shift; therefore, this is an angle-dependent technology.
  - Offers an estimate of mean flow velocities (spatially) at each sampling point within the image field at a given instant in time. To produce a color image, the sampling is performed at a very fast rate.
  - Multiple sampling often causes noise from tissue movement and moving blood cells to be recorded. Filters must be used to eliminate all but the continuously moving signals.
  - Frequency shifts are detected through autocorrelation.
- Power Doppler
  - Color encodement is based on the relative intensity of the Doppler signal rather than the Doppler shift. Because of this feature, the direction of flow cannot be determined.
  - Useful tool for when flow path is off-axis, slow, or perpendicular to the beam.

Doppler Analysis
Audible Sound
- The Doppler-shift frequency falls within the audible range of 200 Hz to 15 KHz.

Spectral Analysis
- The Doppler spectral waveform, generated by fast Fourier transform (FFT) analysis, is a graphic display of the range of frequencies and amplitudes contained within the returned signal throughout each cardiac cycle.
- The frequency shift is displayed on the vertical axis, time on the horizontal axis, and amplitude of the returned signals as shades of gray.

Color Doppler Analysis
- The color display is based on 3 characteristics of color:
  1. Hue: the three primary colors are used to create color maps (red, blue, and green).
  2. Saturation: the amount of white present in a color. This is used to create color shades.
  3. Luminosity: this is used to create the brightness of a color.
- Red hue generally represents flow toward the transducer.
- Blue hue generally represents flow away from the transducer.
- Mosaic color patterns or "desaturation" of a primary color represent high velocity or complex, turbulent flow. Choice of color maps is controlled by the operator.
- With color imaging, spectral broadening may be viewed as "variance."
  - One color is arbitrarily chosen to display a wide range of velocities present within the signals.
  - The color green is frequently chosen to "tag" a threshold velocity. This allows recognition of elevated velocities (i.e., those that exceed the threshold).
- Other color Doppler controls:
  - The number of cycles per color line (often referred to as dwell time, ensemble length, or packet size). As this number is increased, flow sensitivity increases, but frame rate decreases.
  - Gray-scale or color priority: this control determines whether gray-scale or color Doppler information will be emphasized in the display. Increasing this control increases the color saturation. Decreasing it helps decrease the color that may be present because of vessel wall and tissue motion. The control acts as a filter by suppressing color information above a threshold level set by the operator.

Doppler Pitfalls
Aliasing
- Does not occur with continuous-wave Doppler.
- Occurs with PW and color Doppler when the Nyquist limit (½ PRF) is exceeded.
- May be corrected by increasing the PRF (velocity scale), lowering the 0 baseline, changing the angle of insonation, or decreasing the Doppler frequency.

- Appearance: an aliased signal will wrap around the baseline.
- This phenomenon occurs because the pulsed-Doppler system cannot sample often enough.
- Aliasing also may occur with color Doppler. It appears as an abrupt change in high-frequency color codes (i.e., light red to light blue).
- Flow reversal will appear as adjacent deep shades separated by black (0 baseline) on the color image.
- The Doppler signal is backscattered from moving red blood cells (Rayleigh scattering). As frequency increases, Rayleigh scattering increases. As in gray-scale imaging, the operator must choose the incident Doppler frequency for adequate penetration that will allow acceptable resolution and signal amplitude without aliasing.

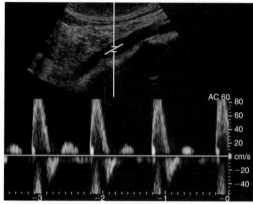

Doppler spectral waveforms demonstrating aliasing of the Doppler signal.

Doppler Mirror Image
- An artifactual display of the Doppler spectral waveform appearing on the opposite side of the zero baseline from the waveform corresponding to the appropriate direction of flow.
- Results from inappropriate angle of insonation or PRF.

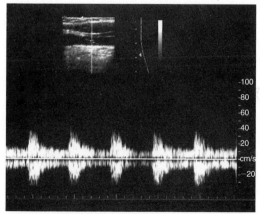

Doppler spectral waveforms illustrating Doppler mirroring. (Courtesy Mary Washington Hospital, Fredericksburg, Va.).

Color Imaging Pitfalls

> **NOTE:** Like PW Doppler, color Doppler is limited by the frame rate, tissue target depth, and PRF of the ultrasound system.

- Color Doppler systems are usually unable to detect flow velocity less than approximately 0.05 meters per second.
  1. Low-velocity signals are often obscured by noise or eliminated by the wall filter (if set too high). This problem may be overcome by using a low color velocity PRF.
  2. Color Doppler system may use frame rates of 4 to 32 frames per second. The frame rate is operator-controlled. Increase for better resolution.
  3. To better detect low-velocity flow, use a higher frequency transducer.
  4. To decrease the effect of tissue or vessel wall vibrations, increase the color wall filter.
- Mirror image artifacts:
  1. To correct range ambiguity artifacts:
     - Decrease the PRF.
     - Increase frequency of the transducer.
     - Decrease far gain.
  2. Grating lobes:
     - Result from decreased lateral resolution because the beam is not perpendicular to the target.
     - To correct, adjust the transducer angle and/or Doppler steering angle.

Biologic Effects
- The American Institute of Ultrasound in Medicine (AIUM) states that for imaging transducers, no known bioeffects have been proven below scanning intensity levels of 100 mW/cm^2 SPTA.
- No known bioeffects have been documented at currently used diagnostic intensity levels.
- All sonographers should be familiar with their equipment and the intensity levels stated in the manufacturer's operator's manual.
- Sonographers should scan conscientiously at all times using the ALARA (as low as reasonable acceptable) principle to adjust power or intensity.
- The AIUM recommends using high power for as brief a period as possible to allow diagnostic studies. This practice ensures that the valuable diagnostic information will still be obtained without introducing any remote risk of harmful biologic effects.

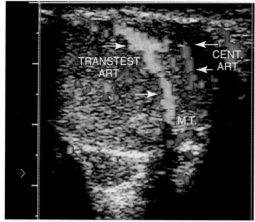

Plate 1 **Testicular Vascular Normal Variant.** The transtesticular artery runs in a direction opposite the centripetal arteries. (See also Figure 14-4, p. 350, Chapter 14.)

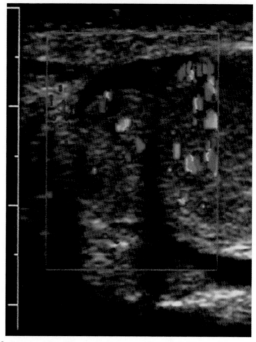

Plate 4 Color flow Image of epididymis. (See also p. 352, Chapter 14.)

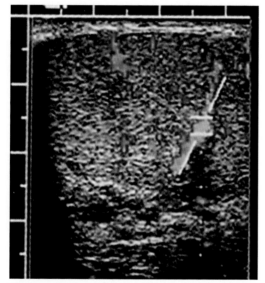

Plate 2 Color flow image and waveform of intra-testicular arteries. (See also p. 350, Chapter 14.)

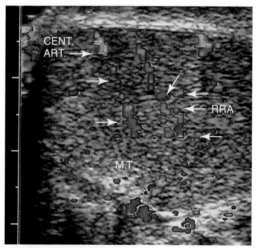

Plate 5 Color flow images of intratesticular arteries. (See also p. 352, Chapter 14.)

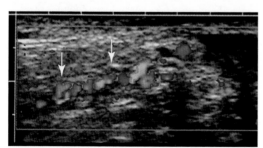

Plate 3 Color flow image of spermatic cord. (See also p. 351, Chapter 14.)

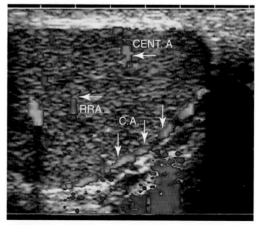

Plate 6 Color flow images of intratesticular arteries (see also p. 352, Chapter 14).

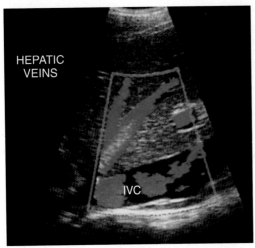

Plate 7 Color flow Doppler image of hepatic veins. (See also p. 472, Chapter 19.)

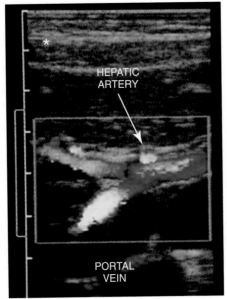

Plate 8 Color Doppler image of flow in the portal vein. (See also p. 472, Chapter 19.)

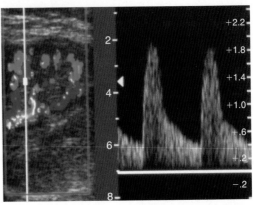

Plate 9 Color flow image and Doppler spectral waveforms recorded from the medullary vessels of a normal renal transplant. (See also p. 486, Chapter 19.)

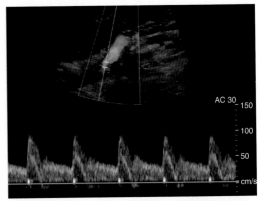

Plate 10 Color Doppler spectral waveforms from the celiac artery origin. (See also p. 487, Chapter 19.)

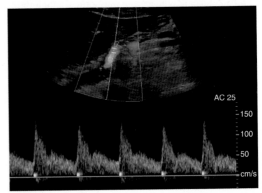

Plate 11 Color Doppler spectral waveforms from the distal celiac trunk. (See also p. 488, Chapter 19.)

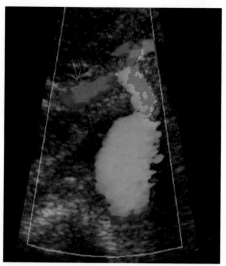

Plate 12 Color flow image of the axial abdominal aorta at the level of the bifurcation of the celiac artery into the common hepatic and splenic arteries. (See also p. 488, Chapter 19.)

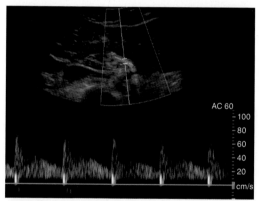

Plate 13 Color Doppler spectral waveforms from the common hepatic artery. (See also p. 489, Chapter 19.)

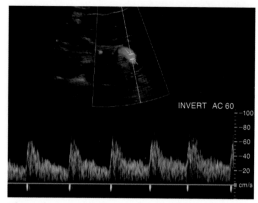

Plate 14 Color Doppler spectral waveforms from the splenic artery. (See also p. 489, Chapter 19.)

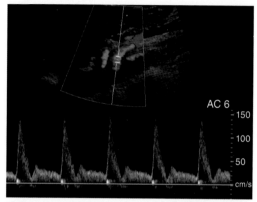

Plate 15 Color Doppler spectral waveforms from the proximal-to-mid section of the superior mesenteric artery. (See also p. 490, Chapter 19.)

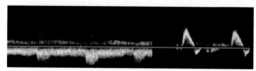

Plate 16 Color Doppler spectral waveforms showing the transition of flow patterns from the aorta through the orifice of the renal artery. (See also p. 492, Chapter 19.)

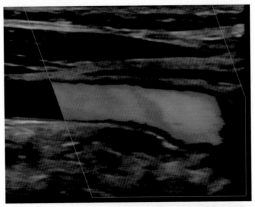

Plate 17 Color flow image of distal innominate artery and common carotid artery. (See also p. 514, Chapter 20.)

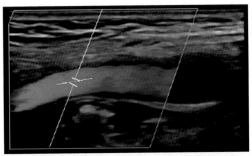

Plate 18 Sagittal color flow image of the carotid bulb and internal carotid artery. (See also p. 515, Chapter 20.)

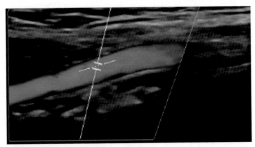

Plate 19 Sagittal color flow image of the external carotid artery. (See also p. 515, Chapter 20.)

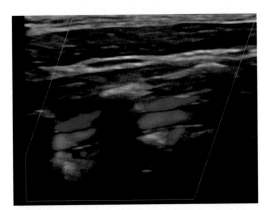

Plate 20 Sagittal color flow image of the vertebral artery and vein in the mid-cervical segment of the neck. (See also p. 516, Chapter 20.)

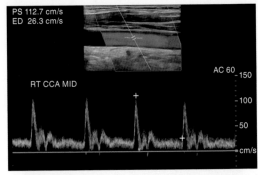

Plate 21 Sagittal color flow image and Doppler spectral waveforms from the mid-common carotid artery. (See also p. 517, Chapter 20.)

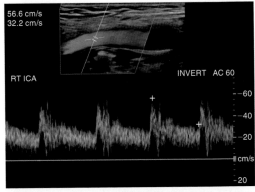

Plate 22 Sagittal color flow image and Doppler spectral waveforms from the internal carotid artery. (See also p. 517, Chap-ter 20.)

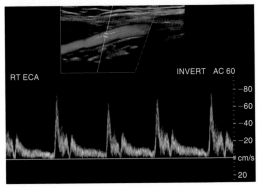

Plate 23 Sagittal color flow image and Doppler spectral waveforms from the external carotid artery. (See also p. 517, Chap-ter 20.)

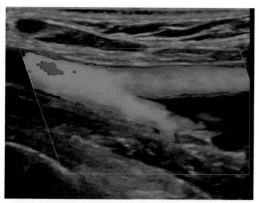

Plate 24 Sagittal color flow image of the common femoral artery bifurcation. (See also p. 538, Chapter 21.)

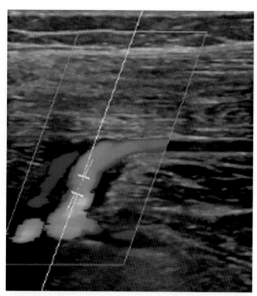

Plate 26 Sagittal color flow image of the proximal anterior tibial artery. (See also p. 539, Chapter 21.)

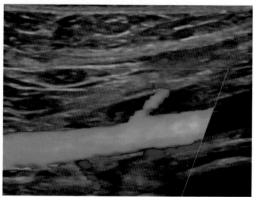

Plate 25 Sagittal color flow image of the popliteal artery. (See also p. 538, Chapter 21.)

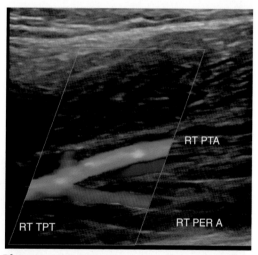

Plate 27 Sagittal color flow image of the tibio-peroneal trunk and origins of the posterior tibial and peroneal arteries. (See also p. 539, Chapter 21.)

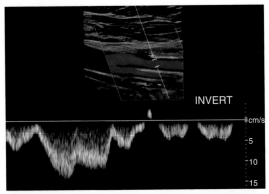

Plate 28 Doppler spectral waveforms demonstrating respira-tory phasicity. (See also p. 558, Chapter 21.)

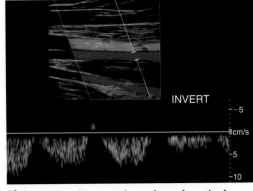

Plate 31 Doppler spectral waveforms from the femoral vein. (See also p. 565, Chapter 21.)

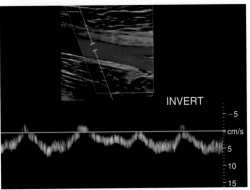

Plate 29 Doppler spectral waveforms from the common femoral vein. (See also p. 564, Chapter 21.)

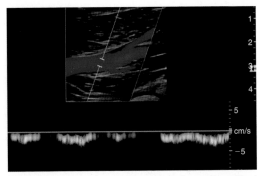

Plate 32 Doppler spectral waveforms from the popliteal vein. (See also p. 566, Chapter 21.)

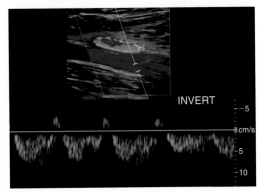

Plate 30 Doppler spectral waveforms from the profunda femoris vein. (See also p. 565, Chapter 21.)

Preparation

Examination Protocol for Abdominal Doppler and Color Flow Imaging

- Abdominal duplex and color flow imaging are performed to confirm patency of vessels, detect the presence and severity of disease, and define the location of disease processes.

Patient Prep

- Patients should fast for 8 to 12 hours or take no food after midnight the evening before the examination. This will decrease abdominal gas, which may interfere with acquisition of image and Doppler flow information.
- Patients with diabetes are made a priority on the early morning schedule. These patients may have dry toast and clear tea before the examination if necessary to prevent hypoglycemia.
- Smoking and gum chewing are discouraged to reduce the amount of swallowed air.
- Morning medications should be taken with sips of water only. No dairy products or citrus juices are allowed because these promote abdominal gas.
- The use of cathartics is usually unnecessary.

Transducer

- A range of transducers from 2.25 MHz to 5.0 MHz, phased or curved linear array probes will be necessary to penetrate to the depth of the abdominal aorta and distal renal arteries.

Patient Position

- The examination is usually initiated with the patient in the supine position with the head resting on a thin pillow.
- Lateral decubitus or prone positions are used as necessary to obtain adequate acoustic windows for visualization of organs and blood vessels.
- The bed is moved to the reverse Trendelenburg position so that the visceral contents can descend into the abdomen. This position facilitates creation of acoustic windows in the upper abdomen.

Arterial Flow Patterns

- Arterial flow pulsates with the cardiac cycle.
- Most arterial flow within the abdomen exhibits a low resistance waveform pattern (celiac, hepatic, splenic, and renal arteries) because these arteries supply end organs with high flow demands.
- Low-resistance Doppler spectral waveforms exhibit constant forward diastolic flow (above the zero baseline).

- Low-resistance arteries or abdominal masses often have a spectral waveform appearance with lower systolic peaks and a more pronounced diastolic component.

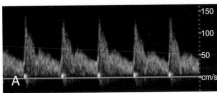 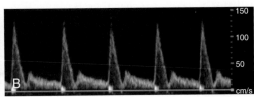

Arterial Flow Patterns. Doppler spectral waveforms demonstrating low-resistance **(A)** and high-resistance **(B)** flow patterns.

- The superior mesenteric and inferior mesenteric arteries supply muscular tissue beds. In the fasting state, these arteries exhibit a high-resistance Doppler spectral waveform.
- High-resistance Doppler spectral waveforms are characterized by low diastolic flow. A reverse flow component may be present at the end of the systolic deceleration phase of the waveform.

> **NOTE:** Each vessel has a characteristic appearance based on the level of **vascular resistance** present in the end organs that they supply or the pathology distal to the sample site.

Examples of Abdominal Arterial Flow
- **Hepatic arteries:**
  - Tend to have a low-impedance flow pattern characterized by forward diastolic flow.
  - Flow-reducing stenosis is suggested by peak systolic velocity greater than 220 cm/sec with poststenotic turbulence.
  - Increased flow in the absence of stenosis may suggest portal hypertension or portal vein thrombosis.
  - Must confirm the presence of hepatic artery flow in patients with liver transplants.
- **Splenic artery:**
  - Low-resistance vascular flow pattern characterized by constant forward diastolic flow.
  - Frequently tortuous; therefore, may demonstrate minimal spectral broadening because of flow disturbance.
  - Flow-reducing stenosis is suggested by peak systolic velocity greater than 220 cm/sec with poststenotic turbulence.
- **Mesenteric arteries:**
  - In normal fasting, the celiac artery exhibits low-resistance Doppler waveforms with constant forward diastolic flow. This is consistent with the flow pattern found in the hepatic and splenic arteries.

- There is no significant change in the normal celiac peak systolic or diastolic velocities postprandially.
- In patients with celiac artery stenosis exceeding 70%, the peak systolic velocity is greater than 200 cm/sec, the end-diastolic velocity exceeds 55 cm/sec, and poststenotic turbulence will be present.
- In normal fasting, the superior mesenteric artery (SMA) Doppler waveform should exhibit low diastolic flow.
- The normal postprandial SMA signal will demonstrate increased systolic flow, at least a 50% increase in diastolic flow, and loss of the reverse flow component. *Exceptions:* patients with diabetic gastroparesis and those with gastric "dumping" syndrome.
- In patients with SMA stenosis exceeding 70%, the peak systolic velocity is greater than 275 cm/sec, the end-diastolic velocity exceeds 45 cm/sec, and poststenotic turbulence is apparent.
- When critical stenosis or occlusion of the SMA and celiac arteries is present, the inferior mesenteric artery may enlarge and course antegrade along the mid-to-lateral abdomen to reconstitute the more proximal mesenteric arteries.
- Retrograde flow may be noted in the common hepatic artery if the celiac artery is occluded.
- **Renal arteries:**
  - The study is performed to detect renal artery stenosis associated with hypertension or decreased renal function.
  - The renal arteries normally exhibit a low-resistance Doppler spectral waveform pattern characterized by constant forward diastolic flow.
  - *Normal:* peak systolic renal artery velocity less than 180 cm/sec, renal–aortic velocity ratio **(RAR)** less than 3.5.

$$RAR = \frac{\text{Renal artery peak systolic velocity}}{\text{Proximal aortic peak systolic velocity}}$$

  - *Flow-reducing renal artery stenosis (>60% to 70%):* peak systolic renal artery velocity greater than 180 cm/sec, renal-aortic ratio greater than 3.5, poststenotic turbulence is present.
  - *Renal artery stenosis that is not yet hemodynamically significant (<60%):* peak systolic renal artery velocity greater than 180 cm/sec, renal-aortic ratio less than 3.5, no poststenotic signal.
  - *Renal artery occlusion:* no flow in imaged renal artery using spectral color and power Doppler optimized for low flow. Doppler waveforms in the renal parenchyma demonstrate low amplitude, low velocity with delayed systolic acceleration, and run-off (tardus-parvus signal). The kidney length is usually less than 9 cm.

- *Renal parenchymal dysfunction (medical renal disease):* vascular resistance increases because of intracellular fluid accumulation, tubular necrosis, and/or narrowing of the small-diameter parenchymal vessels. As resistance to arterial inflow increases, diastolic flow decreases. Increased vascular resistance is often demonstrated by **resistive index (RI)**, **pulsatility index (PI)**, or **diastolic-to-systolic velocity ratio (DSR)**. An RI greater than 0.8 is considered abnormal.

$$RI = \frac{\text{Peak systolic velocity} - \text{End diastolic velocity}}{\text{Peak systolic velocity}}$$

- **Renal transplants:**
  - *Rejection:* diastolic flow decreases as the severity of the rejection episode increases as the result of decreased renal function and increased capillary resistance (often caused by external compression, including compression by the transducer and narrowing of small parenchymal blood vessels).
  - *Renal artery stenosis:* as discussed previously.
  - *Acute tubular necrosis:* in very mild cases, the diastolic flow increases compared to normal. As the necrotic process progresses, the diastolic flow decreases because of increased parenchymal vascular resistance. In very severe cases, the blood flow pattern may be indistinguishable from that associated with severe acute rejection.
  - *Infarction:* spectral, color, and power Doppler must be optimized to detect very low flow signals.

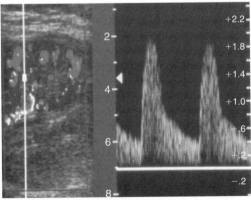

Gray-scale version of color flow image and Doppler spectral waveforms recorded from the medullary vessels of a normal renal transplant.
See Color Plate 9.

- **Miscellaneous**
  - Evaluation of blood supply to any area of interest requires knowledge of normal level of vascular resistance and factors that may alter the normal blood flow pattern.

> **NOTE:** Examination of the abdominal arteries and veins may be performed concurrently for each organ system (e.g., renal, mesenteric).

Mesenteric Arterial Duplex Protocol and Required Images

1. Scan the abdominal aorta in longitudinal and axial sections from the level of the diaphragm to the bifurcation (see Chapter 4). Return to the proximal, longitudinal aorta. Locate the celiac trunk as it arises from the anterior aortic wall just inferior to the level of the diaphragm.
   1. Longitudinal image of the **AORTA** at level of **celiac artery origin**.

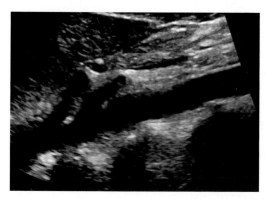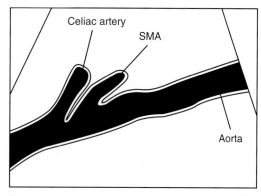

Superior   Inferior

Labeled: **SAG AORTA CELIAC ORIGIN**

- Sample with Doppler throughout the celiac trunk.
   2. Doppler spectral waveform from the **CELIAC ARTERY ORIGIN.**

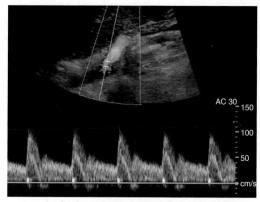

Labeled: **AORTA CELIAC ORIGIN**
Gray-scale version of color Doppler spectral waveforms from the celiac artery origin.
See Color Plate 10.

Mesenteric images courtesy Penn State Hershey Vascular Noninvasive Diagnostic Laboratory, Hershey, Pa.

3. Doppler spectral waveform from the **DISTAL CELIAC TRUNK.**

AC 25

150

100

50

cm/s

Labeled: **CELIAC DIST**
Gray-scale version of color Doppler spectral waveforms
from the distal celiac trunk. See Color Plate 11.

- In a transverse scanning plane, image the axial aorta at the level of the celiac artery origin. Follow the course of the celiac artery to its bifurcation into the common hepatic and splenic arteries. Note that the celiac and splenic arteries may be tortuous.

4. Axial image of the **AORTA** demonstrating longitudinal sections of the celiac artery and the common hepatic and splenic arteries at the **celiac bifurcation.**

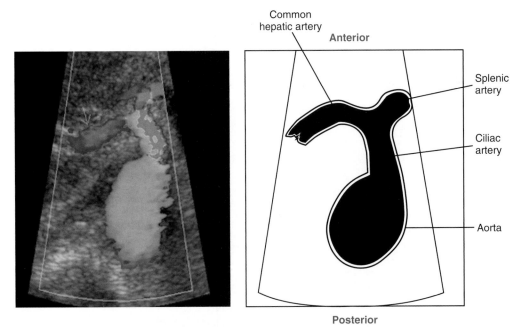

Labeled: **TRV CELIAC BIFURCATION**
Gray-scale version of a color flow image of the axial abdominal aorta at the level of the bifurcation of the
celiac artery into the common hepatic and splenic arteries. See Color Plate 12.

- Sample with Doppler throughout the length of the celiac trunk and the proximal common hepatic and splenic arteries.
    5. Doppler spectral waveforms from the **COMMON HEPATIC** and **SPLENIC ARTERIES.**

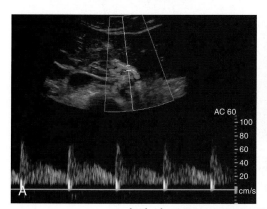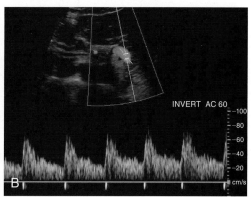

Labeled: **COMM HEP ART (A), SPLENIC ART (B)**

Gray-scale versions of the color Doppler spectral waveforms from the common hepatic **(A)** and splenic **(B)** arteries. See Color Plates 13 and 14.

NOTE: The hepatic artery may be followed from the celiac artery bifurcation to the level of its entry into the liver at the porta hepatis. Images and Doppler spectral waveforms should be documented throughout the proximal, mid, and distal segments of the vessel. In a similar manner, the splenic artery may be examined from its origin at the celiac bifurcation to the level of the splenic hilum. Images and Doppler spectral waveforms are documented throughout the proximal, mid, and distal segments of the vessel. The splenic artery is frequently quite tortuous and color flow imaging may facilitate examination.

- Return to the sagittal scanning plane and image the longitudinal aorta at a level just inferior to the origin of the celiac artery. Now locate the origin of the superior mesenteric artery (SMA), which is usually 1 to 2 cm inferior to the celiac. Note that the celiac and SMA may share a common trunk.

6. Longitudinal image of the **SMA** from its origin to its midsection.

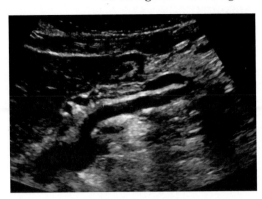 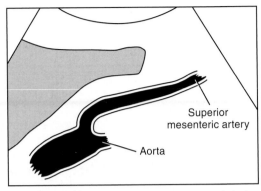

Superior   Inferior

Labeled: **SAG SMA PROX-MID**

- Sample with Doppler throughout the visualized segments of the SMA beginning at its origin.
  7. Doppler spectral waveforms from the **PROXIMAL** to **MID SMA.**

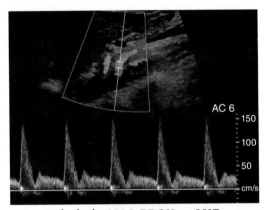

Labeled: **SMA PROX** or **MID**
Gray-scale version of color Doppler spectral waveforms from the
proximal-to-mid section of the superior mesenteric artery.
See Color Plate 15.

NOTE: The inferior mesenteric artery (IMA) is not routinely examined. If the celiac and/or SMA are critically stenosed or occluded, the IMA would be evaluated in a manner similar to the study of the SMA. At present, there are no well-validated diagnostic criteria for IMA imaging, but the presence of post-stenotic turbulence would suggest a hemodynamically significant lesion.

Renal Arterial Duplex Protocol and Required Images

- Scan the abdominal aorta in longitudinal and axial sections from the level of the diaphragm to the bifurcation (see Chapter 4). Obtain an image of the midportion of the longitudinal aorta.
  1. Longitudinal image of the **MID AORTA.**

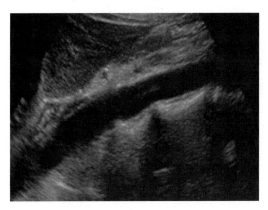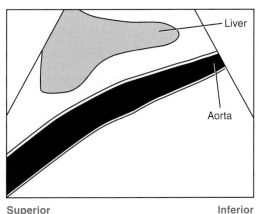

Labeled: **SAG AO**

- In a transverse scanning plane, image the axial aorta at the level of the SMA. Identify the longitudinal section of the left renal vein as it crosses anterior to the aorta immediately posterior to the SMA origin. Locate the long sections of the right and left renal arteries just posterior to the renal veins.
  2. Axial image of the aorta at the level of the left renal vein and **ORIGIN** of the **RENAL ARTERIES.**

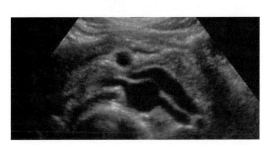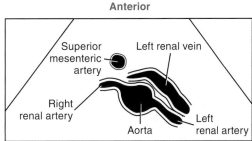

Labeled: **TRV ORIGIN RT** and/or **LT REN ART**

All images courtesy Penn State Hershey Vascular Noninvasive Diagnostic Laboratory, Hershey, Pa.

- Continuously sample with Doppler from within the lumen of the aorta into the orifice of the renal artery by moving the Doppler sample volume slowly along this path. This will allow detection of possible stenosis at the origin of the renal artery.

  3. Transition waveforms from the origin of the **RT** or **LT RENAL ARTERY.**

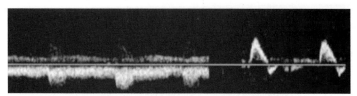

Labeled: **ORIGIN RT** or **LT REN ART**

Gray-scale version of color Doppler spectral waveforms showing the transition of flow patterns from the aorta through the orifice of the renal artery. See Color Plate 16.

- Using gray-scale or color-flow imaging, follow the course of the renal artery from the proximal to the midsegment of the vessel.

  4. Longitudinal image of **PROX-MID RT** or **LT RENAL ARTERY.**

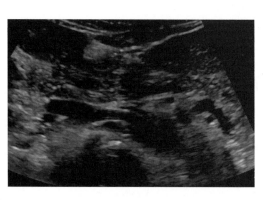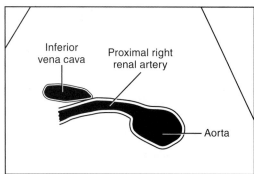

Labeled: **TRV RT** or **LT REN ART PROX – MID**

- Sample continuously with Doppler throughout the visualized length of the renal artery. It is important to avoid "spot-checking" the renal segments because short, focal lesions that do not propagate flow disturbance very far downstream may be present.

   5. Doppler spectral waveforms from the proximal and midsegments of the **RENAL ARTERY.**

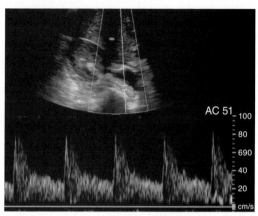

Labeled: **RT** or **LT REN ART PROX – MID**
Gray-scale version of color Doppler spectral waveforms from the proximal to midsegment of the renal artery.

- Move the patient to a lateral decubitus or other position that allows adequate visualization of the kidney and distal to midrenal artery. Image the renal artery from the hilum of the kidney as far proximally as possible.

   6. Axial view of the kidney demonstrating the longitudinal section of the distal to midsegments of the **RENAL ARTERY.**

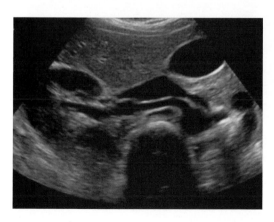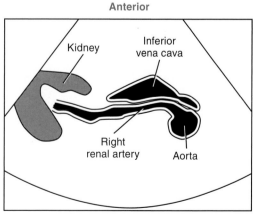

Labeled: **TRV RT** or **LT REN ART DIST – MID**

- Sample continuously with Doppler from the level of the renal hilum throughout the distal to midrenal artery. Take care to use a similar range of Doppler angles as used in to visualize the proximal to midsegments of the artery.
7. Doppler spectral waveforms from the distal and midsegments of the **RENAL ARTERY.**

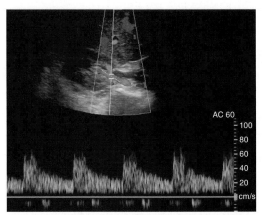

Labeled: **RT** or **LT REN ART DIST – MID**
Gray-scale version of the color Doppler spectral waveforms from the distal to midsegments of the renal artery.

- Obtain a longitudinal view of the kidney. Measure the long axis. Color flow or power Doppler imaging may facilitate demonstration of arterial and venous perfusion of the organ parenchyma.
8. **LONG AXIS** image of the kidney *with measurement.*

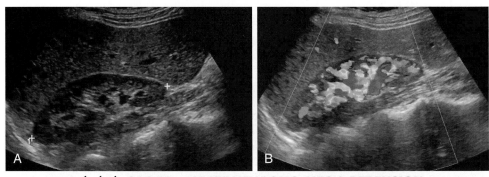

Labeled: **SAG RT** or **LT KIDNEY LONG AXIS & PERFUSION**
Image of the kidney demonstrating long axis measurement **(A)** and the gray-scale version of color perfusion **(B)**.

- Sample with Doppler throughout the intersegmental arteries of the renal medulla (sinus) and the arcuate arteries within the renal cortex. It is not uncommon to obtain both arterial and venous signals within the same sample volume at cortical level because of the small size of the vessels and the arteriovenous shunting that occurs at this location within the organ.

9. Doppler spectral waveforms from the **RENAL MEDULLA** and **CORTEX.**

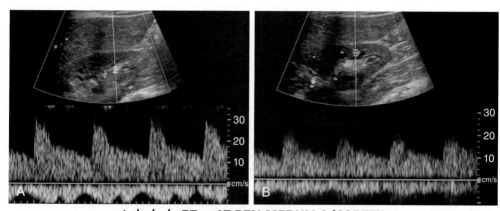

Labeled: **RT** or **LT REN MEDULLA/CORTEX**
Gray-scale versions of the color Doppler spectral waveforms from the renal medulla **(A)** and cortex **(B)**.

NOTE: Approximately 20% of patients will have more than one renal artery on each side. For reasons that are not well understood, this finding is more commonly seen on the left side. These duplicated or accessory polar renal arteries may be detected using several strategies:

• Power Doppler imaging may be useful because this technique relies on the intensity of the signal and is less affected by the angle of insonation than color Doppler imaging.

• Accessory renal arteries usually course to the surface of a pole of the kidney. As a consequence, the Doppler signals from the renal pole with the additional artery may have higher amplitude than signals from other kidney regions.

• Enlarge the Doppler sample volume and scan along the wall of the aorta to locate additional low-resistance renal arterial signals. Additional renal arteries may arise anywhere along the aortic wall from above the primary renal arteries to the level of the common iliac arteries.

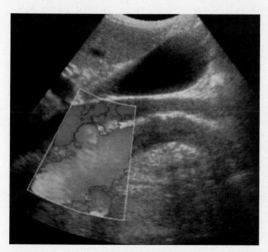 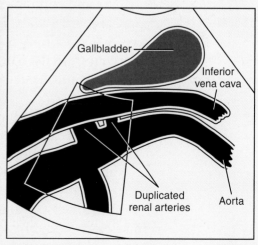

Superior   Inferior

Gray-scale version of a sagittal scanning plane, color flow image of the abdominal aorta and duplicated right renal arteries.

Abdominal Venous Blood Flow Patterns and Duplex Protocols

- Phasicity (the role respiration plays in venous blood flow patterns) varies throughout the abdominal venous system.
  - Portal and splenic veins show minimal respiratory phasicity. In contrast, the hepatic veins and inferior vena caval Doppler spectral waveforms demonstrate both respirophasicity and cardiac influences.

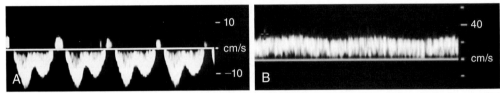

Venous Doppler spectral waveforms demonstrating the pulsatile flow pattern found in a hepatic vein **(A)** and the minimally phasic flow pattern found in the main portal vein **(B)**.

- Absence of respiratory phasicity suggests obstruction to venous outflow or extrinsic compression of the vein distal to the sampling site.

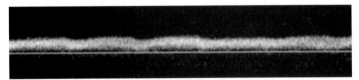

Gray-scale version of the color Doppler spectral waveform demonstrating absence of respiratory phasicity.

- Acute and chronic venous thrombosis normally differ in acoustic properties.
  - Acute thrombus usually has acoustically homogeneous echogenicity. The thrombus is loosely attached to the vein walls and has a smooth surface contour. The vein may be dilated.
  - Chronic thrombus has a continuum of acoustic properties. Initially, the thrombus increases in echogenicity, but over time, the echogenicity fluctuates. The thrombus may have anechoic areas due to necrosis within the clot. The thrombus is usually firmly attached to the vein walls and has an irregular surface contour.
- In cases of venous hypertension, the splanchnic vessels may dilate to exceed 1.5 cm in diameter.

Required Diagnostic Data
- **Inferior vena cava (IVC):**
  - Demonstrate impedance to outflow caused by thrombus or extrinsic compression.
  - Assess for thrombus surrounding IVC clips or filters.
  - Must document patency of the IVC in all patients with a liver transplant.
  - Rule out propagation of tumor thrombus from renal masses.
- **Splenic vein:**
  - See the section on mesenteric ischemia.
  - Confirm patency and flow direction.
- **Superior mesenteric vein:**
  - See the section on mesenteric ischemia.
  - Confirm patency and flow direction.
- **Portal vein:**
  - Normally has steady, minimally phasic flow.
  - Assess for thrombus; if thrombosed, assess for recanalization or evidence of collateral channels.
  - Confirm hepatopetal flow direction.
  - Marked respiratory variations suggest portal hypertension. Such signals are caused by increased hepatic vascular resistance.
  - Portal vein branches should be differentiated from dilated biliary ducts.
- **Renal veins:**
  - Normally have steady, minimally phasic flow.
  - Assess for patency and propagation of renal tumor thrombus.
  - If the renal vein is obstructed, the arterial signals within the renal parenchyma usually exhibit rapid systolic upstroke and rapid systolic deceleration to a reverse, blunted diastolic flow component.

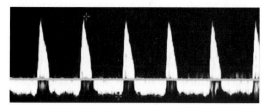

Doppler spectral waveforms recorded within the renal parenchyma demonstrating the blood flow pattern consistent with renal vein thrombosis.

NOTE: Although color flow imaging may facilitate identification of venous anatomic anomalies, collateralization, recanalization, and confirmation of partial venous thrombosis, it is important to recognize that color may overwrite an acute, acoustically homogeneous thrombus. In most cases, it is best to evaluate the venous system using gray-scale imaging and complement the study with color imaging only as needed.

Scanning Tips

- **Vascular tumors:** often have 3 primary characteristics:
  1. High-amplitude signals.
  2. Increased peak systolic velocities.
  3. A "roaring" sound caused by edge motion and interference from the increased vascularity.
- **Hepatomata:** demonstrate high pitched signals due to arteriovenous communications.
- **Pseudoaneurysms:** caused by puncture of two or all three layers of the arterial wall resulting in escape of blood into the surrounding tissue (contained hematoma). They may have disorganized, pulsatile, or circular flow with low velocity signals within the hypoechoic or anechoic blood-filled mass.
  - Are located most often near a vessel branch or surgical anastomosis.
  - A characteristic "to-fro" Doppler flow pattern is noted within the tract, or pedicle, which connects the pseudoaneurysm to the artery.
  - If thrombosed, no Doppler signal should be obtained within the pedicle or the pseudoaneurysm.
- **Arteriovenous fistulae:**
  - The arterial component will demonstrate increased velocity and a decreased resistive index proximal to the arteriovenous communication.
  - The outflow vein should demonstrate pulsatility.
- **Gallbladder cancer versus sludge:**
  - Low flow is usually evident within a malignant tumor.
  - Sludge has no flow.

Gynecologic Studies

- Duplex and color Doppler imaging are routinely used for the following transabdominal and/or endovaginal evaluations.
  - Identification of the dominant follicle or corpus luteal cyst in patients with pelvic pain or suspected ectopic pregnancy.
  - Detection of placental tissue in abnormal intrauterine pregnancy, ectopic pregnancy, or retained products of conception.
  - Diagnosis of ovarian torsion.
  - Detection and characterization of ovarian and adnexal masses.
  - Identification of fibroids, polyps, tumors, arteriovenous fistulae, and/or pelvic congestion syndrome.

- Transabdominal studies are usually performed with transducer frequency ranges of 2.5 to 5 MHz.
- Endovaginal scans are performed with transducer frequency ranges of 5 to 10 MHz.
- A 0-degree angle of insonation is used for small vessels when the direction of flow cannot be determined.

Vascular Anatomy

- The uterine artery is a branch of the internal iliac artery. It enters the uterus at the lower uterine segment and sends branches toward the uterine fundus, cervix, and ovaries in the broad ligament.
- The ovarian arteries originate from the abdominal aorta and course inferiorly to the pelvis. The ovaries also receive branches from the uterine artery.

Blood Flow Patterns

- The uterine artery in a nongravid woman should demonstrate a high-resistance flow pattern with low diastolic flow. A reflected wave (dicrotic notch) is noted on the deceleration phase of systole.

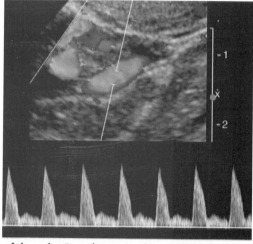

Gray-scale version of the color Doppler spectral waveforms from the uterine artery in a nongravid woman. (Courtesy Philips Medical Ultrasound, Seattle, Wash.)

- During the second trimester of pregnancy, vascular resistance decreases and diastolic flow increases.

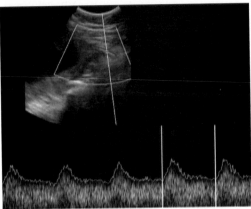

Doppler spectral waveforms from a pregnant woman. (Courtesy Janice Hickey-Scharf, Picton, Ontario, Canada.)

- An active ovary (luteal phase) shows increased peak systolic flow and a diastolic forward flow component. Color Doppler demonstrates a ring of neovascularization around the luteal cyst.
- The diastolic flow component is absent in an inactive ovary.
  - Diastolic flow decreases normally during the follicular phase of ovulation.
  - Spectral Doppler waveforms from postmenopausal ovaries are similar to those observed in inactive ovaries in the follicular state. Power Doppler imaging may facilitate identification of the low-velocity flow.
- Ectopic pregnancies: spectral or color Doppler may help show trophoblastic flow with high diastolic flow components.
- Ovarian torsion: findings include detection of an enlarged ovary in an unusual location (midline superior to the uterus, flank, or cul-de-sac) and absence of arterial and/or venous flow within the ovary. Blood flow may be absent or reversed in the ovarian vessels. Low-velocity flow may be observed around the periphery of the ovary. Color Doppler may facilitate identification of coiling or twisting of the vascular pedicle.
- Infertility: may help to demonstrate the presence of ovarian flow associated with ovulation.

Obstetric Studies

NOTE: Remember to scan prudently.

- Increased vascular resistance within the umbilical artery may be directly related to the presence of intrauterine growth retardation (IUGR).
- The umbilical artery may show the following changes when IUGR is present because of increased placental pressure:
  - Increased vascular resistance.
  - Decreased diastolic flow in the umbilical artery.
- Doppler of the umbilical cord is performed to:
  - Identify a 3-vessel cord.
  - Assess cord insertions.
  - Rule out nuchal cord.

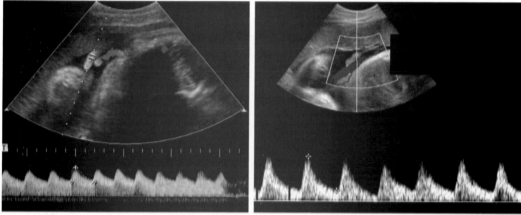

Gray-scale versions of the color Doppler spectral waveforms from umbilical arteries demonstrating variation in the level of vascular resistance. (Courtesy Janice Hickey-Scharf, Picton, Ontario, Canada.)

- Doppler of the fetal heart will help to identify cardiac chambers and flow patterns.
- Doppler of the placenta:
  - Rule out chorioangiomata versus placental lakes.

Breast Sonography

Vascular Anatomy

- The posterior intercostal arteries arise from the thoracic aorta and supply the lateral aspect of the breast.

- The subclavian artery gives rise to the internal thoracic artery, which supplies the medial aspect of the breast.
- A branch of the axillary artery gives rise to the lateral thoracic artery, which supplies blood flow to the posterior aspect of the breast.
  - Current studies are showing an increase in detection of Doppler signals in malignant lesions versus nonmalignant lesions.

Scrotal Sonography

Vascular Anatomy

- The testicular artery originates from the aorta and courses in the retroperitoneum to enter the inguinal canal in the spermatic cord.
- The inferior vesicle artery gives rise to the deferential artery within the spermatic cord. The artery courses to the tail of the epididymis where it divides into a capillary network. Does not supply testicular tissue.

Blood Flow Patterns

- The largest vessels are visualized peripherally.
- The testicular artery has low peripheral resistance with broad systolic peaks and high diastolic flow.
  - Resistive index is generally 0.55 to 0.64, with an accepted range by some of 0.46 to 0.78.
- The deferential artery has high resistance with narrow systolic peaks and low diastolic flow.
- Scrotal veins normally demonstrate low-velocity, phasic flow.

Pathology

- Erectile dysfunction:
  - Doppler evaluation is performed before and injection of vasoactive agents into the intercavernosal tissues:
    - *Preinjection:* peak systolic velocities in the cavernosal arteries are normally greater than 13 cm/sec with a high-resistance flow pattern demonstrating absent or reversed diastolic flow. No flow is evident in the deep dorsal vein.
    - *Postinjection:* a continuum of flow patterns is normally noted. Immediately following injection—increased flow with a low-resistance flow pattern. Three to five minutes postinjection—peak systolic velocity greater than 35 cm/sec with a high-resistance flow pattern. At full tumescence, peak systolic velocities decrease and diastolic flow is absent or reversed. No flow in the deep dorsal vein with color or power Doppler imaging.

- *Dorsal venous incompetence:* presence of flow in the dorsal vein or persistent cavernosal arterial diastolic velocity greater than 5 cm/sec. Absent dorsal venous flow with persistent high diastolic arterial flow suggests leakage of venous blood through the crural veins.
- Inflammatory conditions:
  - Epididymitis.
  - Orchitis.
  - Increased number of blood vessels noted in region of affected area.
  - Increased venous flow in the epididymis.
  - Enlarged; low-gray epididymis.
- Abscesses:
  - Demonstrate hypervascularity.
  - Have decreased resistive indices.
  - Gray-scale image shows decreased echogenicity caused by edema.
- Torsion/ischemia:
  - Complete or near complete absence of flow.
  - Diminished flow may be seen in early or partial torsion.
  - Spontaneous resolution of torsion may demonstrate normal or increased blood flow to testis.
  - Nuclear medicine is still the imaging study of choice.
- Neoplasms:
  - Gray-scale images remain the most helpful in defining masses.
  - Spectral, color, and/or power Doppler may help to confirm vascular tumors.
- Varicoceles:
  - Dilated peritesticular veins that form as sequelae of valvular incompetence.
  - Often easily visible with gray-scale imaging.
  - Flow may be too slow to be detected during normal respiration.
  - A vein larger than 3 mm in diameter apparent during a Valsalva maneuver is considered a varicocele.
  - The study is often facilitated with color Doppler imaging.
  - Check renal veins for tumor and/or thrombus.

Review Questions

Answers on page 630.

1. As the carrier Doppler frequency increases,
   a) blood flow detection decreases.
   b) tissue penetration increases.
   c) resolution increases.
   d) Doppler shift frequency decreases.

2. Aliasing may be corrected by
   a) decreasing the PRF.
   b) changing the angle of insonation.
   c) raising the zero baseline.
   d) increasing the Doppler frequency.

3. Which of the following vessels serves as an excellent landmark for locating the renal arteries?
   a) Left renal vein
   b) Celiac artery
   c) Splenic vein
   d) Aorta

4. The uterine artery in a nongravid woman normally demonstrates
   a) constant forward diastolic flow.
   b) reversed diastolic flow.
   c) blunted diastolic flow.
   d) low diastolic flow.

5. The most accurate estimation of velocity occurs at a Doppler insonation angle of
   a) 0 degrees.
   b) 40 degrees.
   c) 60 degrees.
   d) 90 degrees.

6. Power Doppler is most useful for evaluating
   a) high-velocity flow.
   b) turbulent flow.
   c) laminar flow.
   d) off-axis flow.

7. Minimal respiratory phasicity is normally seen in the
   a) splenic vein.
   b) hepatic veins.
   c) portal veins.
   d) vena cava.

8. In a fasting patient, all of the following exhibit low resistance flow patterns EXCEPT the
   a) hepatic artery.
   b) superior mesenteric artery.
   c) renal artery.
   d) celiac artery.

9. Doppler spectral waveforms from a renal transplant during an episode of acute rejection exhibit
   a) elevated diastolic flow.
   b) increased systolic flow.
   c) low diastolic flow.
   d) turbulent flow.

10. Color Doppler exhibits
    a) mean velocity estimates.
    b) peak flow estimates.
    c) median flow estimates.
    d) peak velocity estimates.

11. Retrograde flow in the common hepatic artery suggests
    a) aberrant anatomy.
    b) portal hypertension.
    c) splenic artery stenosis.
    d) celiac artery occlusion.

12. All of the following statements apply to accessory renal arteries EXCEPT
    a) they course to the surface of a renal pole.
    b) they are more common on the left side.
    c) they occur in more than 40% of the population.
    d) they are often detected with power Doppler.

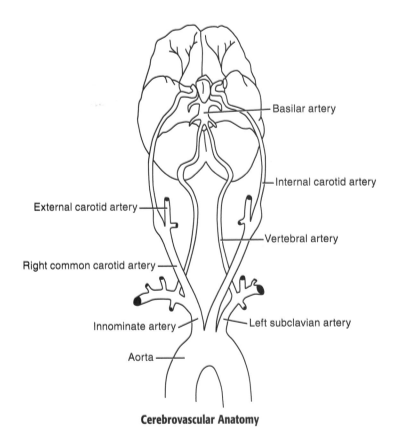

Basilar artery

Internal carotid artery

External carotid artery

Vertebral artery

Right common carotid artery

Innominate artery

Left subclavian artery

Aorta

Cerebrovascular Anatomy

CHAPTER 20

Cerebrovascular Duplex Scanning Protocol

Marsha M. Neumyer

Key Words

Anterior cerebral circulation	Low-vascular resistance beds
Basilar artery	Posterior cerebral circulation
Carotid bulb	Right common carotid artery
High-vascular resistance beds	Vertebral artery
Left common carotid artery	

Objectives

At the end of this chapter, you will be able to:

- Define the key words.
- Describe the normal anatomy of the extracranial cerebrovascular system and indicate common anatomic variations.
- Define the signature blood flow patterns associated with vessels supplying low- and high-resistance vascular beds.
- Explain issues relating to choice of transducer frequency.
- Detail appropriate patient and sonographer positioning for sonographic evaluation of the extracranial cerebrovascular arteries with emphasis on correct application of ergonomics.
- Describe the duplex scanning survey of the extracranial cerebrovascular system and detail the images that are required to ensure an accurate interpretation.
- Answer the review questions at the end of the chapter.

Overview

Location
- Medial to internal jugular vein.
- Lateral to thyroid gland.
- Posteromedial to sternocleidomastoid muscle.

Anatomy
- Right common carotid artery originates from the innominate (brachiocephalic) artery.
- Left common carotid artery originates from the aortic arch.
- At the superior border of the thyroid cartilage (vertebrae C2 to C3), the common carotid artery bifurcates into an anteromedial

507

external carotid artery and a posterolateral internal carotid artery. The level and anatomic configuration of the bifurcation are variable. The carotid bulb, which may be referred to simply as the bifurcation, may not be geometrically distinct. The bulb may be part of the common carotid artery and the internal and/or external carotid artery. The external carotid artery may lie posterior and lateral or posterior and medial to the internal carotid artery.

- The external carotid can be differentiated from the internal carotid artery by the presence of branches within the neck. The internal carotid artery normally has no extracranial branches.
- The internal carotid artery usually has a larger diameter than the external, although this is variable.
- The common, internal, and external carotid arteries form the anterior cerebral circulation.
- The vertebral artery originates from the subclavian artery and courses superiorly and posteriorly, entering the transverse processes of the vertebrae at C6 and exiting between C1-C2. The left vertebral artery is often greater in diameter than the right.
- The vertebral arteries join to form the basilar artery. Together, these vessels make up the posterior cerebral circulation.

Physiology

- The common carotid artery provides blood flow to both low- and high-resistance vascular beds. Approximately 80% of the blood flow from the common carotid artery enters the internal carotid artery to supply blood flow to the low-resistance vascular tissues of the brain and eye. Because of this high-flow demand, the Doppler spectral waveform from the common carotid artery is characterized by a low-resistance blood flow pattern. The remaining 20% of the blood flow volume from the common carotid enters the external carotid artery to supply the high-resistance muscular tissues of the face and scalp.
- The internal carotid artery provides blood flow to the low-resistance anterior cerebral circulation. The blood flow pattern of the internal carotid artery is characterized by constant forward diastolic flow.
- The external carotid artery provides blood flow to the high-resistance vascular bed of the muscles of the face, forehead, and scalp. The blood flow pattern of the external carotid artery is characterized by low diastolic flow.
- The vertebral artery provides blood flow to the low-resistance vascular bed of the posterior cerebral hemispheres. As such, its blood flow pattern is characterized by constant forward diastolic flow.

NOTE: Low-resistance vascular beds consist of tissues that require blood flow throughout the cardiac cycle. They have high metabolic demands and oxygen usage. In addition to the internal carotid and vertebral arteries, examples of low-resistance vascular beds include the renal and hepatic arteries. In contrast, **high-resistance vascular beds** are formed of tissues that normally have a low metabolic demand in the resting state and, as such, exhibit low diastolic flow. In addition to the external carotid artery, examples of high-resistance vascular beds include the lower extremity muscle in a patient at rest and the superior mesenteric artery in a patient who is fasting.

Sonographic Appearance
- In the normal vessel, lumen should be echo-free.
- If viewing the vessel at a perpendicular angle, note that the arterial walls are echogenic. This reflectivity results from acoustic properties of collagen fibers found within the intima and media of the arterial wall and helps to sonographically differentiate arteries and veins.

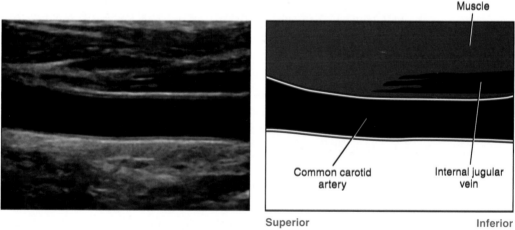

Common carotid artery demonstrating echogenic arterial walls.

- Using multiple scan planes, you should be able to image the common carotid artery, the carotid bulb (bifurcation), and the external and internal carotid and vertebral arteries as separate arterial segments.

Preparation

Patient Prep
- None.

Images in this chapter courtesy Penn State Hershey Vascular Noninvasive Diagnostic Laboratory, Hershey, Pa.

Pulsed Doppler Transducers

- 10.0-MHz to 12.0-MHz linear array: offers better resolution, but may not be able to visualize all anatomy if vessels lie deep within the neck.
- 7.5-MHz linear array: allows slightly better penetration.
- 5.0-MHz linear array: may require use of a standoff pad because of decreased resolution unless using a broadband transducer with auto focusing.
- 2.0-MHz to 4.0-MHz curved array: useful for imaging the innominate and proximal left common carotid artery in some patients.

Patient Position

- Supine with the head resting flat or slightly elevated on a thin pillow, and turned slightly away from the side to be scanned. Hyperextension of the neck must be avoided because this will make it difficult to maintain full transducer contact with the skin and may cause the vessels to lie in an inappropriate anatomic plane.
- As the examiner, you should sit at the head of the examination table with the patient's head directly in front of you. You should be able to rest your elbow on the corner of the table or the end of the pillow. This arm position ensures minimal compression of the carotid vessels by the transducer and an appropriate ergonomic position of your arm and shoulder. You must then scan ambidextrously to be able to reach the ultrasound system easily.
- Alternatively, you may stand beside the examination table and lean one arm across the patient's chest to reach the neck. Care must be taken to ensure that your arm is supported and not at a right angle to your body. A pillow may be placed over the patient's chest to ensure his or her comfort.
- The examination may also be performed with the patient in an erect position if he or she is unable to lie down. Care must be taken to ensure that your arm is supported and not at a right angle to your body.

Cerebrovascular Duplex Survey

1. The purpose of the survey is to identify arterial wall abnormalities, vessel tortuosity, pathology, and anatomic anomalies. The initial survey is performed with gray-scale (B-Mode) imaging to ensure that features of the arterial wall and plaque morphology are accurately characterized.

2. Initiate the survey on the right side of the neck immediately superior to the clavicle with the transducer in a transverse scanning plane anterior to the sternocleidomastoid muscle. Identify the jugular vein. Move medially to detect the proximal common carotid artery and identify the thyroid gland.

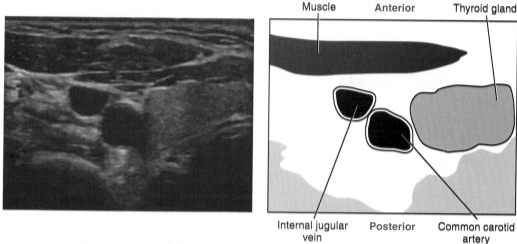

Transverse B-Mode image of common carotid artery with thyroid gland.

3. Return to the transverse view of the proximal common carotid artery. Begin the axial survey of the right common carotid artery.
4. Angle as inferiorly as possible to image the origin of the right common carotid artery.
5. Slowly scan superiorly, noting vessel walls, tortuosity, and anatomic anomalies.
6. At the level of the bifurcation make special note of the carotid bulb, the presence of plaque, and the origin of the bifurcation vessels.
7. Continue to follow the course of the internal and external carotid arteries, imaging as far superiorly as possible.
8. Return to the proximal common carotid artery immediately superior to the clavicle.
9. Rotate the transducer 90 degrees to achieve a sagittal scanning plane. Place the transducer anterior to the sternocleidomastoid muscle (or posterior to the muscle in a sagittal scanning plane or laterally in a coronal imaging plane).
10. Move laterally and identify the jugular vein. Move medially through the common carotid artery and identify the thyroid gland.
11. Return to the longitudinal view of the common carotid artery and angle as inferiorly as possible to view the common carotid artery origin, the distal segment of the innominate artery, and the proximal subclavian artery.

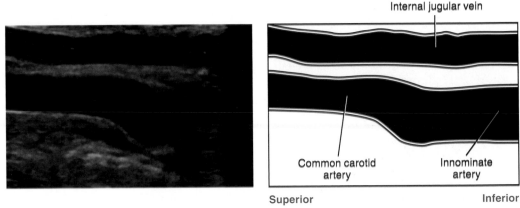

Sagittal B-Mode image of distal innominate artery and proximal common carotid artery.

12. Return to the longitudinal view of the common carotid artery. Slowly move the transducer superiorly, continuously rocking through the vessel medial to lateral to view as much of the vessel wall as possible.

13. While at the level of the midsegment of the common carotid artery, angle the probe in a posterolateral manner and look for the acoustic shadowing indicating the vertebral bodies. Coursing between the vertebral bodies, you should see the vertebral artery, which commonly lies posterior to the vertebral vein. Angle the probe in a very slight medial/lateral manner to ensure the best visualization of the artery. Follow the course of the vertebral artery inferiorly to its origin from the subclavian artery.

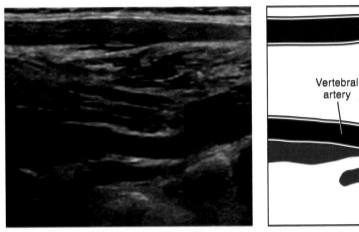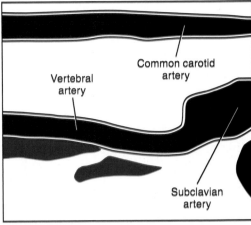

Sagittal B-Mode image of the vertebral artery at its origin from the subclavian artery.

14. Angle the probe anteromedially to return to the common carotid artery survey.
15. Continue to scan superiorly to the level of the bifurcation. Keeping the distal segment of the common carotid artery in view, rock the transducer in an anteromedial/posterolateral motion, and identify the internal and external carotid arteries. Make note of the presence and location of plaque and anatomic abnormalities.

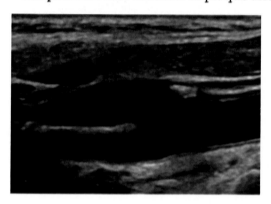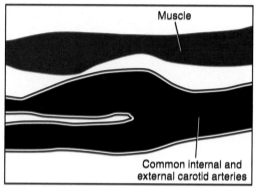

Superior   Inferior

Sagittal B-Mode image of the carotid bifurcation.

NOTE: As you move the transducer superiorly, it may be easier to view a greater length of the internal carotid artery by moving from a more anterior or lateral approach to a more posterior approach.

16. Continue to move the transducer superiorly with a slight posteromedial angle to view the internal carotid artery. Continue to rock the transducer lateral to medial to view the length of the vessel walls completely. Follow the vessel walls as far superiorly as possible.

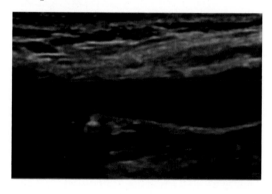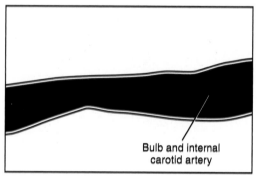

Superior   Inferior

Sagittal B-Mode image of the carotid bulb and internal carotid artery.

17. Return inferiorly to the level of the carotid bulb and rock the transducer anteromedially to identify the external carotid artery. Move the probe superiorly along the length of the external carotid artery, rocking laterally and medially through the vessel to fully visualize the arterial walls.

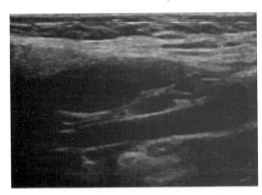 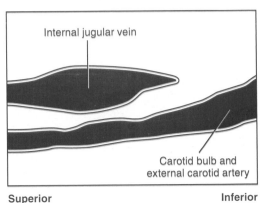

Superior   Inferior

Sagittal B-Mode image of the carotid bulb and external carotid artery.

18. Once you have viewed both the internal and external carotid arteries in a longitudinal plane, return to the level immediately superior to the clavicle to continue the survey with color flow imaging.

19. Maintain a sagittal scanning plane and initiate the color Doppler survey by turning on the color Doppler application (refer to the operator's manual for instrument specifications). Follow the common carotid artery longitudinally, adjusting the color scale, gain, and steering angle as necessary to accurately detail blood flow patterns throughout the vessel segments. You may need to scan more slowly to allow proper color filling of the arterial lumen.

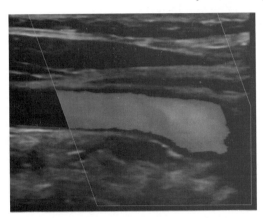 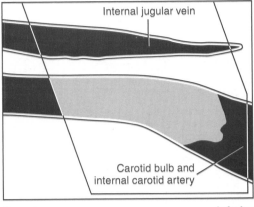

Superior   Inferior

Gray-scale version of the sagittal color flow image of distal innominate artery and common carotid artery. See Color Plate 17.

NOTE: Because the same physical principles apply to color Doppler and spectral Doppler, it is important to keep appropriate angle correction in mind when using color imaging. With color imaging, the pulse lines parallel the sides of the color box. To maintain color angles of insonation that are less than 60 degrees, it is often necessary to change the steering angle as the course of the artery changes.

20. Continuing the color Doppler survey, scan the length of the common carotid artery, bulb, and internal and external carotid arteries. Adjust the color Doppler controls as necessary to assess the quality of flow and to identify regions of disordered, turbulent, or absent flow.

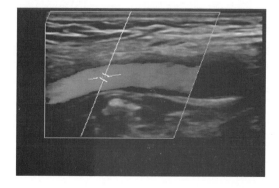 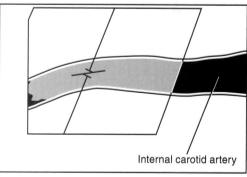

Superior   Inferior

Gray-scale version of the sagittal color flow image of the carotid bulb and internal carotid artery. See Color Plate 18.

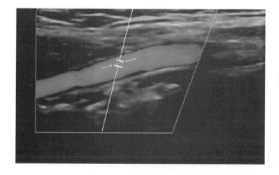 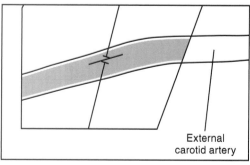

Superior   Inferior

Gray-scale version of the sagittal color flow image of the external carotid artery. See Color Plate 19.

21. Return to the level of the mid–common carotid artery. Angle the probe posterolaterally to image the vertebral artery in the midcervical segment of the neck. Note flow direction.

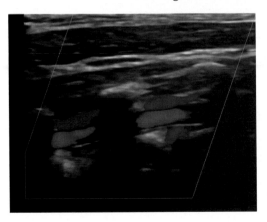

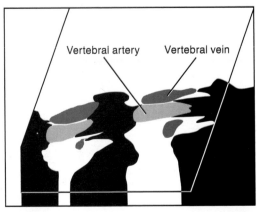

Superior   Inferior

Gray-scale version of the sagittal color flow image of the vertebral artery and vein in the midcervical segment of the neck. See Color Plate 20.

22. Scan the vertebral artery inferiorly to its origin. Note and confirm flow direction and any evidence of disordered or turbulent flow at this location.

> **NOTE:** Power Doppler imaging may be used in a similar manner as a complement to the color Doppler survey.

23. Return to the level immediately superior to the clavicle to continue the survey with spectral Doppler. Begin the survey by turning on the pulsed Doppler application (refer to the operator's manual for instrument specifications). Throughout the examination, adjust the Doppler angle of insonation (always 60 degrees or less with cursor parallel to the vessel wall), the sample volume location, and size as necessary to document blood flow patterns accurately throughout the vessel segments. A low Doppler wall filter should be used throughout the examination.

24. Identify the proximal common carotid artery in the sagittal imaging plane. Angle the probe as inferiorly as possible to view the common carotid artery origin, the distal segment of the innominate artery, and the proximal subclavian artery.

25. If plaque is visualized at the origin of the common carotid artery, sample the distal segment of the innominate artery and the origin of the common carotid artery. The right subclavian artery can be sampled at this location.

26. Continuing the Doppler spectral survey, sample throughout the common carotid artery, bulb, and internal and external carotid arteries. Adjust the Doppler sample size as necessary to assess the quality of flow and to identify regions of disordered or turbulent flow.

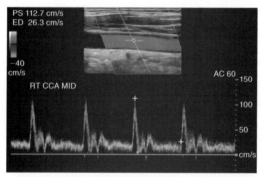

Gray-scale version of the sagittal color flow image and Doppler spectral waveforms from the mid-common carotid artery. See Color Plate 21.

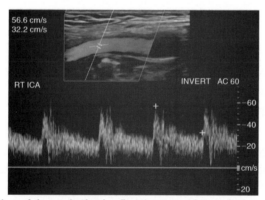

Gray-scale version of the sagittal color flow image and Doppler spectral waveforms from the internal carotid artery. See Color Plate 22.

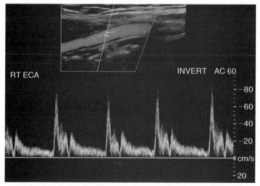

Gray-scale version of the sagittal color flow image and Doppler spectral waveforms from the external carotid artery. See Color Plate 23.

NOTE: Current validated diagnostic criteria for classification of disease severity in the internal carotid artery use a ratio of the highest angle-corrected velocity in the internal carotid to the systolic velocity recorded in the common carotid artery (CCA) 2 to 4 cm proximal to the carotid bulb (mid-to-distal CCA).

27. Return to the level of the mid–common carotid artery. Angle the probe posterolaterally to sample the vertebral artery in the mid-cervical segment of the neck. Note flow direction.
28. Scan the vertebral artery inferiorly to its origin. Note and confirm flow direction and any evidence of disordered or turbulent flow at this location.

NOTE: If plaque is present in any vessel segment, sample at sites proximal, within, and distal to the lesion(s) to determine the presence of disturbed flow or significant stenosis or to confirm occlusion.

29. Once flow has been assessed thoroughly in all vessels, return to the level of the clavicle and the proximal common carotid artery and obtain required images and Doppler spectral waveforms.

NOTE: A high or deep carotid bifurcation may make it very difficult to differentiate vessels by appearance alone. Always use spectral Doppler waveforms.
NOTE: Long-standing occlusions of the internal carotid artery may result in enlargement of the external carotid artery and its branches, which may cause erroneous vessel identification.
NOTE: Flow disturbance may be present in tortuous or kinked vessels that are otherwise normal. The cause of flow disturbance should be determined because it may not be associated with pathology. Turbulent flow is not normal.
NOTE: It is best to use color Doppler after a thorough gray-scale survey in longitudinal and axial planes.

Cerebrovascular Duplex Required Images

1. Longitudinal image of the right proximal **COMMON CAROTID ARTERY.**

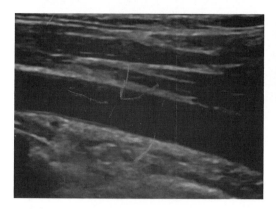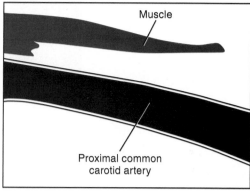

Superior   Inferior

Labeled: **SAG RT PCCA**

2. Spectral waveforms from the right proximal **COMMON CAROTID ARTERY** *with peak systolic and end-diastolic velocities measured.*

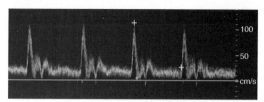

Labeled: **RT PCCA**

3. Longitudinal image of the right middle **COMMON CAROTID ARTERY.**

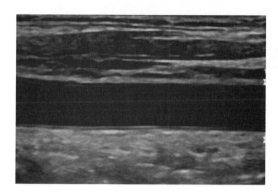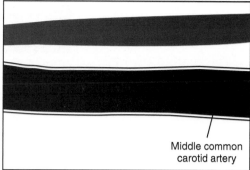

Superior   Inferior

Labeled: **SAG RT MCCA**

4. Spectral waveforms from the right middle **COMMON CAROTID ARTERY** *with peak systolic and end-diastolic velocities measured.*

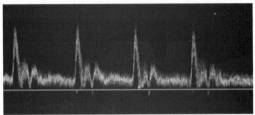

Labeled: **RT MCCA**

5. Longitudinal image of the right distal **COMMON CAROTID ARTERY.**

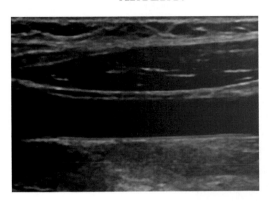 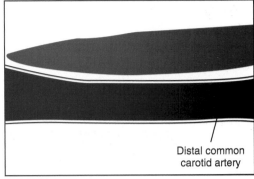

Distal common carotid artery

Superior   Inferior

Labeled: **SAG RT DCCA**

6. Spectral waveforms from the right distal **COMMON CAROTID ARTERY** *with peak systolic and end-diastolic velocities measured.*

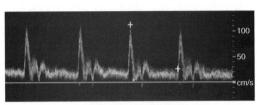

Labeled: **RT DCCA**

7. Longitudinal B-Mode image of the right **CAROTID BULB** (bifurcation).

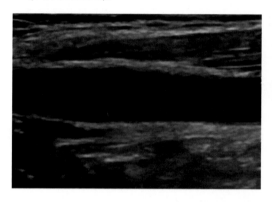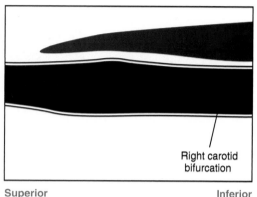

Superior   Inferior

Labeled: **SAG RT BIFURCATION**

8. Spectral waveforms from the right **CAROTID BULB** *with peak systolic and end-diastolic velocities measured.*

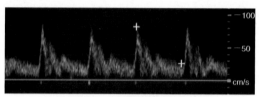

Labeled: **RT BIFURCATION**

9. Longitudinal B-Mode image of the right proximal **INTERNAL CAROTID ARTERY** at its origin.

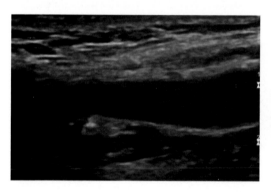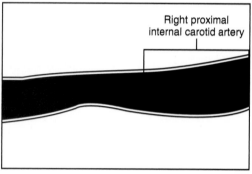

Superior   Inferior

Labeled: **SAG RT PICA**

10. Spectral waveforms from the right proximal **INTERNAL CAROTID ARTERY** *with peak and end-diastolic velocities measured.*

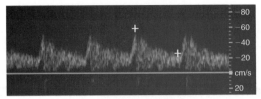

Labeled: **RT PICA**

11. Longitudinal B-Mode image of the right midsegment of the **INTERNAL CAROTID ARTERY.**

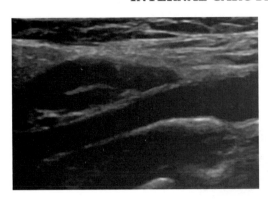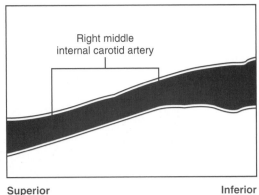

Right middle
internal carotid artery

Superior   Inferior

Labeled: **SAG RT MICA**

12. Spectral waveforms from the right midsegment of the **INTERNAL CAROTID ARTERY** *with peak and end-diastolic velocities measured.*

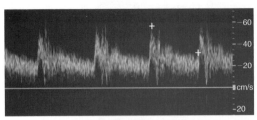

Labeled: **RT MICA**

13. Longitudinal B-Mode image of the right distal **INTERNAL CAROTID ARTERY.**

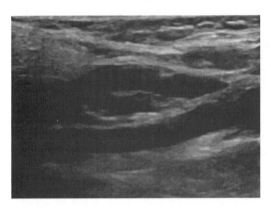 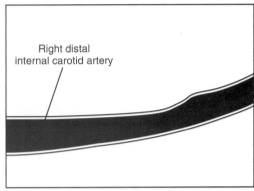

Right distal
internal carotid artery

Superior   Inferior

Labeled: **SAG RT DICA**

14. Spectral waveforms from the right distal internal carotid artery *with peak and end-diastolic velocities measured.*

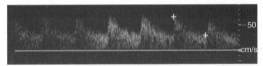

Labeled: **RT DICA**

15. Longitudinal B-Mode image of the right **EXTERNAL CAROTID ARTERY.**

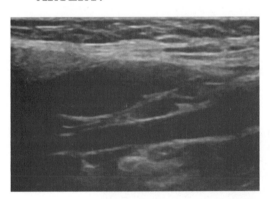 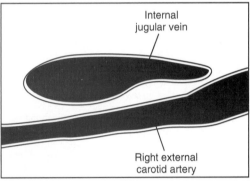

Internal
jugular vein

Right external
carotid artery

Superior   Inferior

Labeled: **SAG RT ECA**

16. Spectral waveforms representing the right **EXTERNAL CAROTID ARTERY** flow pattern *with peak and end-diastolic velocities measured.*

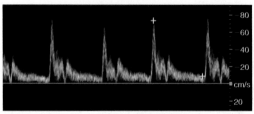

Labeled: **RT ECA**

17. Optional longitudinal B-Mode image of the right **VERTEBRAL ARTERY** in the midcervical segment of the neck.

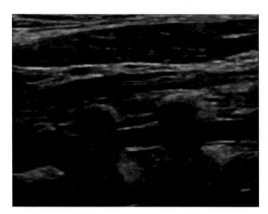
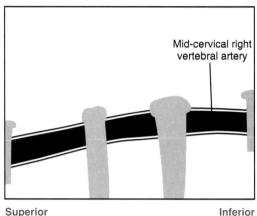

Labeled: **SAG MID-CERVICAL RT VERT**

18. Spectral waveforms from the right midcervical segment of the **VERTEBRAL ARTERY** *with peak systolic and end-diastolic velocities measured.*

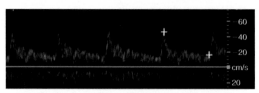

Labeled: **MID-CERVICAL RT VERT**

19. Longitudinal B-Mode image of the right **VERTEBRAL ARTERY** at its origin from the right subclavian artery.

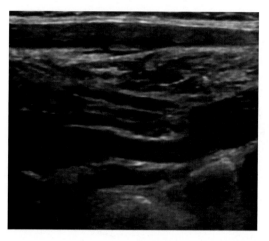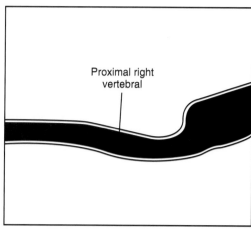

Superior   Inferior

Labeled: **SAG PROX RT VERT**

20. Spectral waveforms from the right proximal **VERTEBRAL ARTERY** *with peak systolic and end-diastolic velocities measured.*

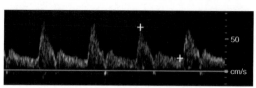

Labeled: **PROX RT VERT**

NOTE: Repeat the required images on the left side, beginning with a thorough survey.

NOTE: Even in the absence of visible pathology, it is important to carefully image the carotid bulb. This area is likely most prone to atherosclerosis because of shear forces imposed on the arterial wall by the moving blood and by the geometry of this region of the bifurcation. Stenotic lesions often remain asymptomatic until they produce a pressure-flow gradient (reducing the diameter of the arterial lumen by more than 60%). Lesser lesions may be detected only with careful, thorough scanning in the transverse and longitudinal planes.

Data Documentation

NOTE: Although the primary diagnostic criteria are based on velocity parameters, the study may be complemented with measurement of arterial plaque in the axial and sagittal image planes.

NOTE: Additional images of plaque may be necessary to define its acoustic properties (homogeneous, heterogeneous) and surface characteristics (smooth, irregular). Ulcerated lesions should be identified and measured in multiple image planes, and depth and width exceeding 2 mm should be noted.

Table 20-1   Current Diagnostic Criteria

| Degree of Stenosis | Primary Parameters | | Additional Parameters | |
	ICA PSV (cm/sec)	Plaque Estimate (%)	ICA/CCA PSV Ratio	ICA EDV (cm/sec)
Normal	<125	None	<2.0	<40
<50%	<125	<50	<2.0	<40
50%-69%	125-230	≥50	2.0-4.0	40-100
>70% but less than near occlusion	>230	≥50	>4.0	>100
>80% but less than near occlusion	>230	≥50	>4.0	>140
Near occlusion	High, low, or undetectable	Visible	Variable	Variable
Total occlusion	Undetectable	Visible, no detectable lumen	N/A	N/A

CCA, Common carotid artery; *EDV*, end-diastolic volume; *ICA*, internal carotid artery; *PSV*, peak systolic velocity.

Modified from Grant EG, Benson CB, Moneta GL, et al: Carotid artery stenosis: Gray-scale and Doppler US diagnosis—Society of Radiologists in Ultrasound Consensus Conference. *Radiology* 2003;229:340–346.

NOTE: The severity of internal carotid artery stenosis is commonly divided into the clinically relevant categories of >70% or >80% diameter reduction. The primary differentiation of the two categories is based on the end-diastolic velocity. The criteria from the Society of Radiologists in Ultrasound use an end-diastolic velocity >100 cm/sec to distinguish >70% stenosis, whereas the criteria from University of Washington employ an end-diastolic velocity >140 cm/sec to signify arterial diameter reduction >80%.

Review Questions

Answers on page 631.

1. Which of the following characterizes blood flow to a low-resistance vascular bed?
   a) Minimal spectral broadening
   b) Reversed diastolic flow
   c) Forward diastolic flow
   d) High amplitude

2. All of the following are points to remember when scanning the carotid arteries EXCEPT
   a) you may need to use a variety of scan planes.
   b) increased transducer pressure may be required to see deeper arterial segments.
   c) multiple transducer frequencies may be required.
   d) you may need to make slight rocking motions with the transducer to see vessel segments.

3. Which of the following is suggested by diastolic flow of 0 in a common carotid artery?
   a) Normal common carotid artery flow
   b) Proximal common carotid artery stenosis
   c) Proximal common carotid artery occlusion
   d) Distal carotid stenosis or occlusion

4. Atherosclerotic disease in the extracranial carotid arteries is most common
   a) within the carotid bulb and mid–common carotid artery.
   b) at points of bifurcations and within the carotid bulb.
   c) within the proximal common carotid artery and the origin of the internal carotid artery.
   d) in the internal and external carotid arteries.

5. Turbulent flow
   a) always occurs at vessel bifurcations.
   b) is associated with vessel bends and kinks.
   c) indicates stenosis exceeding 60%.
   d) should not be mistaken for pathology.

6. All of the following are associated with a normal vertebral artery EXCEPT
   a) low diastolic flow.
   b) antegrade flow.
   c) side-to-side diameter difference.
   d) rapid systolic upstroke.

7. The common carotid artery lies
   a) lateral to the internal jugular vein.
   b) medial to the superior thyroid cartilage.
   c) anterior to the sternocleidomastoid muscle.
   d) lateral to the thyroid gland.

8. The most accurate way to confirm the identity of the internal carotid artery is
   a) to look for absence of branches in the neck.
   b) to find low-resistance Doppler spectral waveforms.
   c) to note a larger diameter than the external carotid artery.
   d) to confirm its posterolateral course.

9. To obtain Doppler spectral waveforms the angle of insonation should be ≤60 degrees. The Doppler cursor should be
   a) aligned perpendicular to the vessel wall.
   b) aligned parallel to the color flow jet.
   c) aligned perpendicular to the color flow jet.
   d) aligned parallel to the vessel wall.

10. What is the best angle of insonation to use when examining the arterial wall?
    a) 0 degrees
    b) 40 degrees
    c) 60 degrees
    d) 90 degrees

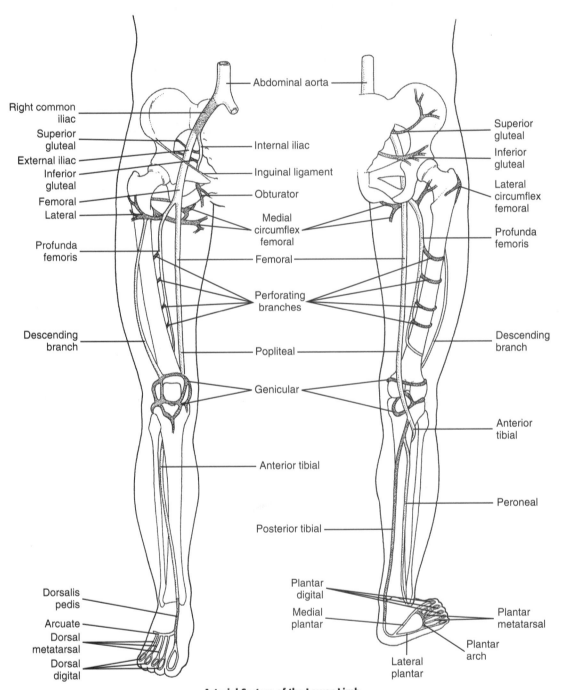

Right common iliac

Superior gluteal

External iliac

Inferior gluteal

Femoral

Lateral

Profunda femoris

Descending branch

Dorsalis pedis

Arcuate

Dorsal metatarsal

Dorsal digital

Abdominal aorta

Internal iliac

Inguinal ligament

Obturator

Medial circumflex femoral

Femoral

Perforating branches

Popliteal

Genicular

Anterior tibial

Posterior tibial

Plantar digital

Medial plantar

Lateral plantar

Superior gluteal

Inferior gluteal

Lateral circumflex femoral

Profunda femoris

Descending branch

Anterior tibial

Peroneal

Plantar metatarsal

Plantar arch

Arterial System of the Lower Limb

CHAPTER 21

Peripheral Arterial and Venous Duplex Scanning Protocols

Marsha M. Neumyer

Key Words

Augmentation	Respiratory phasicity
Coaptation	Soleal sinuses
Compressibility	Spontaneous flow
High vascular resistance	Sural veins
Lateral malleolus	Valves
Low vascular resistance	Valvular competence
Medial malleolus	Venous reflux

Objectives

At the end of this chapter, you will be able to:

- Describe the normal anatomy of the lower extremity arterial system and indicate common anatomic variations.
- Define the blood flow patterns associated with arteries supplying the high resistance vascular bed of the lower limb muscles.
- Explain issues relating to choice of transducer frequency.
- Detail appropriate patient and sonographer positioning for sonographic evaluation of the lower extremity arteries and veins with emphasis on correct application of ergonomic principles.
- Describe the duplex scanning survey of the lower extremity arterial and venous systems and detail the images that are required to ensure an accurate interpretation.
- Describe the normal anatomy of the lower extremity deep, superficial, and perforator venous systems and indicate common anatomic variations.
- Define normal and abnormal venous blood flow patterns.
- Answer the review questions at the end of the chapter.

Lower Extremity Arterial Duplex Ultrasonography Overview

Location

- *Abdominal aorta:* originates at the aortic hiatus of the diaphragm, courses left of midline, anterior to the vertebrae, and terminates at the fourth lumbar vertebra.
- *Aortic bifurcation:* originates approximately at level of the umbilicus to form the common iliac arteries.

- *Common iliac arteries:* terminate at the origin of the internal iliac (hypogastric) and external iliac arteries.
- *External iliac arteries:* originate at the common iliac artery bifurcation; form the common femoral artery just proximal to the inguinal ligament.
- *Lower extremity arterial system:* originates with common femoral artery just inferior to the inguinal ligament.

Anatomy

- *Abdominal aorta:* lies to the left of the midline and courses along the lower abdomen with a slight posterior-to-anterior angulation. The aorta tapers as it moves toward its bifurcation where it has a diameter of approximately 1.5 cm in a normal adult. It gives rise to the iliac arteries, which course through the pelvis to form the common femoral artery at the level of the inguinal ligament.
- *Common femoral artery:* lies lateral to the common femoral vein and bifurcates into the profunda femoris (deep femoral) artery and the superficial femoral artery.
- *Profunda femoris artery:* lies lateral to the superficial femoral artery and gives rise to branches that supply the region of the femoral head and the deep thigh muscles. In a small percentage of patients, the profunda femoris will originate medially from the common femoral artery.
- *Superficial femoral artery:* lies anterior to the femoral vein and courses along the anteromedial aspect of the thigh. It courses deep as it enters the adductor canal in the distal thigh where it becomes the popliteal artery.
- *Popliteal artery:* within the popliteal fossa lies anterior and medial to the popliteal vein and gives rise to small geniculate branches. It branches into the anterior tibial artery and the tibioperoneal trunk.
- *Anterior tibial artery:* passes superficial to the interosseous membrane and courses anteriorly along the membrane. Distally, the anterior tibial artery courses along the anterior aspect of the tibia and becomes the dorsalis pedis artery after crossing the ankle joint.
- *Tibioperoneal trunk:* gives rise to the posterior tibial and peroneal arteries that supply the calf muscles.
- *Posterior tibial artery:* originates between the tibia and the fibula and courses along the medial aspect of the calf to a midpoint between the medial malleolus (ankle bone) and the heel.
- *Peroneal artery:* originates from the tibioperoneal trunk and courses obliquely along the medial aspect of the fibula. The peroneal artery lies deep to the posterior tibial artery and in close apposition to the fibula.

Physiology

- The lower extremity arteries supply blood to the muscles of the thigh and calf. Normal resting muscle has a low flow demand. In contrast exercising muscle requires a significant increase in flow volume to oxygenate the tissues and carry away exercise-related toxins.
- In the resting state, normal muscle will exhibit a high-resistance blood flow pattern characterized by low diastolic flow. In contrast, exercising muscle has a low-resistance blood flow pattern, exhibiting constant forward diastolic flow.

Sonographic Appearance

- The normal vessel lumen should be echo-free.
- Using multiple scan planes, you should be able to image the vessel bifurcations, which may be off-axis.

Preparation

Patient Prep

- None.

Pulsed Doppler Transducers

- 5.0-MHz to 7.5-MHz linear array for thigh and calf in majority of patients.
- 2.0-MHz to 4.0-MHz curved array for abdominal aorta and iliac arteries and may be required to image upper thigh vessels in patients of large body habitus.

Patient Position

- Beginning with the patient in a supine position, obtain bilateral brachial systolic blood pressures using an appropriately sized blood pressure cuff (the width of the cuff bladder should exceed 20% of the limb diameter) and a continuous-wave Doppler transducer. Record the pressures on the worksheet (see the section on Data Documentation: Using Blood Pressures). In a similar manner, obtain bilateral ankle systolic pressure measurements from the dorsalis pedis and posterior tibial arteries by placing an appropriately sized blood pressure cuff immediately above the ankle. Record all tibial pressures on the worksheet and calculate the ankle/brachial index for both legs.
- Continue with the patient lying supine with the leg rotated outward and the knee slightly flexed in a frog-leg position to allow access to the common femoral artery and the popliteal fossa.
- Or have the patient lie prone with the feet slightly elevated on a pillow or rolled towel to allow access to the popliteal fossa.

• You may stand beside the examination table to scan the limb nearest to you. To ensure appropriate ergonomic positioning, make sure that your arm is supported and not at a right angle to your body and that the examination table has been raised to a height that is comfortable for you.

Lower Extremity Arterial Duplex Survey

1. The purpose of the survey is to identify arterial wall abnormalities, vessel tortuosity, pathology, and anatomic anomalies. The initial survey is performed with gray-scale (B-Mode) imaging to ensure that features of the arterial wall and plaque morphology are accurately characterized.

2. As clinically indicated or requested, initiate the survey superior to the umbilicus to image the mid-to-distal abdominal aorta. Beginning with the transducer in a transverse imaging plane, locate the axial section of the inferior vena cava lying to the right of the abdominal midline. Move the transducer left lateral to image the aorta.

3. Begin the axial survey of the mid-to-distal abdominal aorta. Scan inferiorly, noting vessel walls, tortuosity, diameter changes, and anatomic anomalies.

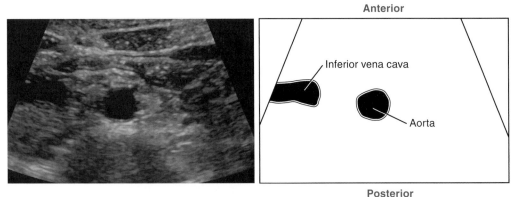

Axial image of the mid-to-distal abdominal aorta.

4. Locate the aortic bifurcation and identify the right and left common iliac arteries. Make special note of the presence of plaque and/or aneurysmal dilation.

5. Continue to scan inferiorly along the course of the right common iliac artery, noting its bifurcation into the internal and external iliac arteries and the curving deep to superficial course of the external iliac artery. The internal iliac artery commonly lies deep to the

external iliac artery. The external iliac artery lies superior to the external iliac vein.

NOTE: In many patients it may be difficult to image the common and external iliac arteries in the transverse imaging plane due to body habitus. In such cases, complete the survey of the iliac arteries using a sagittal imaging plane.

NOTE: The examination of the iliac arteries may be facilitated by having the patient lie in a lateral decubitus position and by placing the transducer medial to the anterior iliac spine and parallel to the iliac wing.

6. Continue to scan inferiorly to follow the external iliac artery to the level of the inguinal ligament where it becomes the common femoral artery.

NOTE: The aorta and iliac arteries are not routinely evaluated as part of the lower extremity arterial examination. The sonographic examination would be extended into the iliac arteries and the aorta if the Doppler spectral waveforms from the common femoral artery demonstrated delayed systolic upstroke consistent with proximal flow-limiting disease or if the patient's presenting symptoms indicated the likelihood of an aortoiliac lesion.

7. Immediately inferior to the inguinal ligament, confirm the identity of the common femoral artery by identifying the common femoral vein. If the iliac arteries have been scanned in the sagittal plane, rotate the transducer 90 degrees to assume a transverse imaging plane. Apply firm compression of the tissues over the vein with the transducer held perpendicular to the anterior vessel wall to distinguish the compressible vein from the noncompressible artery (see the section on Peripheral Venous Duplex Sonography in this chapter).

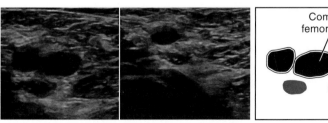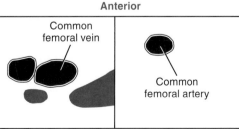

Transverse scanning plane, split-screen axial images of the common femoral artery and vein demonstrating venous compression.

8. Move the transducer laterally to identify the common femoral artery.

9. Continue the axial survey of the right common femoral artery. Angle as superiorly as possible to image the proximal right common femoral artery.

10. Scan inferiorly, noting vessel walls, tortuosity, and anatomic anomalies.

11. At the level of the bifurcation, make special note of the presence of plaque and the origin of the bifurcation vessels.

12. Scan the proximal to mid profunda femoris artery.

13. Return to the common femoral artery bifurcation.

14. Continue to follow the course of the superficial femoral artery, imaging as far inferiorly as possible.

15. At the level of the distal thigh, in the region of the adductor canal, the superficial femoral artery courses deeper into the tissues to become the popliteal artery. Visibility of the artery may be compromised at this level of the limb.

16. Move the transducer behind the knee into the popliteal fossa. With your free hand placed over the patella (knee cap), apply counterpressure to the knee. Angle the transducer superiorly and slightly medially to image the popliteal artery and vein. Confirm the identity of the artery by using a venous compression maneuver. Scan as superiorly into the distal thigh as possible.

17. Continue to follow the course of the popliteal artery, noting the presence of small geniculate branches and any diameter changes that would signify aneurysmal dilation.

18. Approximately 6 to 8 cm below the knee, the popliteal will give rise to the anterior tibial artery and the tibioperoneal trunk.

19. Follow the course of the proximal anterior tibial artery, noting the presence of plaque.

20. Return to the popliteal artery and follow the course of the tibioperoneal trunk. Note its bifurcation into the posterior tibial artery and the peroneal artery.

NOTE: Visibility of the posterior tibial and peroneal arteries may be facilitated by imaging the vessels from the medial side of the calf. In many patients, the peroneal artery can best be seen by imaging from the lateral aspect of the calf as the artery lies close to the fibula.

21. Follow the more superficial posterior tibial artery to the level of the medial malleolus (ankle) as it courses along the medial aspect of the calf.

22. Return to the bifurcation of the tibioperoneal trunk.
23. Follow the deeper lying peroneal artery to the level of the ankle as it courses along the medial aspect of the calf.

> **NOTE:** To image the popliteal and tibioperoneal arteries, it may be useful to place the patient in a prone position with the foot slightly elevated.

24. Return to the level of the umbilicus to complete the survey of the mid-to-distal abdominal aorta in the sagittal imaging plane.
25. Locate the inferior vena cava and the abdominal aorta. Rotate the transducer 90 degrees into the sagittal scanning plane to obtain a longitudinal view of these vessels.
26. Follow the course of the mid-to-distal aorta to the level of the bifurcation into the common iliac arteries. Obtain appropriately angle-corrected (angle of insonation 60 degrees or less with the cursor parallel to the vessel wall) Doppler spectral waveforms from the distal aorta, making careful note of regions of flow disturbance or turbulence.
27. Identify the right common iliac artery. Follow the longitudinal course of this vessel in the sagittal imaging plane. Obtain representative angle-corrected Doppler spectral waveforms from this vessel segment.

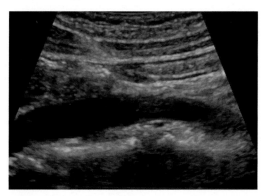 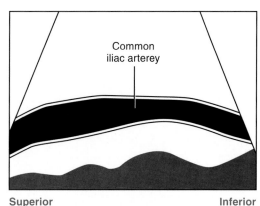

Common iliac arterey

Superior   Inferior

Sagittal scanning plane image of the right common iliac artery.

28. Continue to follow the course of the common iliac artery into the external iliac artery. Obtain representative Doppler spectral waveforms from this vessel segment.
29. Continue to move inferiorly to identify the longitudinal section of the common femoral artery. Obtain representative Doppler spectral waveforms from this vessel segment.

30. Identify the common femoral artery bifurcation. Scan the proximal to midsegment of the profunda femoris artery. Obtain representative Doppler spectral waveforms from this vessel segment.

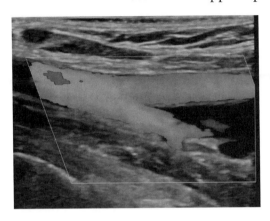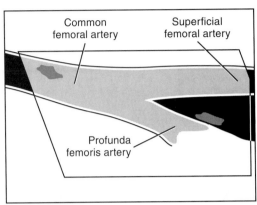

Gray-scale version of the sagittal scanning plane, color flow image of the longitudinal section of the common femoral artery bifurcation. See Color Plate 24.

31. Return to the common femoral artery bifurcation. Identify the origin of the superficial femoral artery. Obtain longitudinal images of this vessel segment and record representative Doppler spectral waveforms.
32. Continue to follow the course of the superficial femoral artery. Obtain longitudinal images of the mid and distal segments and record representative Doppler spectral waveforms from these vessel segments.
33. Place the transducer in the popliteal fossa to obtain longitudinal images of the popliteal artery. Obtain representative Doppler spectral waveforms from this vessel segment.

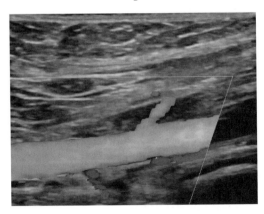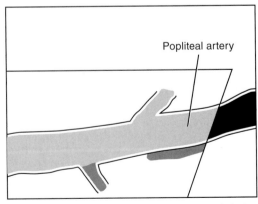

Gray-scale version of the sagittal scanning plane, color flow image of the longitudinal section of the popliteal artery. See Color Plate 25.

34. Locate the proximal anterior tibial artery. Obtain longitudinal images of the vessel origin and proximal segment. Record representative Doppler spectral waveforms from this vessel segment.

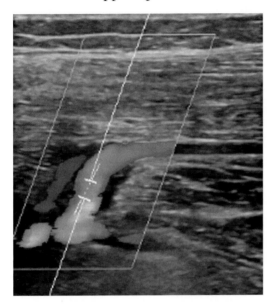
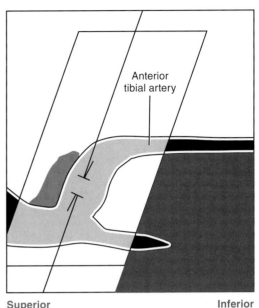

Gray-scale version of the sagittal scanning plane color flow image of the longitudinal section of the proximal anterior tibial artery. See Color Plate 26.

35. Return to the popliteal artery and identify the tibioperoneal trunk. Obtain longitudinal images of the origin and proximal segment of the peroneal artery. Record representative Doppler spectral waveforms from this vessel segment.

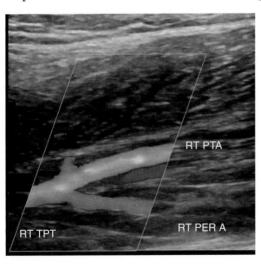
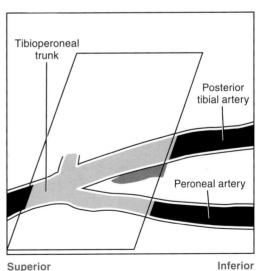

Gray-scale version of the sagittal scanning plane, color flow image of the longitudinal sections of the tibioperoneal trunk and origins of the posterior tibial and peroneal arteries. See Color Plate 27.

36. Continue to follow the course of the peroneal artery in the sagittal imaging plane. Obtain images of the mid and distal segments of the artery and record representative Doppler spectral waveforms from these vessel segments.

37. Return to the popliteal artery and identify the tibioperoneal trunk. Obtain longitudinal images of the origin and proximal segment of the posterior tibial artery. Record representative Doppler spectral waveforms from this vessel segment.

38. Continue to follow the course of the longitudinal section of the posterior tibial artery in the sagittal imaging plane. Obtain images of the mid and distal segments of the artery and record representative Doppler spectral waveforms from these vessel segments.

39. Repeat the survey on the contralateral limb.

> **NOTE:** The longitudinal image survey of the lower limb arteries may be complemented with color-flow imaging as necessary to confirm the presence and location of anatomic anomalies and pathology that produces disordered or turbulent flow patterns.

Lower Limb Arterial Duplex Required Images

1. Longitudinal image of the **MID-TO-DISTAL ABDOMINAL AORTA.**

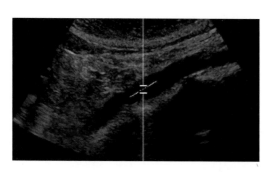 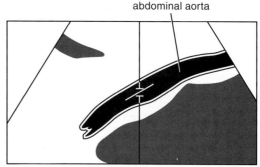

Mid-to-distal abdominal aorta

Superior   Inferior

Labeled: **SAG MID-TO-DIST AO**

2. Doppler spectral waveform from the **MID-TO-DISTAL ABDO-MINAL AORTA.**

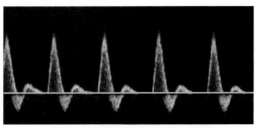

Labeled: **MID-TO-DISTAL AO**

3. Longitudinal image of the **COMMON ILIAC ARTERY.**

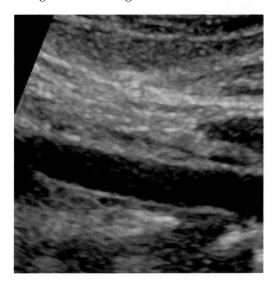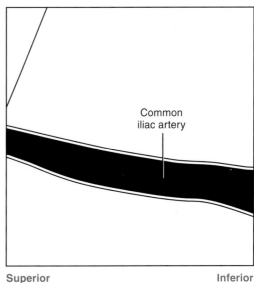

Superior   Inferior

Labeled: **SAG RT** or **LT CIA**

4. Doppler spectral waveform from the **COMMON ILIAC ARTERY.**

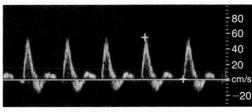

Labeled: **RT** or **LT CIA**

5. Longitudinal image of the **EXTERNAL ILIAC ARTERY.**

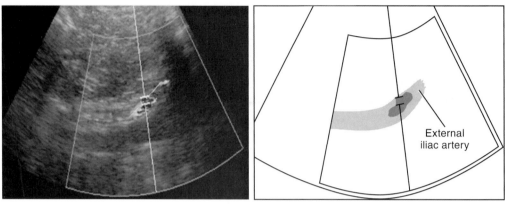

Labeled: **SAG RT** or **LT EIA**

6. Doppler spectral waveform from the **EXTERNAL ILIAC ARTERY.**

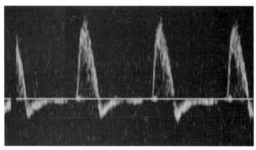

Labeled: **RT** or **LT EIA**

7. Longitudinal image of the **COMMON FEMORAL ARTERY.**

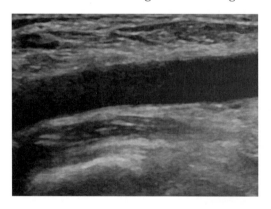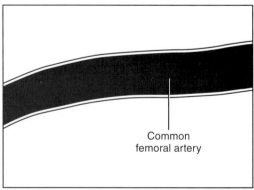

Superior   Inferior

Labeled: **SAG RT** or **LT CFA**

8. Doppler spectral waveform from the **COMMON FEMORAL ARTERY.**

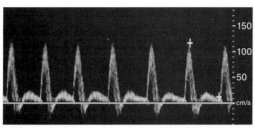

Labeled: **RT** or **LT CFA**

9. Longitudinal image of the **PROXIMAL PROFUNDA FEMORIS ARTERY.**

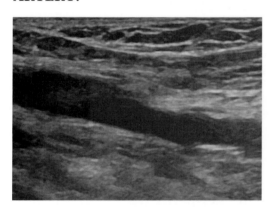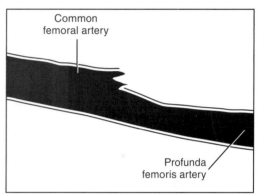

Labeled: **SAG RT** or **LT PFA**

10. Doppler spectral waveform from the **PROXIMAL PROFUNDA FEMORIS ARTERY.**

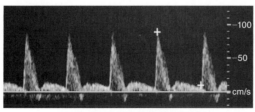

Labeled: **RT** or **LT PF**

11. Longitudinal image of the **PROXIMAL SUPERFICIAL FEMORAL ARTERY.**

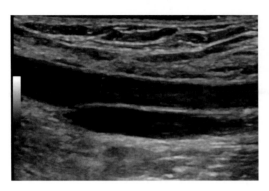 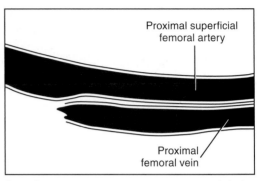

Labeled: **SAG RT** or **LT PROX SFA**

12. Doppler spectral waveform from the **PROXIMAL SUPERFICIAL FEMORAL ARTERY.**

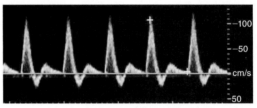

Labeled: **RT** or **LT PROX SFA**

13. Longitudinal image of the **MID SUPERFICIAL FEMORAL ARTERY.**

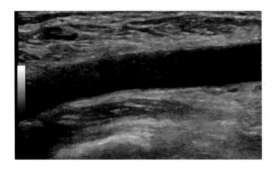 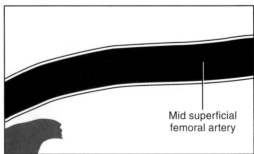

Labeled: **SAG RT** or **LT MID SFA**

14. Doppler spectral waveform from the **MID SUPERFICIAL FEMORAL ARTERY.**

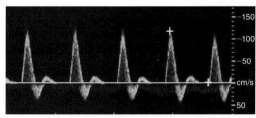

Labeled: **RT** or **LT MID SFA**

15. Longitudinal image of the **DISTAL SUPERFICIAL FEMORAL ARTERY.**

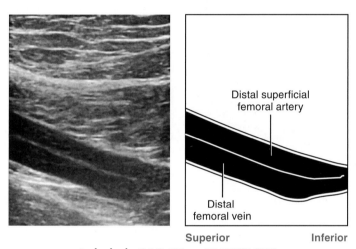

Labeled: **SAG RT** or **LT DIST SFA**

16. Doppler spectral waveform from the **DISTAL SUPERFICIAL FEMORAL ARTERY.**

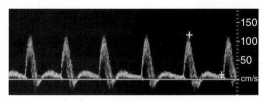

Labeled: **RT** or **LT DIST SFA**

17. Longitudinal image of the **POPLITEAL ARTERY.**

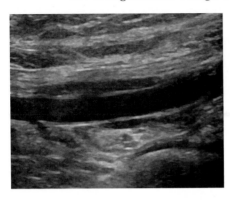
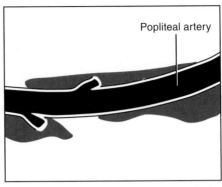

Superior   Inferior

Labeled: **SAG RT** or **LT POP**

18. Doppler spectral waveform from the **POPLITEAL ARTERY.**

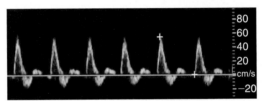

Labeled: **RT** or **LT POP**

19. Longitudinal image of the **PROXIMAL ANTERIOR TIBIAL ARTERY.**

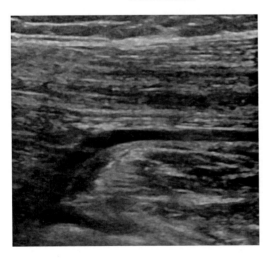
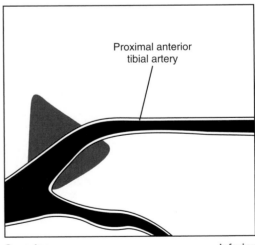

Superior   Inferior

Labeled: **SAG RT** or **LT PROX AT**

20. Doppler spectral waveform from the **PROXIMAL ANTERIOR TIBIAL ARTERY.**

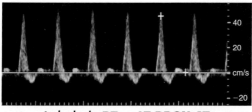

Labeled: **RT** or **LT PROX AT**

21. Longitudinal image of the **PROXIMAL PERONEAL ARTERY.**

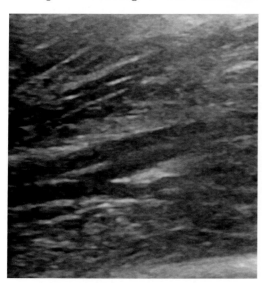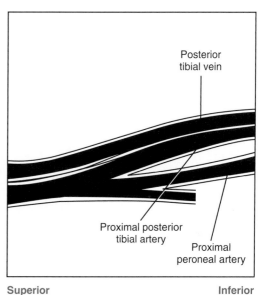

Posterior
tibial vein

Proximal posterior
tibial artery

Proximal
peroneal artery

Superior   Inferior

Labeled: **SAG RT** or **LT PROX PER**

22. Doppler spectral waveform from the **PROXIMAL PERONEAL ARTERY.**

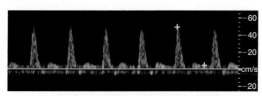

Labeled: **RT** or **LT PROX PER**

23. Longitudinal image of the **MID PERONEAL ARTERY.**

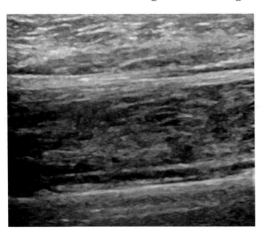
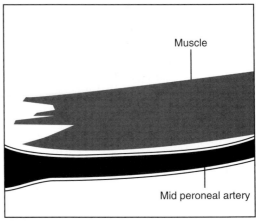

Superior   Inferior

Labeled: **SAG RT** or **LT MID PER**

24. Doppler spectral waveform from the **MID PERONEAL ARTERY.**

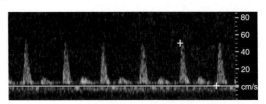

Labeled: **RT** or **LT MID PER**

25. Longitudinal image of the **DISTAL PERONEAL ARTERY.**

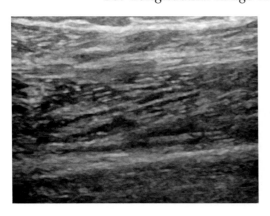
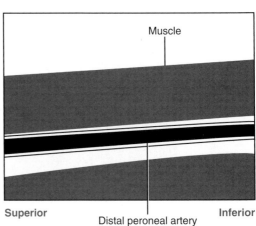

Superior   Distal peroneal artery   Inferior

Labeled: **SAG RT** or **LT DIST PER**

26. Doppler spectral waveform from the **DISTAL PERONEAL ARTERY.**

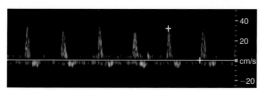

Labeled: **RT** or **LT DIST PER**

27. Longitudinal image of the **PROXIMAL POSTERIOR TIBIAL ARTERY.**

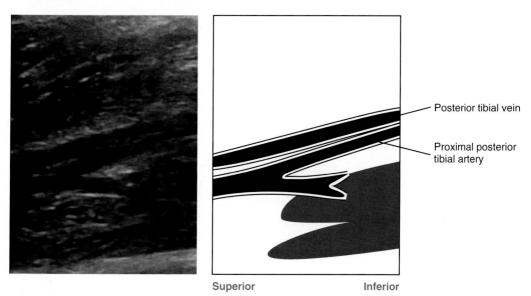

Labeled: **SAG RT** or **LT PROX PT**

28. Doppler spectral waveform from the **PROXIMAL POSTERIOR TIBIAL ARTERY.**

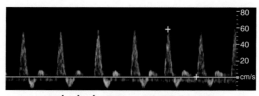

Labeled: **RT** or **LT PROX PT**

29. Longitudinal image of the **MID POSTERIOR TIBIAL ARTERY.**

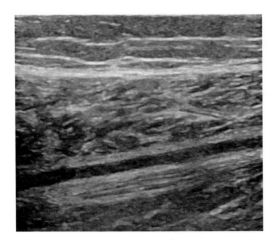 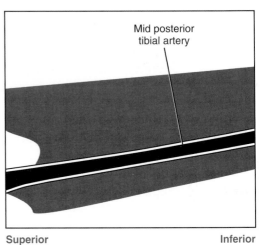

Labeled: **SAG RT** or **LT MID PT**

30. Doppler spectral waveform from the **MID POSTERIOR TIBIAL ARTERY.**

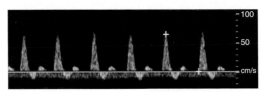

Labeled: **RT** or **LT MID PT**

31. Longitudinal image of the **DISTAL POSTERIOR TIBIAL ARTERY.**

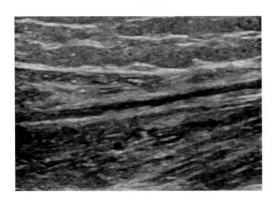 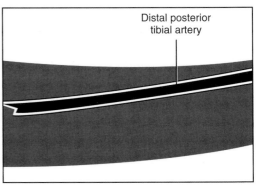

Labeled: **SAG RT** or **LT DIST PT**

32. Doppler spectral waveform from the **DISTAL POSTERIOR TIBIAL ARTERY.**

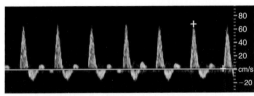

Labeled: **RT** or **LT DIST PT**

Data Documentation

Using Blood Pressures

- The severity of blood flow compromise in the lower extremities may be assessed by using the ankle-brachial index.
- Blood pressure is measured in both brachial arteries and in the dorsalis pedis and posterior tibial arteries of both lower limbs. For reimbursement, in addition to pressure measurements, waveforms must be obtained from both tibial arteries using continuous-wave Doppler or from the ankle using pulse volume recording.
- The equation for calculating the ankle-brachial index is:

$$\frac{\text{The highest brachial pressure}}{\text{The higher of the two tibial artery pressures}}$$

Table 21-1	Ankle-Brachial Index
>1.3	Arterial calcification
1.0-1.3	Normal
0.9-1.0	Mild arterial compromise with only mild symptoms
0.5-0.9	Mild to moderate ischemia with mild to moderate claudication
0.3-0.5	Moderate to severe ischemia with severe claudication or rest pain
<0.3	Severe ischemia with rest pain or gangrene

NOTE: Artifactually elevated tibial artery pressures may be found in patients with stiff, calcified vessels. In such cases, the systolic pressures may be measured in the great toe because the digital arteries infrequently calcify. The blood pressure may be obtained by using a photoplethysmographic sensor or continuous-wave Doppler probe. The toe brachial index is calculated by dividing the toe pressure by the highest brachial pressure. The blood pressure in the great toe is usually 80% of the brachial pressure. Therefor, a normal toe-brachial index exceeds 0.8.

Doppler Waveform Morphology

- **Triphasic (multiphasic) waveforms:** have a rapid systolic upstroke and deceleration from peak systole to a brief period of late systolic flow reversal followed by diastolic forward flow. The reverse flow component is caused by vasoconstriction in the arteriolar capillary bed of the normal resting lower extremity.
- **Biphasic waveforms:** two variations are described and used clinically. Biphasic (A) is found in normal arteries and arteries with lesions that are not yet flow reducing (<50% to 60% stenosis). This waveform has a rapid systolic upstroke and deceleration from peak systole to a brief period of late systolic flow reversal. **The forward diastolic flow component is absent.** This waveform morphology is frequently seen in geriatric patients or patients with arterial wall calcification or loss of vessel wall elasticity and compliance. Biphasic (B) is found in arteries with flow-reducing lesions (>50% to 60% diameter reduction). It is characterized by rapid systolic upstroke and systolic deceleration. **The reversed diastolic flow component is absent** and is followed by forward diastolic flow.
- **Monophasic waveforms:** exhibit delayed systolic upstroke and run-off. This waveform morphology is most often noted distal to a flow-limiting lesion or site of extrinsic arterial compression.

Normal Lower Extremity Arterial Velocities

Common femoral artery	80-100 cm/sec
Popliteal artery	60-80 cm/sec
Tibial arteries	40-60 cm/sec

NOTE: The peak systolic velocity range for each artery is given as a guide only. Most often, a ratio of the prestenotic velocity to the stenotic velocity is used to determine the hemodynamic significance of a lesion. A velocity ratio >2.0 suggests at least a 50% diameter-reducing stenosis, whereas a ratio >4.0 suggests at least a 75% stenosis.

Table 21-2	Lower Extremity Arterial Duplex Diagnostic Criteria			
% Stenosis	**Waveform**	**Spectral Broadening**	**Velocity/Ratio**	**Distal Waveform**
Normal	Triphasic or biphasic	None	None	Normal
1%-19%	Triphasic or biphasic	Minimal	<30% increase in PSV compared with proximal segment	Normal
20%-49%	Triphasic or biphasic	Pansystolic	30%-100% increase in PSV compared with proximal segment	Normal
50%-74%	Biphasic or monophasic	Pansystolic; possible turbulence	>100% increase in PSV compared with proximal segment; 2:1 ratio	Monophasic distally
75%-99%	Biphasic or monophasic	Pansystolic; possible turbulence	Four-fold increase in PSV compared with proximal segment; 4:1 ratio	Monophasic distally
Occluded	No flow	None	None	Collaterals are monophasic with reduced PSV

Classification of Disease Severity Based on Doppler Waveform Morphology

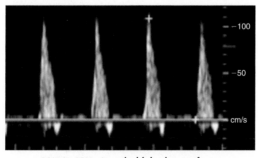

20% to 49% stenosis: biphasic waveform.

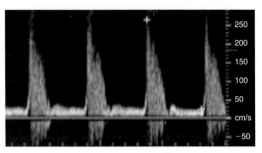

50% to 74% stenosis.

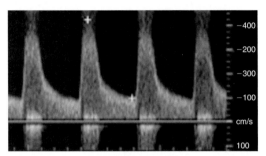

75% to 99% stenosis.

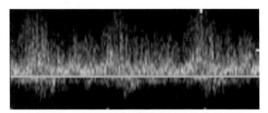

Poststenotic turbulence.

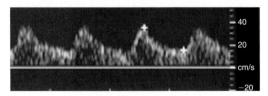

Monophasic waveform.

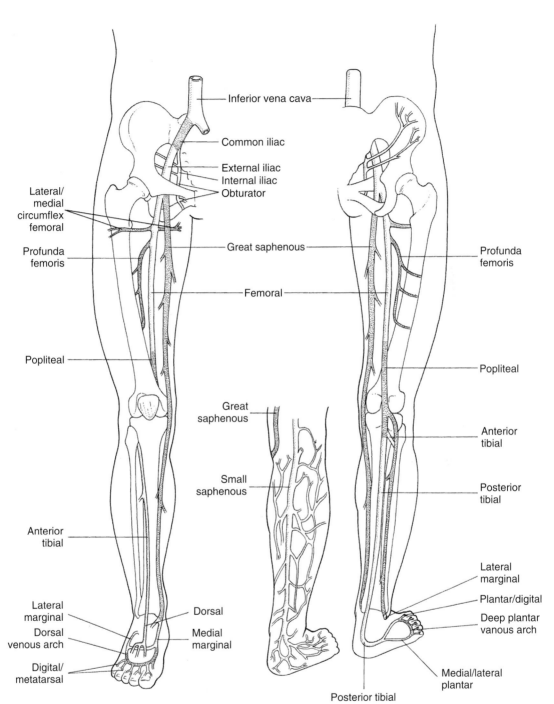

Venous System of the Lower Limb. Normal deep and superficial venous anatomy of the legs.

Lower Extremity Peripheral Venous Duplex Sonography Overview

Anatomy

* *Common femoral vein (CFV):* lies medial to the common femoral artery (CFA).

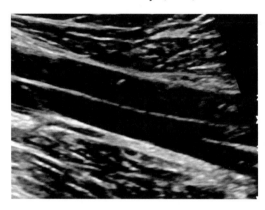
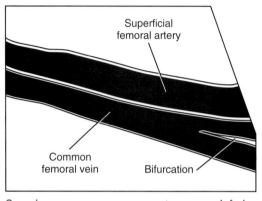

Sagittal plane image of the superficial femoral artery and common femoral vein bifurcation.

* *Femoral vein:* lies posterior to the superficial femoral artery (SFA) superiorly and follows a medial course along the inner curve of the thigh. At its inferior aspect, just superior to the knee, it lies posterior to the SFA. The femoral vein is duplicated in approximately 20% to 30% of the population.
* *Profunda femoris vein (deep femoral vein):* is found posterior to the FV with its insertion at approximately the same level.
* *Popliteal vein:* lies posterior and lateral to the popliteal artery and is formed by the anterior tibial trunk and the tibioperoneal trunk.
* *Gastrocnemius (sural) veins:* accompany the sural artery in the gastrocnemius muscle of the proximal calf and insert into the popliteal vein.
* *Anterior tibial veins:* originate as the dorsalis pedis veins and course on top of the interosseous membrane, lateral to the tibia. Just below the knee they penetrate the proximal end of the membrane to unite with the tibioperoneal trunk and insert into the popliteal vein.
* *Tibioperoneal trunk:* is formed by the union of the common tibial trunk and the common peroneal trunk.
* *Peroneal veins:* course along the lateral aspect of the calf lying in close proximity to the fibula. The paired veins converge to form the common peroneal trunk.
* *Posterior tibial veins:* are formed by the plantar veins of the foot. They accompany the posterior tibial artery posterior to the medial

malleolus (ankle) and course superiorly along the medial calf to form the common tibial trunk.

- *Great saphenous vein:* originates inferiorly on the dorsum of the foot and ascends along the leg medial to the FV and usually inserts into the CFV at the level of the FV insertion.
- *Small saphenous vein:* courses superiorly and laterally just anterior to the **lateral malleolus** (ankle) along the midline of the calf. The level of its insertion is variable but is most commonly noted at the level of the popliteal vein.
- *Soleal sinuses:* are venous reservoirs within the soleal muscles of the calf. They drain into the posterior tibial and peroneal veins.
- With the exception of the soleal veins, **valves** are located in all of the lower extremity veins to prevent retrograde venous flow. The number of valves is greatest in the tibial veins of the calf.
- All veins are thin walled and collapse easily with minimally applied pressure.

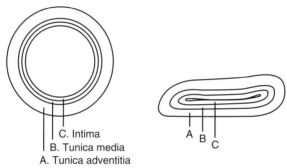

C. Intima
B. Tunica media
A. Tunica adventitia
Noncompressed and compressed sections of a vein.

- Venous duplication is common in the deep and superficial venous systems.

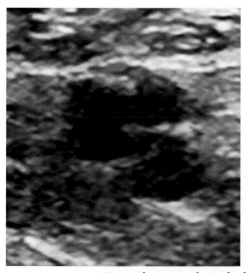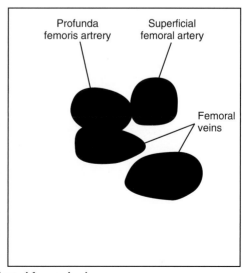

Image demonstrating a duplicated femoral vein.

Normal Sonographic Findings

- The normal vein lumen should be echo free.
- If viewing the vein at a perpendicular angle, you should be able to visualize the dilated vein valve cusps and the valve leaflets.

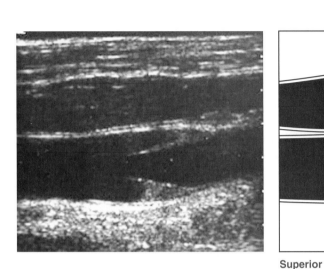
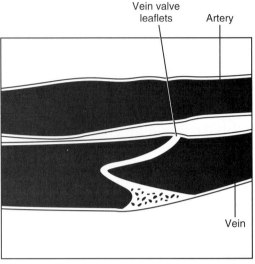

Image of vein segment demonstrating vein valve leaflets.

- There are 5 normal lower extremity blood flow patterns seen sonographically:
  1. **Spontaneous flow**: Doppler interrogation of the veins should demonstrate flow without use of manual augmentation or the Valsalva maneuver. Absence of flow may suggest thrombosis or extrinsic compression of the vein.
  2. **Respiratory phasicity**: Doppler flow patterns vary because of changes in intraabdominal and intrathoracic pressure associated with respiration. Flow decreases during inspiration due to increased intraabdominal pressure. Flow increases with expiration because intraabdominal pressure decreases. Continuous flow with no noticeable respiratory variation suggests a proximal obstruction.

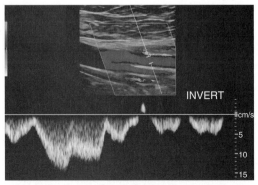

Gray-scale version of Doppler spectral waveforms demonstrating respiratory phasicity.
See Color Plate 28.

3. **Augmentation**: With distal limb compression, there should be a rush of venous flow superiorly. This finding indicates the absence of complete vein thrombosis between the transducer and the point of compression.

4. **Valvular competence**: With proximal compression of the veins, the presence of competent valves should prevent significant retrograde (inferior) venous flow.

  - If retrograde flow (reflux) is noted with firm, extended proximal compression or release of distal compression of the limb, valvular incompetence is suggested. In an upright patient, duration of retrograde flow in the deep veins >1.0 sec suggests clinically significant valvular incompetence. This value decreases to >0.5 sec when applied to the great saphenous vein. Incompetence most often results from venous varicosities or the presence of residual thrombus that has caused the valve leaflets to become stiff and nonpliable.

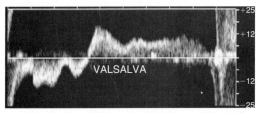

Doppler spectral waveforms from common femoral vein demonstrating valvular incompetence (retrograde flow, reflux) occurring with the Valsalva maneuver.

  - A minimal amount of retrograde flow may be noted if quick, hard compressions are applied to the limb. Such compressions do not allow enough time for the valve leaflets to close adequately.

  - An appropriately performed Valsalva maneuver may also be used to assess valvular competence at the level of the thigh veins.

5. **Nonpulsatility**: Venous flow variations occur with respiratory cycles, not with each heartbeat. Pulsatile venous flow suggests congestive heart failure, fluid overload, or tricuspid insufficiency.

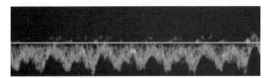

Gray-scale version of Doppler spectral waveforms demonstrating venous pulsatility.

Preparation

Patient Prep
- None.

Transducer
- 5.0-MHz to 7.5-MHz linear array with spectral and color Doppler capabilities for imaging the lower limb veins.
- 2.0-MHz to 4.0-MHz curved array with spectral and color Doppler capabilities for imaging the pelvic and abdominal veins.

Patient Position
- Supine with the examination table placed in the reversed Trendelenburg position to promote venous pooling.

Lower Extremity Venous Duplex Survey

1. The purpose of the survey is to identify deep venous thrombosis and superficial thrombophlebitis, venous duplication, and venous reflux. The initial survey is performed with gray-scale (B-Mode) imaging to ensure that features of the vein are accurately characterized.
2. In a transverse scanning plane, the axial survey is initiated with the patient lying supine with the lower limb rotated outward and the knee slightly flexed in a frog leg position to gain access to the common femoral and popliteal veins.
3. Locate the common femoral vein and common femoral artery at the level of the inguinal ligament. Assess compressibility of the vein by applying slow, firm pressure over the vein and confirm that the vein walls coapt. The walls of the CFA should not deform with adequate compression of the vein.
4. Continue to scan inferiorly to the level of the CFV bifurcation. Note the insertions of the profunda femoris and femoral veins.
5. Follow the course of the profunda femoris vein, confirming compressibility every 1 to 2 cm.
6. Return to the CFV bifurcation and locate the FV. Follow the course of the FV along the medial aspect of the thigh. Confirm compressibility of the FV in the proximal, mid-, and distal thigh or at more frequent intervals as indicated by the clinical presentation.
7. Place the transducer in the popliteal fossa to obtain an axial image of the popliteal vein. Using your free hand to apply counterpressure to the patella (knee cap), assess compressibility of the popliteal vein in the distal thigh and behind the knee.
8. Identify the gastrocnemius veins and follow them into the upper calf, taking care to note duplication if present. Assess compressibility of the gastrocnemius veins.

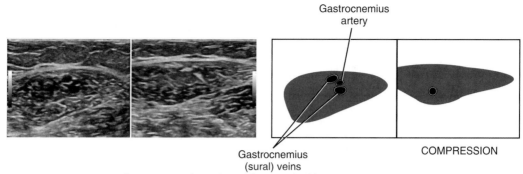

Image of gastrocnemius veins without and with compression maneuver.

9. Return to the popliteal vein. Follow the popliteal inferiorly and note the insertion of the anterior tibial veins. Assess compressibility of the anterior tibial veins as far along their visible course as possible.

10. Return to the popliteal vein and follow it inferiorly to the tibioperoneal trunk. Assess compressibility of the trunk.

11. Continue to follow the tibioperoneal trunk. Note the insertion of the peroneal veins and posterior tibial veins.

12. As far as possible, follow the peroneal veins into the proximal calf. If visibility of the veins is compromised, move the transducer to the medial aspect of the upper calf and locate the fibula. With the acoustic shadow of the fibula to the right or left of the image, locate the echogenic interosseous membrane. The peroneal and posterior tibial veins and their accompanying arteries lie inferior to the membrane with the peroneal veins being deeper than the posterior tibial veins.

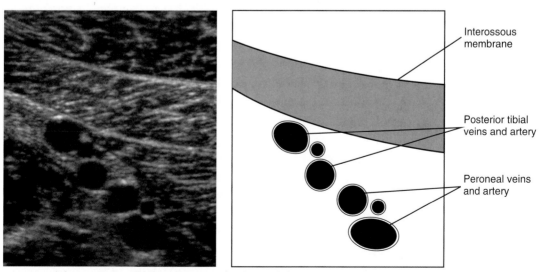

Image of the posterior tibial and peroneal veins and their accompanying arteries lying inferior to the interosseous membrane in the calf.

13. Follow the peroneal veins to the level of the ankle. Assess compressibility, as a minimum, in the proximal, mid, and distal calf regions.

14. Return to the tibioperoneal trunk and identify the posterior tibial veins. Follow the course of the posterior tibial veins to the level of the ankle. Assess compressibility, at a minimum, in the proximal, mid, and distal calf regions.

15. Return to the popliteal vein. Identify the insertion of the small saphenous vein. Follow its course toward the skin line and confirm its location between the fascial borders. Scan the vein as inferiorly as possible, performing compressions every 1 to 3 cm.

16. Return to the thigh and the CFV. Identify the insertion of the great saphenous vein. Follow the course of the saphenous vein toward the skin line and confirm its location between the fascial borders. Continue to scan inferiorly, assessing compressibility of the great saphenous vein in the proximal, mid, and distal thigh, at the level of the knee, and in the proximal, mid, and distal calf. Take care to note duplication of the vein, which may occur over short or long vein segments.

17. Return to the level of the CFV. Rotate the transducer 90 degrees to image the CFV in the sagittal plane. Obtain Doppler spectral waveforms. Assess for respiratory phasicity.

> **NOTE:** Although velocities are not usually of diagnostic importance for extremity venous examinations, if you choose to angle-correct, use an insonation angle <60 degrees with the cursor aligned parallel to the vessel wall at center stream.

18. Have the patient perform the Valsalva maneuver or apply manual compression to the patient's abdomen to assess for venous reflux and augmentation. Record representative Doppler spectral waveforms from the CFV.

19. Identify the profunda femoris vein. Record representative Doppler spectral waveforms from the profunda femoris vein.

20. Return to the CFV and identify the insertion of the FV. Obtain Doppler spectral waveforms just before the insertion and assess for respiratory phasicity and augmentation.

21. Follow the FV along its course in the thigh. Obtain Doppler spectral waveforms. Assess for respiratory phasicity.

22. Perform proximal and distal limb compressions in the upper, mid-, and lower thigh. Record representative Doppler spectral waveforms from these limb segments to demonstrate augmentation and evidence of valvular incompetence.

23. Place the transducer in the popliteal fossa and obtain a sagittal image of the popliteal vein. Obtain Doppler spectral waveforms and assess for respiratory phasicity.

24. Perform limb compression of the proximal calf and distal thigh to assess augmentation and look for evidence of valvular incompetence. Record representative Doppler spectral waveforms.

25. Locate the peroneal veins in either the proximal calf or at ankle level. Obtain Doppler spectral waveforms from the proximal, mid, and distal calf segments and assess for respiratory phasicity.

26. Perform limb compression at the proximal, mid, and distal calf to assess augmentation and look for evidence of valvular incompetence. Record representative Doppler spectral waveforms.

27. Locate the posterior tibial veins in either the proximal calf or at ankle level. Obtain Doppler spectral waveforms from the proximal, mid, and distal calf segments and assess for respiratory phasicity.

28. Perform limb compression at the proximal, mid, and distal calf to assess augmentation and for evidence of valvular incompetence. Record representative Doppler spectral waveforms.

NOTE: A low spectral Doppler velocity scale should be used for examination of the small tibial veins.

NOTE: In the calf veins, absence of spontaneous flow can be a normal finding. The study may be facilitated by using color Doppler optimized for slow flow.

NOTE: For patients with pain and tenderness in the calf, it is helpful to examine the calf muscle in the region of pain. Thrombus originates in the soleal veins in the calf. Look for large, swollen soleal veins filled with thrombus. The soleal veins normally drain into the posterior tibial and peroneal veins.

29. Return to the CFV in the proximal thigh. Locate the insertion of the great saphenous vein. Obtain Doppler spectral waveforms from the proximal, mid, and distal thigh segments, at the level of the knee and in the proximal, mid, and distal calf segments and assess for respiratory phasicity.

30. Perform limb compression at the same levels on the limb to assess augmentation and look for evidence of valvular incompetence. Record representative Doppler spectral waveforms.

NOTE: The Intersocietal Accreditation Commission requires calf vein imaging for accreditation in peripheral venous evaluations. When performing a unilateral venous examination, the Commission also requires Doppler spectral waveforms and images demonstrating compression at the level of the CFV on the contralateral limb.

Lower Limb Venous Duplex Required Images

1. Split-screen axial images of noncompressed and compressed **COMMON FEMORAL VEIN.**

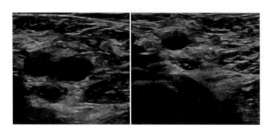 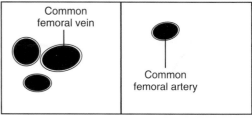

NONCOMPRESSED   COMPRESSED

Labeled: **RT** or **LT CFV**

2. Doppler spectral waveform from the **COMMON FEMORAL VEIN.**

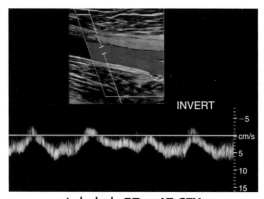

Labeled: **RT** or **LT CFV**
Gray-scale version. See Color Plate 29.

3. Split-screen axial images of noncompressed and compressed **PROFUNDA FEMORIS VEIN.**

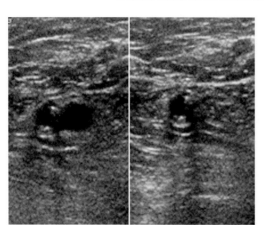 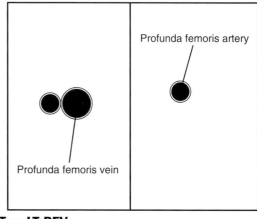

Labeled: **RT** or **LT PFV**

4. Doppler spectral waveform from the **PROFUNDA FEMORIS VEIN.**

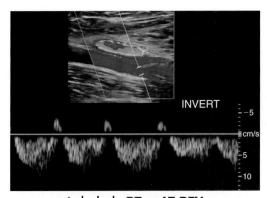

Labeled: **RT** or **LT PFV**
Gray-scale version. See Color Plate 30.

5. Split-screen axial images of noncompressed and compressed proximal, mid, or distal **FEMORAL VEIN.**

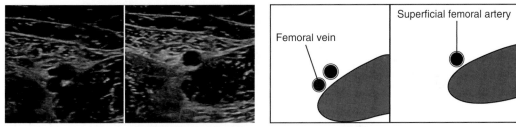

Labeled: **RT** or **LT PROX, MID,** or **DIST FV**

6. Doppler spectral waveform from the proximal, mid, or distal **FEMORAL VEIN.**

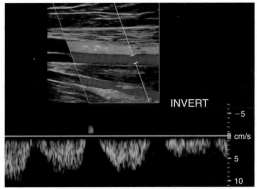

Labeled: **RT** or **LT PROX, MID,** or **DIST FV**
Gray-scale version. See Color Plate 31.

7. Split-screen axial images of noncompressed and compressed **POPLITEAL VEIN.**

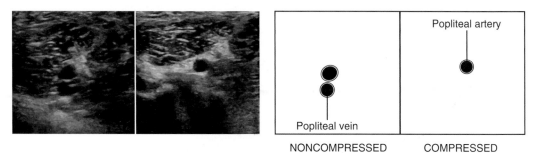

NONCOMPRESSED   COMPRESSED

Labeled: **RT** or **LT POPLITEAL V**

8. Doppler spectral waveform from the **POPLITEAL VEIN.**

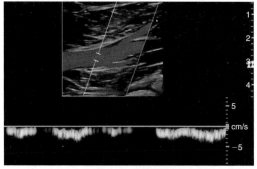

Labeled: **RT** or **LT POPLITEAL V**

Gray-scale version. See Color Plate 32.

9. Split-screen images of noncompressed and compressed **GASTROCNEMIUS VEINS.**

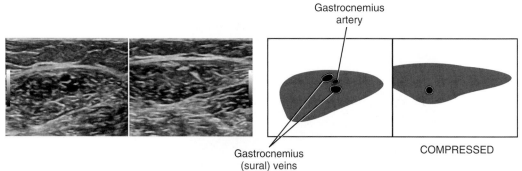

Labeled: **RT** or **LT GASTROC VV**

10. Split-screen axial images of noncompressed and compressed proximal **ANTERIOR TIBIAL VEINS.**

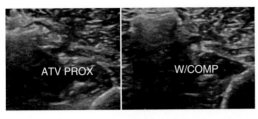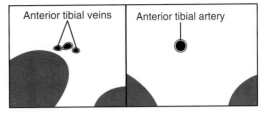

NONCOMPRESSED   COMPRESSED

Labeled: **RT** or **LT PROX ATIB VV**

11. Split-screen axial images of noncompressed and compressed **TIBIOPERONEAL TRUNK.**

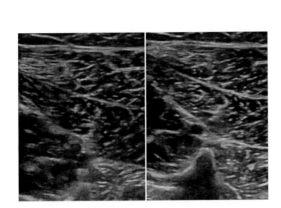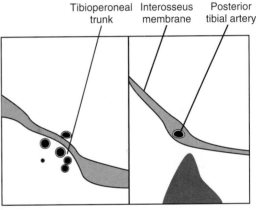

NONCOMPRESSED   COMPRESSED

Labeled: **RT** or **LT TIBPER TRUNK**

12. Split-screen axial images of noncompressed and compressed proximal, mid, or distal **PERONEAL VEINS.**

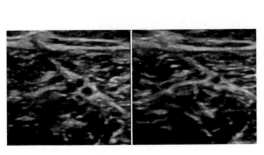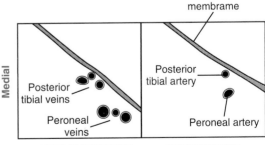

NONCOMPRESSED   COMPRESSED

Labeled: **RT** or **LT PROX, MID,** or **DIST PER VV**

13. Doppler spectral waveform from the proximal, mid, or distal **PERONEAL VEINS.** (gray-scale version).

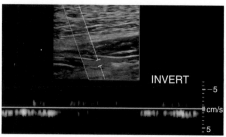

Labeled: **RT** or **LT PROX, MID,** or **DIST PER VV**

14. Split-screen axial images of noncompressed and compressed proximal, mid, or distal posterior **TIBIAL VEINS.**

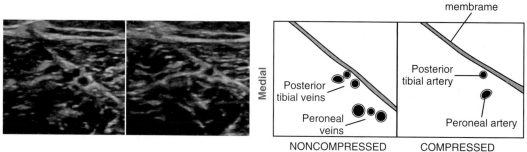

Labeled: **RT** or **LT PROX, MID,** or **DIST PT VV**

15. Doppler spectral waveform from the proximal, mid, or distal **POSTERIOR TIBIAL VEINS** (gray-scale version).

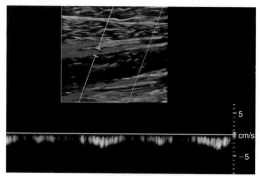

Labeled: **RT** or **LT PROX, MID,** or **DIST PT VV**

16. Split-screen axial images of noncompressed and compressed proximal, mid, or distal **SMALL SAPHENOUS VEIN.**

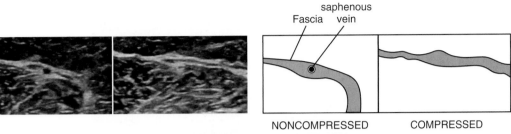

Labeled: **RT** or **LT PROX, MID,** or **DIST SSV**

17. Doppler spectral waveform from the proximal, mid, or distal **SMALL SAPHENOUS VEIN** (gray-scale version).

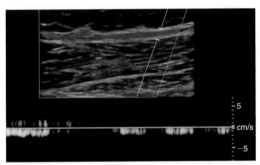

Labeled: **RT** or **LT PROX, MID,** or **DIST SSV**

18. Split-screen axial images of noncompressed and compressed proximal, mid, or distal thigh segments of the **GREAT SAPHE-NOUS VEIN.**

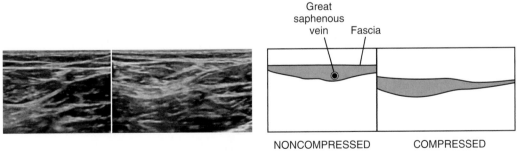

Labeled: **RT** or **LT PROX, MID,** or **DIST THIGH GSV**

19. Doppler spectral waveform from the proximal, mid, or distal thigh and calf segments and at the knee of the **GREAT SAPHENOUS VEIN.** (gray-scale version).

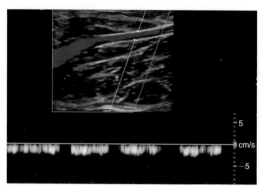

Labeled: **RT** or **LT PROX, MID,** or **DIST THIGH GSV**

Data Documentation

Normal Examination

- **Compressibility:** if the vein walls coapt completely with moderate probe compression, and there is no evidence of intraluminal echoes.
- **Flow pattern:** the Doppler spectral waveforms demonstrate spontaneous flow with respiratory phasicity in all venous segments. There is no evidence of significant retrograde flow with proximal compression.

Abnormal Examination

- **Compressibility:** the vein walls are not compressible or are partially compressible and there is evidence of intraluminal echoes. Veins may be partially compressible with both acute and chronic thrombosis and both acute and chronic processes may exist in the same vein. The presence of recanalization and/or collateralization does not exclude an acute thrombosis. Outflow obstruction is suggested if the vein is noncompressible but the lumen of the vein is echo-free. Respiratory phasicity is absent. Check for extrinsic compression of the proximal veins.

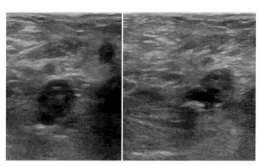
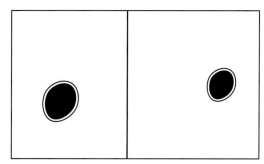

NONCOMPRESSED   COMPRESSED

Split-screen axial images of noncompressed and compressed thrombus-filled vein showing lack of compressibility.

- **Flow pattern:** the Doppler spectral waveforms demonstrate continuous, nonphasic flow. Pulsatility may be noted when congestive heart failure, a distal arteriovenous fistula, or fluid overload is present.

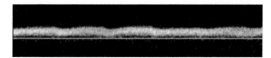

Gray-scale version of Doppler spectral waveform demonstrating continuous nonphasic flow pattern consistent with obstruction to venous outflow.

- **Venous dilation:** significant venous dilation compared with proximal venous segments suggests venous aneurysm.
- **Acute** versus **chronic thrombus** (see Table 21-3).

Table 21-3   Characterization of Venous Thrombus

Acute	Chronic
Acoustically homogeneous or anechoic	Continuum of acoustic changes from heterogeneous to homogeneous to anechoic in necrotic areas of thrombus
Spongy texture on compression	Firm texture on compression
Poorly attached to vein wall or free-floating	Well attached to vein wall
Vein may be dilated if occluded	Small, contracted; recanalization and/or collateralization may be apparent

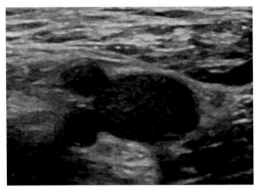 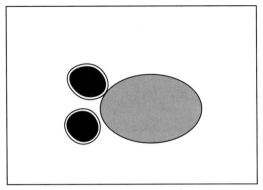

Axial image of acute deep venous thrombosis demonstrating the homogeneous echo pattern of the thrombus.

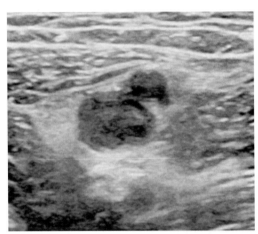 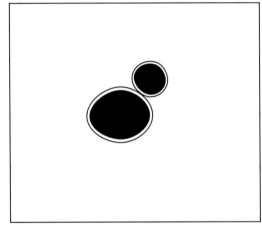

Axial image of chronic deep venous thrombosis demonstrating the echogenicity of the thrombus.

Review Questions

Answers on page 630.

1. The popliteal artery divides into the
   a) anterior tibial and posterior tibial arteries.
   b) tibioperoneal trunk and posterior tibial artery.
   c) anterior tibial artery and tibioperoneal trunk.
   d) peroneal artery and tibioperoneal trunk.

2. The primary diagnostic criterion for venous duplex evaluations is
   a) compressibility.
   b) competence.
   c) augmentation.
   d) spontaneity.

3. The acoustic properties of chronic thrombus are
   a) homogeneous.
   b) spongy and heterogeneous.
   c) heterogeneous and homogeneous.
   d) contracted and homogeneous.

4. In the adductor canal, the femoral vein lies posterior to the
   a) profunda femoris vein.
   b) common femoral artery.
   c) superficial femoral artery.
   d) common femoral vein.

5. Which of the following would facilitate confirmation of collateralization and/or recanalization of a thrombosed vein?
   a) Increase the wall filter.
   b) Decrease the color Doppler velocity scale.
   c) Increase the spectral Doppler velocity scale.
   d) Decrease the echo-write priority.

6. The majority of valves are found in the
   a) proximal deep veins.
   b) saphenous veins.
   c) perforating veins.
   d) calf veins.

7. A continuous, nonphasic venous flow signal indicates
   a) deep vein thrombosis.
   b) venous reflux.
   c) obstruction to venous outflow.
   d) superficial thrombophlebitis.

8. The common femoral artery lies lateral to the
   a) common femoral vein.
   b) profunda femoris vein.
   c) gastrocnemius vein.
   d) common iliac vein.

9. In a resting patient, the normal lower extremity artery will exhibit a
   a) monophasic waveform pattern.
   b) disordered outer frequency envelope.
   c) reversed flow component.
   d) minimally phasic flow pattern.

10. Deep venous thrombosis of the calf veins commonly originates in the
    a) anterior tibial veins.
    b) gastrocnemius veins.
    c) soleal sinuses.
    d) peroneal veins.

PART VII

ECHOCARDIOGRAPHY

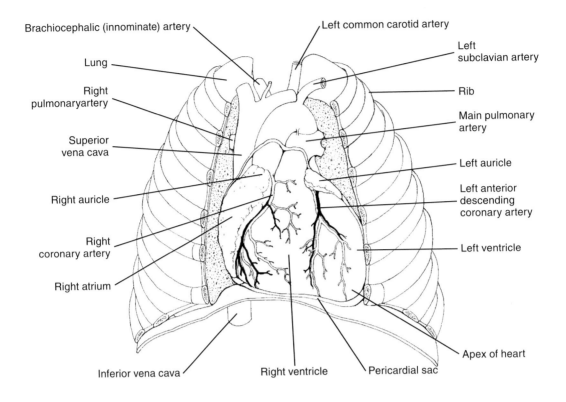

Brachiocephalic (innominate) artery

Left common carotid artery

Left subclavian artery

Lung

Right pulmonaryartery

Rib

Main pulmonary artery

Superior vena cava

Left auricle

Left anterior descending coronary artery

Right auricle

Right coronary artery

Left ventricle

Right atrium

Apex of heart

Inferior vena cava

Right ventricle

Pericardial sac

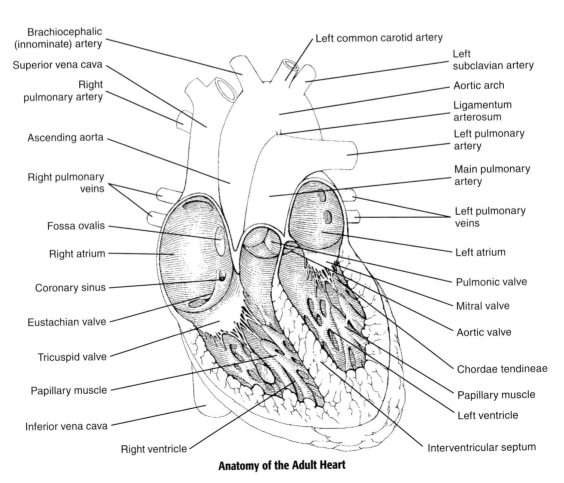

Brachiocephalic (innominate) artery

Left common carotid artery

Left subclavian artery

Superior vena cava

Aortic arch

Right pulmonary artery

Ligamentum arterosum

Ascending aorta

Left pulmonary artery

Right pulmonary veins

Main pulmonary artery

Fossa ovalis

Left pulmonary veins

Right atrium

Left atrium

Coronary sinus

Pulmonic valve

Eustachian valve

Mitral valve

Tricuspid valve

Aortic valve

Papillary muscle

Chordae tendineae

Inferior vena cava

Papillary muscle

Left ventricle

Right ventricle

Interventricular septum

Anatomy of the Adult Heart

CHAPTER 22

Adult Echocardiography Scanning Protocol

Maureen E. McDonald

Key Words

Annulus fibrosus	Mitral valve
Aortic valve	Moderator band
Appendage	Myocardium
Atria	Papillary muscles
Atrioventricular (AV) node	Pectinate muscle
Atrioventricular (AV) valves	Pericardium
Bundle of His	Pulmonic valve
Chordae tendineae	Purkinje fibers
Coronary sinus	Semilunar valves
Diastole	Sinoatrial (SA) node
Endocardium	Superior vena cava (SVC)
Epicardium	Systole
Eustachian valve	Thebesian valve
Fossa ovalis	Trabeculae carneae
Inferior vena cava (IVC)	Tricuspid valve
Interventricular septum (IVS)	Ventricles
Ligamentum arteriosum	

Objectives

At the end of this chapter, you will be able to:

- Define the key words.
- Distinguish the sonographic appearance of the adult heart and the terms used to describe it.
- Describe the transducer options for scanning the adult heart.
- Name the various suggested breathing techniques for patients when scanning the adult heart.
- List the suggested patient position (and options) when scanning the adult heart.
- Describe the patient prep for an adult heart study.
- Name the survey steps and explain how to evaluate the entire adult heart and associated structures.
- List the order and exact locations to take representative images of the adult heart aorta.
- Answer the review questions at the end of the chapter.

Overview

Location
- The heart is found within the thoracic cavity in a space called the middle mediastinum.
- Posterior to the ribs and lungs, it is located between the third to fifth intercostal spaces.
- The upper portion, or **base** of the heart, lies closer to the sternum than the lower portion, or **apex,** which lies inferior and to the left of midline.
- The apex is slightly more anterior than the base.

Anatomy
- The heart is a muscle consisting of 3 layers:
  1. Epicardium (smooth, thin outer layer).
  2. Myocardium (thicker, muscular layer).
  3. Endocardium (smooth, thin inner surface).
- The heart sits within a sac called the **pericardium** and is surrounded by a small amount of serous fluid to prevent friction as the heart beats.
- The heart has 4 chambers:
  - Two upper chambers, the right and left **atria.**
  - Two lower chambers, the right and left **ventricles.**
- The upper portion of both atria have a small triangular extension called an **appendage** (also called *auricle*) that is tightly lined with muscle called **pectinate muscle.**
- The lining of the right atrium (RA) is mostly smooth with some pectinate muscle on the free wall. It receives unoxygenated blood from 3 major sources:
  1. **Superior vena cava (SVC):** enters the chamber from above.
  2. **Inferior vena cava (IVC):** enters from below.
  3. **Coronary sinus:** found between the IVC and the opening to the right ventricle (RV).
- The IVC and coronary sinus have prominent edges that represent remnants of valves that once covered them during fetal days. These are the **eustachian valve** and the **thebesian valve** respectively.
- The midposterior RA wall is also the interatrial septum. It has a thinner area in the midportion representing the **fossa ovalis.**

NOTE: During fetal circulation, the fossa ovalis serves as a passage to the left heart, allowing most of the blood to bypass the undeveloped lungs.

- The left atrium (LA) is also smooth walled and receives oxygenated blood from four pulmonary veins. This is the most posterior chamber.
- The right ventricle (RV) is the most anterior chamber whose inner surface is lined with bands of muscle called **trabeculae carneae.** There is a dense band of tissue in the distal part of the chamber that runs perpendicular to the interventricular septum called the **moderator band.**
- The **interventricular septum (IVS)** separates the RV from the LV and consists of mostly muscular tissue with the exception of a small portion of membranous tissue near the insertion of the valves.
- The left ventricle (LV) is more trabeculated than the RV and the walls are also much thicker. The LV makes up the apex of the heart.
- The heart also has 4 valves that control blood flow in and out of the chambers:
  - 2 **atrioventricular (A-V) valves** that control the blood flow from the atria to the ventricles
  - 2 **semilunar valves** that control blood flow from the ventricles to the great vessels.
- The mitral and tricuspid valves are the A-V valves. Their leaflets attach to a ring of dense tissue between the chambers called the **annulus fibrosus.** From the free edges of the leaflets are multiple strong, thin fibers called **chordae tendineae.** These chordae attach to cone-shaped projections of muscle from the ventricular walls called **papillary muscles.**
- The **mitral valve** is located between the LA and LV and has 2 leaflets: the anterior leaflet and the posterior leaflet. Also known as the bicuspid valve, its cords attach to the anterolateral and posteromedial papillary muscles.
- The **tricuspid valve** is found between the RA and RV and has 3 leaflets: the anterior, posterior, and septal. There are 3 papillary muscles in the RV where the tricuspid cords attach: the anterior, posterior, and septal papillary muscles.
- The semilunar valves are the aortic and pulmonic valves. They are crescent shaped and have no cords or papillary muscles associated with them.
- The **aortic valve** is found in the left heart between the LV and the aortic root and has 3 cusps:
  1. Right coronary
  2. Left coronary
  3. Noncoronary
- The **pulmonic valve** is located between the RV and the main pulmonary artery. It has 3 cusps:
  1. Anterior
  2. Right
  3. Left

- The main pulmonary artery and the aorta comprise the great vessels. These are found at the base or superior aspect of the heart. A short ligament, the ligamentum arteriosum, connects the two.

  NOTE: The ligamentum arteriosum was once the ductus arteriosus in the fetus. Blood would flow through the duct from the pulmonary artery to the aorta, bypassing the lungs.

- The *aorta* arises from the ventricle and is divided into three regions: the ascending, arch, and descending aorta. There are 3 vessels that originate from the arch: the brachiocephalic (also called *innominate*), left common carotid, and left subclavian arteries. The brachiocephalic branch is directed rightward and bifurcates into the right common carotid and right subclavian arteries.
- The *main pulmonary artery* (PA) begins at the infundibular region of the RV and moves anteriorly before it bifurcates into the right and left pulmonary arteries. The right PA is directed toward the right lung and moves posterior to the aortic arch. The left PA branches in the direction of the left lung.
- Just beyond the aortic valve are 3 small, crescent-shaped pouches called the *sinus of Valsalva*. Each is associated with one of the aortic cusps. The right coronary artery originates from the right cusp sinus and the left coronary artery from the left cusp sinus. The remaining sinus has no coronary artery associated with it, hence the name noncoronary cusp.
- The left main coronary artery bifurcates shortly after its origin into the left anterior descending (LAD) and the left circumflex artery. These are found embedded in fat on the exterior surface of the heart. The fat is there to protect the vessels. The LAD runs inferiorly down the anterior interventricular sulcus which is a groove separating the RV from the LV. The left circumflex is located posterolateral to the LAD and runs partly in the atrioventricular groove (also called coronary sulcus), which is the separation between the RA and RV on the external surface of the heart.
- The right coronary artery (RCA) eventually bifurcates but not so quickly as the left, and is also embedded in fat wrapping around the heart in the right atrioventricular groove. The branches of the RCA are the right posterior descending and the marginal artery. The posterior descending artery is found in the posterior interventricular sulcus.
- The cardiac veins drain into the coronary sinus, which is found in the left atrioventricular groove (coronary sulcus) on the posterior surface of the heart between the LA and LV.

Physiology

- The heart is the center of the circulatory system responsible for directing the flow of deoxygenated blood to the lungs and then distributing the reoxygenated blood to the rest of the body.
- The heart has its own intrinsic conduction system consisting of specialized tissue called *nodes*. The nodes create the impulse that regulates the heart's rate of contraction. The sinoatrial (SA) node, found in the upper portion of the RA near the SVC, is considered the initial pacemaker of the heart. When it fires, an impulse is sent by way of internodal pathways across the atria, causing them to depolarize and contract. The atrioventricular (AV) node, found in the lower portion of the right interatrial septum, is then stimulated and directs the pulse toward the ventricles by way of the Bundle of His, which then bifurcates into the right and left bundle branches. These extend towards the apex of the heart by way of the interventricular septum. Multiple small bands called Purkinje fibers branch off the main bundle branches, across the ventricles, and into the muscle cells, spreading the impulse through the ventricles and causing them to depolarize and contract simultaneously.
- The conduction system emits an electrical impulse that can be detected on the surface of the body, which is how we get an electrocardiogram (ECG). The ECG consists of 3 distinct phases:
  1. The P wave is a small bump corresponding to atrial contraction and depolarization.
  2. The QRS complex, which is a series of downward and upward deflections, relates to ventricular contraction and depolarization.
  3. The T wave is a small bump representing ventricular repolarization. Atrial repolarization is not observed on the ECG because it occurs at the same time as the QRS complex.

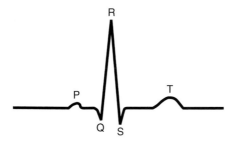

- There are 2 parts to the cardiac cycle: systole (muscular contraction) and diastole (muscular relaxation).

Sonographic Appearance

*   The *pericardium* is the most reflective structure and appears almost white.
*   The *papillary muscles* and *myocardium* are medium gray and homogeneous in echo texture.
*   The *valves* are slightly more echogenic than the walls when perpendicular to the ultrasound beam.
*   The area *within the chambers* and *great vessels,* as well as any other *fluid space,* is anechoic.

Preparation

Patient Prep

*   A basic ECG is attached to the patient to assist with the timing of the cardiac cycle. Leads are attached to the right chest, left chest, and left hip region—avoiding hair, if possible.

Patient Position

*   Left lateral decubitus for most views with the left arm extended above the head and the right arm at the patient's side.
*   *Subxiphoid:* left lateral decubitus or supine. Bend the knees to relax the stomach muscles if needed.
*   *Suprasternal:* the patient is supine with the neck extended. A pillow can also be placed under the shoulders allowing the head to drop back, hyperextending the neck even further.

Transducer

*   **2.5 MHz.**
*   3.5 MHz recommended for smaller, thinner patients.
*   Use a 5.0-MHz transducer when structures in the near field need to be further evaluated (e.g., LV apex).

Breathing Techniques

*   For the majority of patients, **normal respiration.**
*   When ribs or lungs interfere, having the patient either hold his or her breath or expel all air and not breathe, may improve the image. You may also need to slide an interspace to follow the movement of the heart. Experiment to find the best possible picture.

Transducer Orientation

*   Images are taken from 4 routine positions on the chest wall:
    1. Parasternal
    2. Apical
    3. Subxiphoid (also called *subcostal*)
    4. Suprasternal

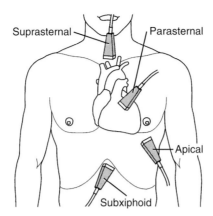

NOTE: Hold the transducer like a pencil, keeping two fingers on the patient at all times. This contact helps to prevent unintentional sliding and allows the sonographer to know how much pressure he or she is applying.

NOTE: To simplify the discussion of transducer orientation, imagine a clock on the patient's chest. The indicator on the transducer, which is some type of mark or indentation, will be directed anywhere from 1 to 12 o'clock. (To check indicator orientation, put gel on the transducer and touch the face on the indicator side. There should be movement on the left side of the sector. Adjust L/R invert if necessary.)

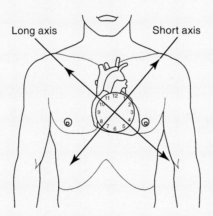

NOTE: Most movements are very slight once the proper interspace is found.

NOTE: Remember that the heart sits on an angle between the right shoulder and the left hip.

Adult Heart Survey • 2D Examination

The purpose of the 2D examination is to:
- Identify the chambers and walls and valves of the heart, and evaluate their size, thickness, and motion.
- Assess the anatomical relationships of structures to rule out congenital defects.
- Document the presence of any pathology including tumors or fluid surrounding the heart, or thrombi within.

Parasternal Views

1. Begin with parasternal long axis by placing the transducer to the left side of the sternum in the second to third intercostal space with the indicator on the transducer directed towards 10 o'clock. Evaluate the sizes of the LA, LV, aortic root, and the RV. Assess for thickness and motion of the AV, MV, IVS, and posterior wall of the LV.

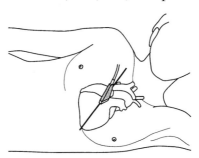

2. Maintaining the same interspace and 10 o'clock orientation, angle the transducer inferior and medial towards the umbilicus. This produces the right ventricular inflow view and visualizes the more anterior structure of the heart: the RA, TV, and RV. A remnant of the eustachian valve (a normal variant) may also be observed in the RA.

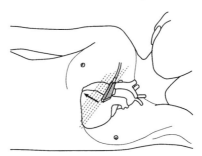

3. To obtain the right ventricular outflow view, the transducer is now angled superior and lateral towards the left shoulder. The indicator is still directed towards 10 o'clock. This will open the pulmonary artery and allow for assessment of the pulmonic valve.

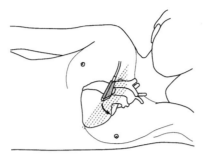

4. Rotate the transducer 90 degrees clockwise towards 1 o'clock, maintaining the same interspace as above and keeping the transducer close to the sternum. The parasternal short-axis views are observed here, beginning with the aortic valve level. Tilt the transducer towards the right shoulder. Start by visualizing the area above the aortic valve for the presence of pathology, then slowly sweep towards the level of the aortic valve. The AV should be in the center of the screen with the LA, RA, RV, and PA surrounding it. Evaluate for the presence of 3 aortic cusps and note the thickness and motion of all the valves.

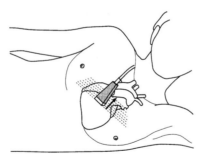

5. Continue to slowly sweep laterally through the left ventricular outflow tract region towards the mitral valve. Only the angle of the transducer has changed and the ultrasound beam is now pointing almost directly anterior to posterior. Both leaflets of the mitral valve should be observed as well as its biphasic motion.

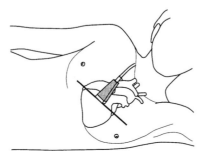

6. Slowly angle the transducer further lateral, towards the left hip. The cross section of the LV appears round with the papillary muscles indenting the inner surface, giving the cavity a mushroom like appearance. Assess LV function for focal or global abnormalities. Continue to sweep laterally, beyond the papillary muscles as deep into the ventricle as possible allowing for further assessment of LV function.

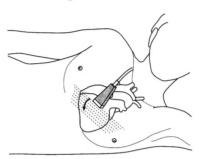

NOTE: Occasionally, you may need to slide an interspace to obtain the different levels of short axis, though angling is usually sufficient.

Apical Views

1. Place the transducer on the left flank, lateral to the left breast and point upwards, in the direction of the right shoulder. The indicator is oriented to 3 o'clock. The heart is transected from apex to base and the four chambers, MV, TV, interventricular septum, and lateral wall of the LV are seen. In addition, the walls in the apical region are now visualized. Each structure is evaluated in respect to its size, thickness, and motion. This is known as the apical 4-chamber view.

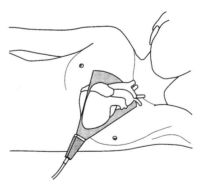

NOTE: If unable to find the proper apical interspace, locate the PMI (point of maximal impulse) by placing 2 fingers on the left side of the chest and feeling for the heartbeat. The transducer is placed at this position. This is the apex of the heart.

NOTE: It is important to visualize the endocardium of the LV to assess function. Evaluate the walls to see if they are thickening and whether there are any focal or global ischemic abnormalities. When estimating motion, it is easiest to segmentalize the ventricle, looking first at the proximal, mid, then distal walls, and then to check overall function.

2. For the apical 5-chamber view, angle the transducer slightly superior to open the LVOT and the aortic valve. The MV and TV become obscured. Evaluate for the presence of any obstruction in the outflow tract region.

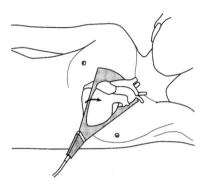

3. Rotate the transducer counterclockwise towards 12 o'clock while still pointing towards the right shoulder. The MV, LA, and LV are observed and thus called the apical 2-chamber view. The inferior, anterior, and apical walls of the LV can now be assessed.

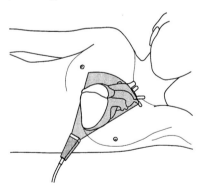

4. Rotate the transducer further counterclockwise towards 11 o'clock, opening up the apical long axis view. The structures seen in the parasternal long axis are visualized again in this view, but because of the different orientation, the apical region of the heart is now observed.

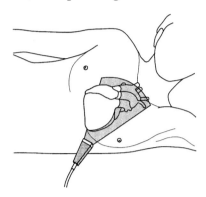

Subxiphoid Views

1. To obtain the subxiphoid long axis, place the transducer below the xiphoid process and slightly to the right of midline away from the stomach on a softer portion of the abdomen. Using the liver as a window, point the transducer toward the left shoulder. Hold the hand above the transducer, rather than like a pencil. This enables the transducer to be angled under the ribs and prevents the hand from interfering with the scan. The indicator is pointed towards 3 o'clock. The 4 chambers of the heart are observed and assessed for relative sizes. If the chambers appear foreshortened, the transducer should be rotated accordingly. The area around the heart should also be evaluated for the presence of pericardial fluid, tumors, and masses. The interatrial septum is also best evaluated in this view.

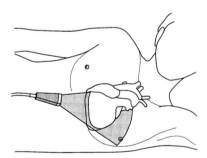

2. For the subxiphoid short axis views, rotate the transducer 90 degrees counterclockwise towards 12 o'clock. Sweeping the transducer from the direction of the left shoulder to the direction of the right shoulder produces the same 3 levels as the parasternal short-axis views (papillary muscles, mitral valve, and aortic valve levels) but with the heart on a slightly different tilt. In addition, the hepatic veins and IVC can be seen to enter the RA by pointing more rightward, beyond the aortic valve level. Make sure the IVC is clear with no thrombi.

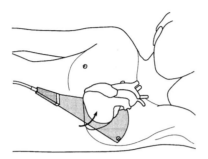

Suprasternal View

1. With the patient in the supine position, neck extended, place the transducer at the sternoclavicular groove and angle inferior toward the heart. This will visualize the aortic arch and its branches, along with a cross section of the right pulmonary artery. The transducer is oriented towards 12 o'clock.

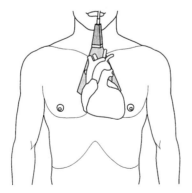

2. For a short axis of the aorta, rotate the transducer 90 degrees clockwise to 3 o'clock. A longitudinal section of the right pulmonary artery may also be seen anterior to the LA.

NOTE: This view should be used when questions involving the aorta arise, such as in dissection or Marfan syndrome.

Adult Heart Required Images

> **NOTE:** The study is videotaped allowing for real-time assessment of structures. At least 6 to 10 beats of each view should be recorded with additional images of any pathology.

1. Parasternal **LONG AXIS.**

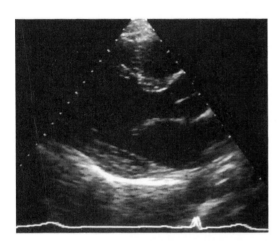 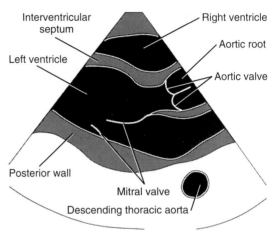

> **NOTE:** The anterior portion of the aortic root and the interventricular septum should be continuous and as perpendicular to the ultrasound beam as possible. The posterior portion of the aortic root runs continuous with the anterior mitral valve leaflet.

2. **RIGHT VENTRICULAR INFLOW** view.

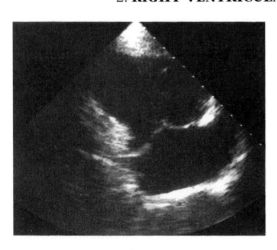 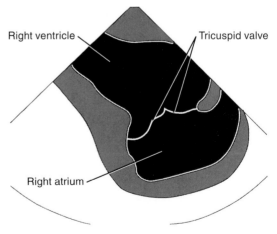

3. **RIGHT VENTRICULAR OUTFLOW** view.

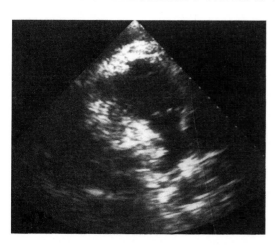
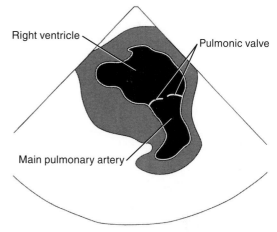

4. Parasternal short axis at the level of the **AORTIC VALVE.**

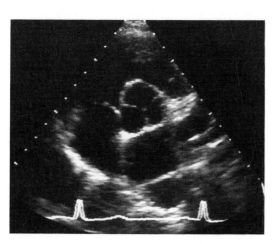
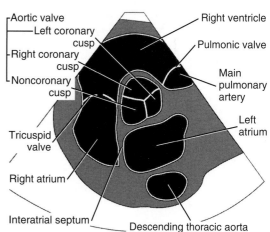

5. Parasternal short axis at the level of the **MITRAL VALVE.**

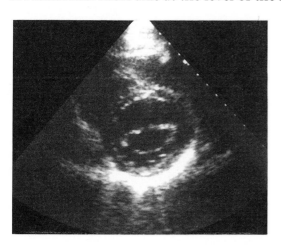
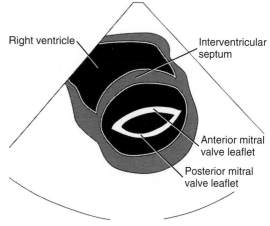

6. Parasternal short axis at the level of the **PAPILLARY MUSCLES.**

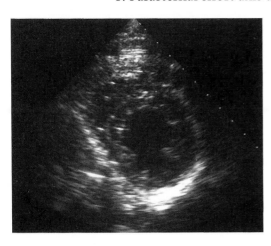
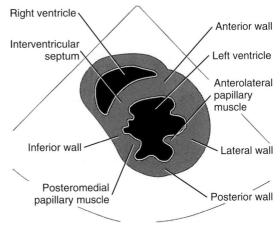

7. **APICAL 4-CHAMBER** view.

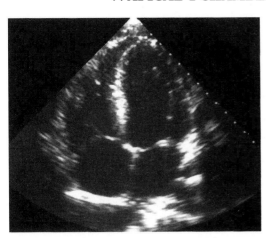
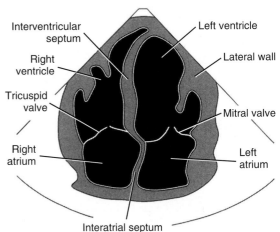

8. **APICAL 5-CHAMBER** view.

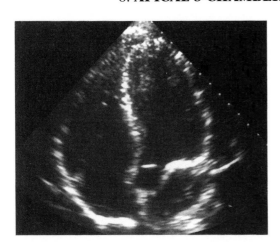
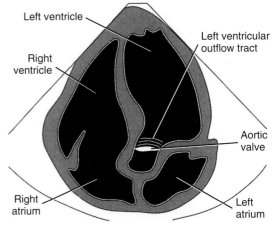

9. **APICAL 2-CHAMBER** view.

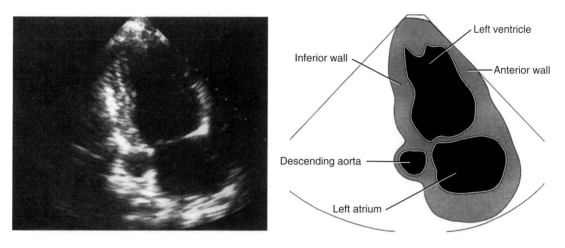

NOTE: When questions involving the aorta arise, a portion of the descending thoracic aorta can be visualized posterior to the 2-chamber view, and it should be evaluated for pathology.

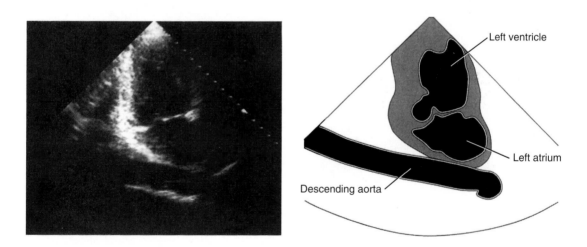

10. Apical **LONG AXIS.**

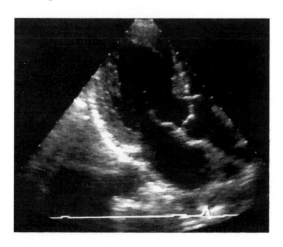
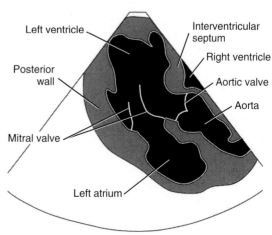

11. **SUBXIPHOID 4-CHAMBER** view.

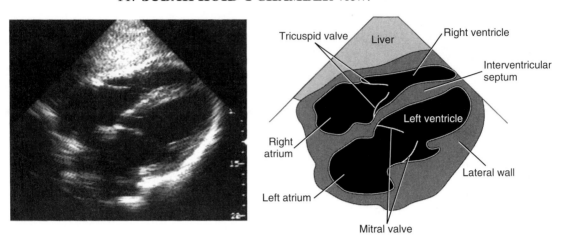

12. Subxiphoid short axis **PAPILLARY MUSCLE** level.

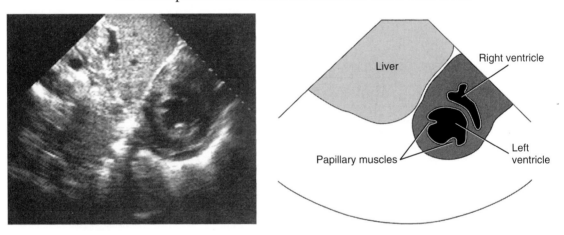

13. Subxiphoid short axis at the level of the **MITRAL VALVE.**

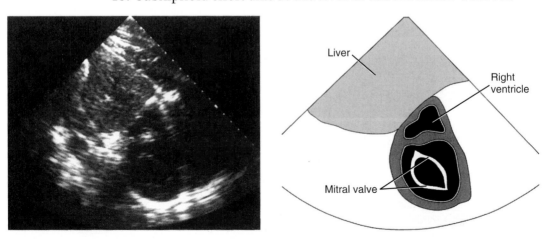

14. Subxiphoid short axis at the level of the **AORTIC VALVE.**

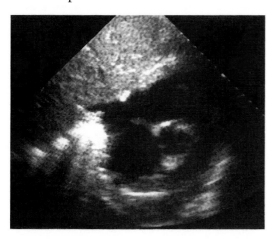 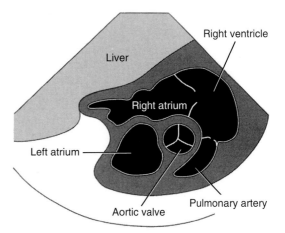

15. Subxiphoid short axis viewing the **IVC ENTERING THE RA.**

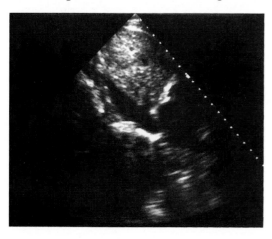 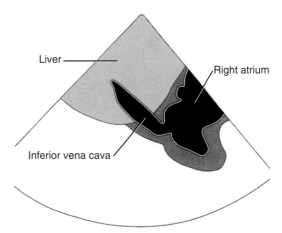

16. Suprasternal notch viewing the **LONG AXIS** of the aorta.

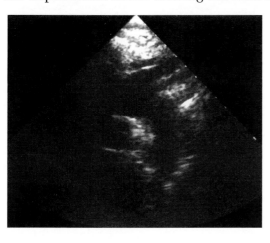 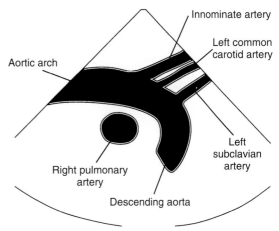

> **NOTE:** This view should be used when questions arise that involve the aorta, such as dissection or Marfan syndrome. A short axis of the aorta should also be evaluated in these cases.

M-Mode Evaluation

The M-Mode is a one-dimensional graphic drawing of the heart used to measure distance over time. An M-Mode is useful for obtaining dimensions of the heart and assessing fine movements too subtle for the eye to see.

> **NOTE:** Minimum of 6 beats should be recorded at each level demonstrating both systolic and diastolic motion.
>
> **NOTE:** The M-Mode may be documented on either videotape or strip chart recorder. If the strip chart is used, begin with a frozen image of the parasternal long axis view to demonstrate the orientation of the heart.
>
> **NOTE:** The 2D image must be as perpendicular to the ultrasound beam as possible, lessening the chance for inaccurate measurements. (A tipped ventricle will yield exaggerated numbers.) When measuring, if unsure of a dimension, omit it.

Aortic Valve Level

- The cursor is placed so that it transects the RV, aorta, and LA in either the parasternal long or short axis view.

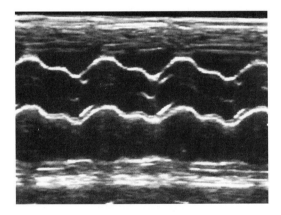
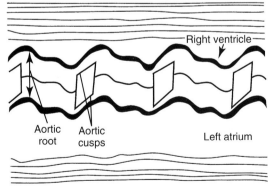

- Measurements*:
  1. *Aortic root:* from the anterior wall of the root to the posterior wall of the root, at the level of the Q wave on the ECG; normally 1.9 to 4 cm.
  2. *Aortic valve cusp separation:* normally has the shape of a box when open with the right coronary cusp more anterior and the noncoronary cusp posterior. Measured at the onset of systole (when the valve first opens); normally 1.5 to 2.6 cm.
  3. *Left atrium:* measured at the largest dimension (end systole); normally 1.9 to 4 cm.

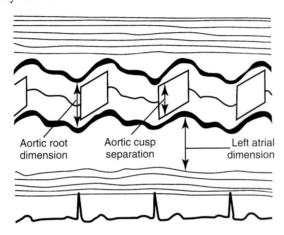

NOTE: Always measure structures from leading edge to leading edge.

Mitral Valve Level

- Slowly sweep the cursor through the LVOT region to the tip of the mitral valve leaflets. This sweep will demonstrate structural continuity. The biphasic opening of both mitral leaflets should then be documented.

*Normal values used in the laboratory at Thomas Jefferson University, Philadelphia, Pa.

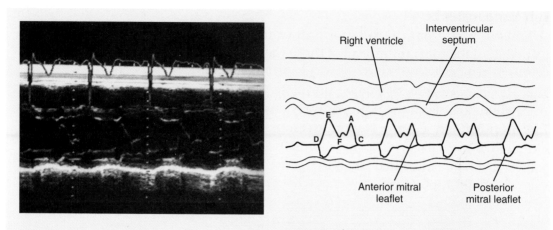

NOTE: The mitral valve is labeled to describe the different phases of its motion.

D: Beginning of diastole.

E: Maximal excursion of the valve.

F: Point to which the valve had closed following the passive filling phase.

A: Atrial contraction (P wave on the ECG).

B: Extra bump between A and C (occurs only when pathology, such as diastolic dysfunction, is present).

C: Closure of the valve and the beginning of systole.

- Measurements*:
    1. D to E excursion; normally greater than 1.6 cm.
    2. E to F slope over the period of 1 second (expressed in mm/sec); normally greater than 70 mm/sec.
    3. E point to septal separation; normally no greater than 1 cm.

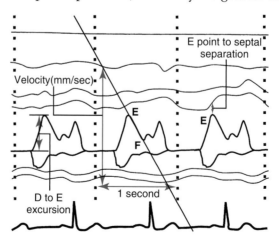

*Normal values used in the laboratory at Thomas Jefferson University, Philadelphia, Pa.

Left Ventricular Level

Slowly sweep the cursor just beyond the mitral leaflets but stopping before the papillary muscles. Both systolic and diastolic dimensions of the LV should be documented.

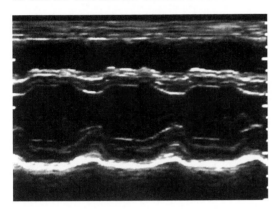 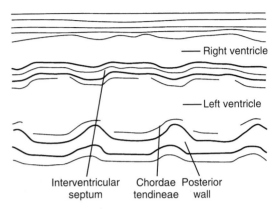

- Measurements*:
  1. All of the following are measured at the level of the Q wave on the ECG: RV (not greater than 2.7 cm); IVS, posterior LV wall (both normally between 0.6 and 1.2 cm); and LV end diastolic dimension (LVEDD) (normal range 3.5 to 5.7 cm).

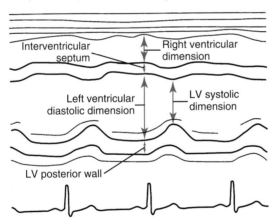

NOTE: Often the free wall of the RV is not visualized because of its close proximity to the transducer, making it difficult to determine the true size of the chamber. The measurement is therefore taken from the point where motion is first observed, to the leading edge of the interventricular septum. Then subtract 0.5 cm from the total to compensate for the RV wall thickness.

  2. LV end systolic dimension (LVESD): measure at the smallest dimension.

*Normal values used in the laboratory at Thomas Jefferson University, Philadelphia, Pa.

NOTE: The LVEDD and the LVESD should be measured on the same beat.

NOTE: Be careful not to include chordae tendineae in the thickness of the LV walls.

Tricuspid and Pulmonic Valves

An M-Mode of the tricuspid or pulmonic valve is used to demonstrate thickness and motion and are not necessarily a routine part of the examination. No standard measurements are obtained.

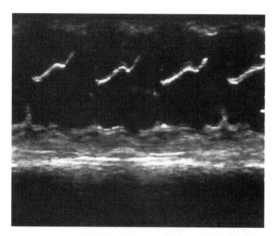
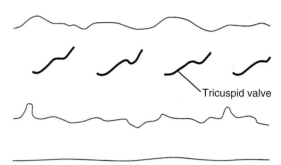

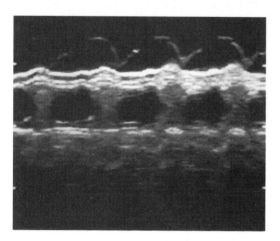
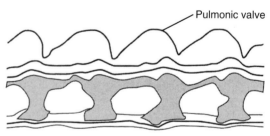

Doppler Evaluation

- Used to assess blood flow through the heart, including increased velocities, stenosis, regurgitation, and shunts.
- Both continuous-wave (CW) and pulsed-wave (PW) Doppler are used in conjunction with each other. In addition, color Doppler simplifies the mapping process and gives a visual representation of the size and direction of blood flow disturbances.

Normal Valve Profiles

Mitral Valve

- The flow profile is shaped like an M and is best sampled in the apical 4-chamber view. Here, blood flow moves towards the transducer during diastole; therefore, the waveform appears above the baseline. Peak velocity should not exceed 1.3 m/sec.*

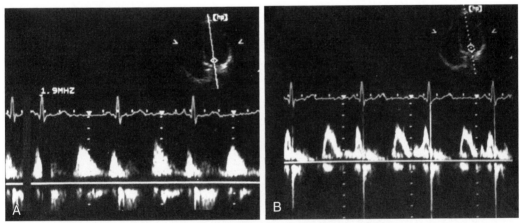

A, Continuous-wave mitral valve Doppler. **B,** Pulsed-wave mitral valve Doppler.

NOTE: Pulsed-wave Doppler has an envelope (whiter outline) and window (darker interior) versus the filled-in profile of continuous wave. In cases of turbulent flow, this PW window can become filled in and is called spectral broadening.

Tricuspid Valve

- The flow profile also looks like an M and occurs during diastole. It is best sampled in either the right ventricular inflow view or the apical 4-chamber view. Blood flow moves towards the transducer; therefore, the profile appears above the baseline. Peak velocity should not exceed 0.7 m/sec.*

*Hatle L, Angelsen B: *Doppler ultrasound in cardiology,* ed 2. Philadelphia, 1985, Lea & Febiger, p 93.

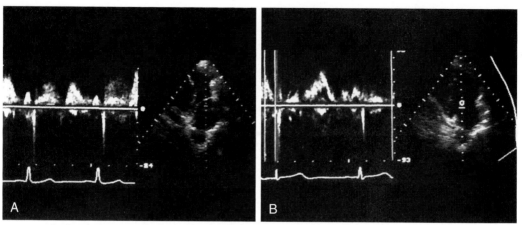

A, Continuous-wave tricuspid valve Doppler. **B,** Pulsed-wave tricuspid valve Doppler.

Aortic Valve

- A sample is best taken from the apical 5-chamber view and the profile has the shape of a bullet. In this case, blood flow is moving away from the transducer during systole and therefore appears below the baseline. Peak velocity should not exceed 1.7 m/sec.*

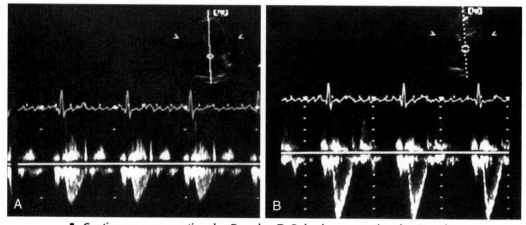

A, Continuous-wave aortic valve Doppler. **B,** Pulsed-wave aortic valve Doppler.

Pulmonic Valve

- The profile is also shaped like a bullet, but is best sampled in parasternal short axis at the level of the aortic valve. Flow moves away from the transducer during systole; therefore, it appears below the baseline. Peak velocity should not exceed 0.9 m/sec.*

*Hatle L, Angelsen B: *Doppler ultrasound in cardiology,* ed 2. Philadelphia, 1985, Lea & Febiger, p 93.

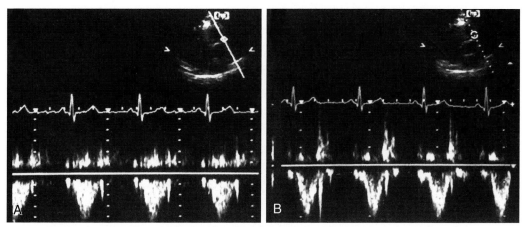

A, Continuous-wave pulmonic valve Doppler. **B,** Pulsed-wave pulmonic valve Doppler.

Left Ventricular Outflow Tract

- Systolic flow sampled in this region is also shaped like a bullet and appears below the baseline. It is best sampled in the apical five-chamber view and peak velocity should not exceed 1.1 m/sec.*

> **NOTE:** Doppler is best when flow is parallel to the ultrasound beam. In contrast, 2D is best when perpendicular. Therefore, the best Doppler image is not necessarily the best 2D image.

Valve Survey

> **NOTE:** The following sequence should be used in the evaluation of each valve: color Doppler, continuous-wave (CW) Doppler, then pulse-wave (PW) Doppler. Assess each value separately beginning with the mitral valve. Repeat this process on the aortic, tricuspid, and pulmonic valves, and the left ventricular outflow tract (LVOT) if necessary.

Color Doppler Survey

> **NOTE:** Flow moving towards the transducer appears as various shades of red. Flow moving away is blue. A lower velocity would be deeper in color and gradually lighten as the velocity increases to almost yellow or white. At times, a variance map is used. This is usually green tagged on the end of the color spectrum. The green makes the higher velocities or turbulent flows stand out.

---

*Hatle L, Angelsen B: *Doppler ultrasound in cardiology,* ed 2. Philadelphia, 1985, Lea & Febiger, p 93.

- The color sector should be placed so that the valve or area being assessed is in the center of the sample. Normally, mitral and tricuspid flow appear red, and pulmonic and aortic flow are blue. When the valves are closed, no color (regurgitation) should be seen below them. Mitral and tricuspid regurgitation appear blue; aortic and pulmonic regurgitation are usually red.
- Slowly angle the transducer back and forth across the valve plane to locate any eccentric areas of turbulence. Demonstrate the size and location of any regurgitation or turbulent flow.
- Color can also be used to locate the peak flow velocity across the valve allowing for easy placement of the CW Doppler cursor.

NOTE: Regurgitation or any pathology should be demonstrated in more than one view.

Continuous-Wave Doppler Survey

- CW Doppler is best for determining peak flow velocities. Place the cursor so it bisects the opening of the valve that is to be sampled. If the peak velocity across a valve exceeds its normal velocity, the peak should then be measured. Three profiles are measured and averaged. Do not measure post PVC beats. If the patient is in atrial fibrillation, average at least 5 or 6 beats.
- The peak velocity of tricuspid regurgitation is also measured to help with the evaluation of pulmonary hypertension.

NOTE: If unable to find a peak velocity on any valve, tricuspid or aortic regurgitation, a nonimaging, stand-alone CW probe should be used. Because of the smaller footprint of the transducer and the lower frequency, the peak velocity can be easily found.

Pulsed-Wave Doppler Survey

- PW Doppler demonstrates exactly where a flow disturbance occurs and is then used to map out the direction and size of the disturbance. Place the cursor or Doppler "gate" slightly above the valve opening. Slowly move below the valve, then across the valve plane in both directions. If regurgitation is detected, follow the flow into the chamber as far back as it goes, mapping the length and also the width of the turbulent area.

NOTE: If any additional flow disturbances (e.g., ASD, VSD) are visualized, they too should be evaluated with color, CW, and PW Doppler.

Table 22-1 Standard Doppler Positions	
View	**Structure**
Parasternal long axis	Interventricular septum
Parasternal short axis:	
Aortic valve level	Tricuspid valve, pulmonic valve, right ventricular outflow tract (RVOT), pulmonary artery, ductal flow
Mitral to left ventricle	Interventricular septum
Right ventricular inflow	Tricuspid valve
Right ventricular outflow	Pulmonic valve, RVOT
Right parasternal	Aortic valve flow
Apical 4-chamber	Mitral valve, tricuspid valve
Apical 5-chamber	Aortic valve, left ventricular outflow tract (LVOT)
Apical 2-chamber	Mitral valve
Apical long axis	Mitral valve, aortic valve, LVOT
Subcostal 4-chamber	Interatrial and interventricular septums, IVC
Suprasternal	Ascending, arch and descending aorta, pulmonary flow

Review Questions

Answers on page 631.

1. The adult heart is located between the _____ intercostal spaces.
   a) first and fifth
   b) fourth and seventh
   c) third and fifth
   d) fourth and fifth

2. The right atrium receives blood from the
   a) superior vena cava, inferior vena cava, and coronary sinus.
   b) superior vena cava and inferior vena cava.
   c) superior vena cava and pulmonary veins.
   d) superior vena cava and coronary sinus.

3. The _____ is the sac around the heart.
   a) epicardium
   b) endocardium
   c) myocardium
   d) pericardium

4. The _____ is the muscular layer of the heart.
   a) epicardium
   b) endocardium
   c) myocardium
   d) pericardium

5. The _____ is the smooth inner layer of the heart.
   a) epicardium
   b) endocardium
   c) myocardium
   d) pericardium

6. The _____ is the smooth, outer layer of the heart.
   a) epicardium
   b) endocardium
   c) myocardium
   d) pericardium

7. An appendage or auricle is found at
   a) the upper portion of both ventricles.
   b) the inferior portion of both ventricles.
   c) the inferior portion of both atria.
   d) the upper portion of both atria.

8. The _____ is the most anterior heart chamber.
   a) right atrium
   b) left atrium
   c) left ventricle
   d) right ventricle

9. The _____ valve is located between the left atrium and left ventricle.
   a) tricuspid
   b) thebesian
   c) mitral
   d) eustachian

10. The _____ valve is located between the right atrium and right ventricle.
    a) tricuspid
    b) thebesian
    c) mitral
    d) eustachian

11. The four routine positions to image the heart are
    a) subxiphoid, subcostal, parasternal, and apical.
    b) intercostal, subcostal, parasternal, and suprasternal.
    c) subxiphoid, subcostal, suprasternal, and apical.
    d) subxiphoid, parasternal, suprasternal, and apical.

12. The heart sits at an angle between the
    a) left shoulder and left hip.
    b) right shoulder and right hip.
    c) right shoulder and left hip.
    d) right shoulder and sternum.

13. The _____ view should be used to rule out abnormalities of the aorta.
    a) apical
    b) subcostal
    c) suprasternal
    d) parasternal

14. At least _____ beats of each view should be recorded when video-taping a study.
    a) 10 to 12
    b) 10
    c) 6
    d) 6 to 10

15. The _____ is a one-dimensional graphic presentation of the heart.
    a) M-mode
    b) Doppler
    c) gray-scale image
    d) B-mode

16. The _____ obtains dimensions of the heart and assesses fine movements too subtle for the eye to see.
    a) M-mode
    b) Doppler
    c) gray-scale image
    d) B-mode

17. The _____ assesses blood flow through the heart.
    a) M-mode
    b) Doppler
    c) gray-scale image
    d) B-mode

18. Pulsed-wave Doppler and continuous-wave Doppler are _____ to evaluate the heart.
    a) used in conjunction with each other
    b) used in lieu of each other
    c) converted to gray-scale
    d) not used

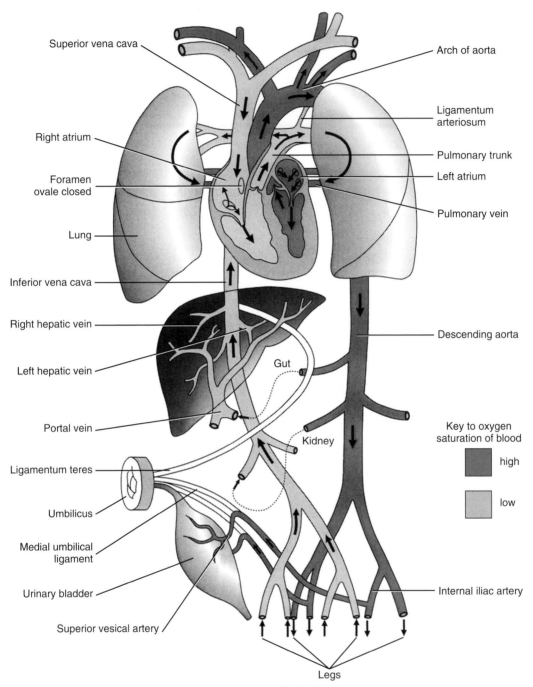

Superior vena cava

Arch of aorta

Ligamentum arteriosum

Right atrium

Pulmonary trunk

Foramen ovale closed

Left atrium

Pulmonary vein

Lung

Inferior vena cava

Right hepatic vein

Descending aorta

Left hepatic vein

Gut

Portal vein

Kidney

Key to oxygen saturation of blood

high

Ligamentum teres

low

Umbilicus

Medial umbilical ligament

Urinary bladder

Internal iliac artery

Superior vesical artery

Legs

Anatomy of the Pediatric Heart

CHAPTER 23

Pediatric Echocardiography Scanning Protocol

Maureen E. McDonald

Objectives
At the end of this chapter, you will be able to:

- Distinguish the sonographic appearance of the pediatric heart and the terms used to describe it.
- Describe the transducer options for scanning the pediatric heart.
- List the imaging planes of the pediatric heart.
- Name the various suggested breathing techniques for the pediatric patient when scanning the heart.
- List the suggested patient position (and options) when scanning the pediatric heart.
- Describe the patient prep for a pediatric heart study.
- Name the survey steps and explain how to evaluate the entire pediatric heart and associated structures.
- List the order and exact locations to take representative images of the pediatric heart aorta.
- Answer the review questions at the end of the chapter.

Overview

Anatomy and Physiology
- See Chapter 22, Adult Echocardiography Scanning Protocol.

Sonographic Appearance
- The pericardium is the brightest structure and appears almost white.
- The valves tend to be the next brightest, appearing light gray to almost white depending upon how perpendicular the valve is to the ultrasound beam.
- The myocardium has a homogeneous texture and appears gray.
- The area within the chambers, vessels, and any fluid appear anechoic.

Preparation

Patient Prep
- An infant or young child may need to be sedated if he or she is uncooperative with the examination. Special arrangements should

be made to have a physician administer chloral hydrate before the examination.

- ECG leads should be attached to the right shoulder, left shoulder, and left hip regions.

Transducer

- 7.5 MHz used for premature infants.
- 5.0 MHz to 7.5 MHz used for neonates to infants.
- 5.0 MHz to 3.5 MHz for toddlers (depending on the body surface area).
- 3.5 MHz to 2.5 MHz used for children and teenagers (depending on body habitus).

Patient Position

- Neonates and infants may remain supine.
- Children (classified as anyone under the age of 17 years) should be in the left lateral decubitus position.

Breathing Techniques

- Normal respiration.

Transducer Orientation

- Images are obtained from the following 4 windows:
  1. Parasternal
  2. Apical
  3. Subcostal
  4. Suprasternal

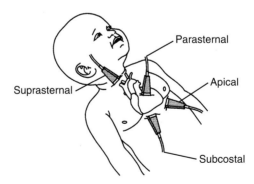

- Scanning is performed in the anatomically corrected position; therefore, the sector is inverted for the subcostal and apical views. The study thus provides an anatomic reference for the surgeon.

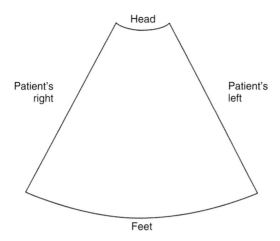

- The ECG rate is increased to 100% for neonates because of the higher infant heart rate. This allows for easier interpretation of the Doppler and ECG.

Pediatric Heart Survey

1. Begin by placing the transducer midline on the abdomen, below the xiphoid process. Flip the sector, so the point appears at the bottom of the screen. Looking at the monitor, the image should be oriented so the structures on the patient's left appear to the right of the screen. Point directly anterior to posterior, visualizing the liver and cross sections of **the inferior vena cava (IVC)** (found on the patient's right) and aorta (to the patient's left). This establishes normal situs of the abdominal structures.

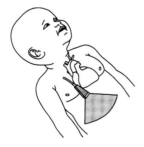

2. Slowly angle superiorly, demonstrating the entry of the hepatic veins into the IVC and eventually the IVC into the right atrium (RA). Continue to angle superiorly until the 4 chambers of the heart are observed. Verify the orientation of the heart, its chambers, and valves. The apex should appear to the right of the screen. Look for the 4 pulmonary veins to enter the left atrium (LA). Use color Doppler and pulsed-wave (PW) Doppler to assess the flow across the **mitral (MV)** and **tricuspid (TV) valves**. Use color Doppler for the interatrial septum and interventricular septums to

assess for the presence of a shunt. Pulse any turbulence observed. Use continuous-wave (CW) Doppler to evaluate any high veloci-ties (e.g., ventricular septal defect, tricuspid regurgitation).

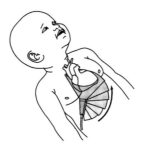

3. Continue to angle the transducer more superiorly, opening the left ventricular outflow tract (LVOT) and the aorta. Use color and PW Doppler for these, looking for the presence of regurgitation or turbulence.
4. Tilting the transducer even more superiorly will open the right ventricular outflow region, **pulmonic valve (PV)**, and pulmonary artery (PA). Use color and PW Doppler to assess the PV for turbu-lence and for the presence of a patent ductus arteriosus (PDA).
5. Slowly tilt inferiorly to return to the 4-chamber view, then rotate the transducer clockwise 90 degrees. This is the orientation for the subcostal short axis views. Begin by directing the transducer toward the right shoulder, demonstrating the entry of the supe-rior vena cava and inferior vena cava into the right atrium. Use color Doppler to scan the IVC and superior vena cava (SVC). Use PW to establish normal flow profiles.

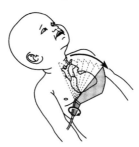

6. Slowly begin to angle the transducer toward the left shoulder, first observing the interatrial septum, then the PA, PV, and **aor-tic valve (AV).** Use color Doppler and PW for any turbulence observed. Continue to sweep leftward through the mitral and tricuspid valves, assessing thickness and motion, to the cross section of the left (LV) and right (RV) ventricles. Slowly sweep beyond the papillary muscles to the apical region, all the while assessing thickness and contractility. Repeat using color Doppler, looking for any shunts.

7. Move the transducer to the left flank, directing the beam towards the right shoulder. This will dissect the heart from apex to base, and the apical 4-chamber view is visualized. The left side of the heart should appear to the right of the screen. The LA, LV, RA, and RV are observed as well as the mitral and tricuspid valves. Assess the chamber sizes and valves. Use color and PW Doppler for both the valves, and use CW Doppler for any high-velocity flow.

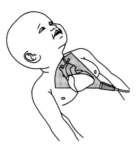

8. Angle the transducer slightly anterior to open the LVOT and aorta. This is the apical 5-chamber view. Use color and PW Doppler for the aortic valve and LVOT.

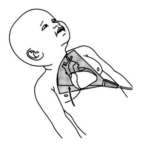

9. Rotate the transducer clockwise to open the outflow tract even more. This produces the apical long axis. In addition, the AV, LA, LV, and MV are seen. Again, use color Doppler for the LVOT region and PW Doppler up the IVS, looking for a step-up in velocity or any turbulence.

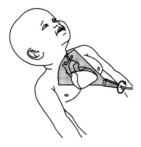

10. Flip the sector to its original position, with the point at the top of the screen. Move the transducer to the left of the sternum to the parasternal region. The image should be oriented so a long

axis of the left ventricle appears to the left of the screen and the aorta to the right. The anterior portion of the aortic root and the interventricular septum (IVS) should run continuous and the posterior part of the aortic root and the anterior mitral valve leaflet are continuous. Evaluate the size of the LA, MV, LV, posterior LV wall, IVS, and the RV for anatomic relationships, size, thickness, and motion. Use color Doppler to evaluate the valves and IVS. Use CW Doppler for any high velocities.

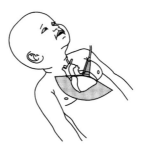

11. Slowly angle the transducer inferior and medial to open the right ventricular inflow view. This will visualize the RA, RV, and TV, which are the most anterior structures of the heart. Assess the tricuspid valve with color Doppler and CW Doppler for any high velocities. Slowly return to the parasternal long axis view, using color Doppler to evaluate the IVS. Use CW Doppler for any high velocities.

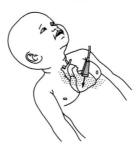

12. Angle the transducer towards the left shoulder to open the right ventricular outflow region. This includes the RV outflow tract, PV, and main PA. Use color Doppler and PW Doppler for any turbulence. Again return to the long axis view.

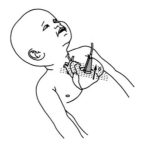

13. Rotate the transducer clockwise 90 degrees to obtain the short-axis parasternal views. Begin by directing the beam towards the right shoulder, demonstrating the aortic valve, LA, RA, PV, and PA. Assess the number of cusps of the aortic valve. Slowly angle slightly above the level of the leaflets to evaluate for the presence of the right and left coronary arteries. Use color Doppler for the interatrial septum, tricuspid, and pulmonic valves. Angle slightly anterior and leftward to open the right and left pulmonary arteries and use PW Doppler for each. Use color Doppler to check for the presence of a PDA, and PW and CW Doppler if PDA is present.

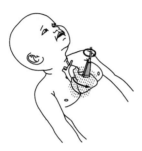

14. Slowly begin sweeping the transducer to the left, moving through the level of the mitral valve to the left ventricle and as far towards the apex as possible, all the while assessing thickness and contractility. Repeat the sweep, this time using color Doppler, looking for any turbulence across the septum. Use CW Doppler for any high velocities.

15. Move the transducer near the sternoclavicular notch in the suprasternal region. Direct the beam inferiorly, looking for a long axis of the aortic arch. Identify the branching vessels and establish aortic orientation. Look for any areas of narrowing, using color Doppler to identify areas of turbulence. Use PW Doppler for the ascending, arch, and descending aorta, and CW Doppler for any increased velocities. Evaluate the LA posterior to the right pulmonary artery and look for the presence of pulmonary veins.

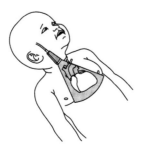

16. Rotate the transducer clockwise 90 degrees, opening the branching PAs. Use color and PW Doppler for each branch. A cross section of the aorta is also visualized.

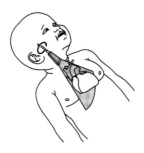

Pediatric Heart Required Images

NOTE: The following views are all recorded on videotape, allowing for real-time assessment of cardiac structures. At least 8 to 10 beats of each view is recorded with additional images for color, PW, and CW Doppler.

Subcostal Views

1. **AORTA** and **IVC** orientation.

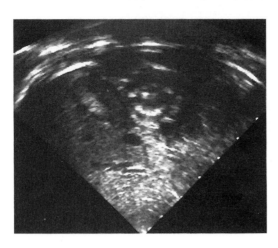
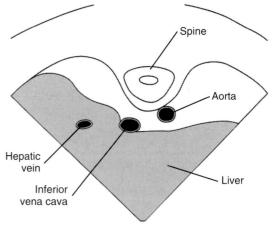

2. Subcostal **4-CHAMBER** view.

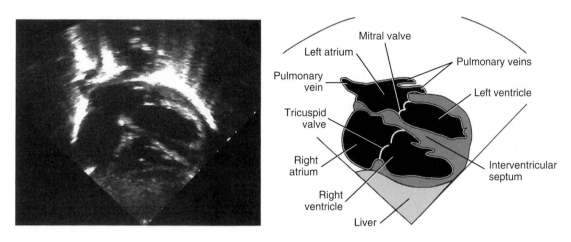

3. **5 CHAMBER** with **AORTA** and **LVOT** (left ventricular outflow tract).

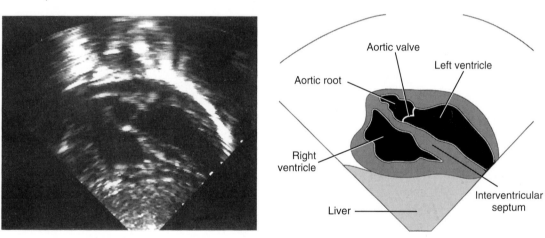

4. Anterior angled long axis with **RVOT** (right ventricular outflow tract), **PULMONIC VALVE,** and **PULMONARY ARTERY.**

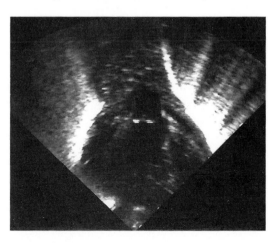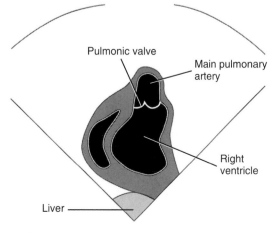

5. Short axis with **IVC** and **SVC** entering the **RIGHT ATRIUM.**

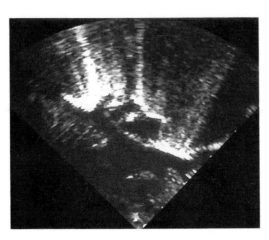
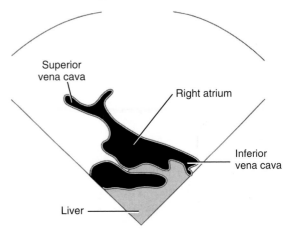

6. Short axis with **AORTIC VALVE, PULMONARY,** and **INTER-ATRIAL SEPTUM.**

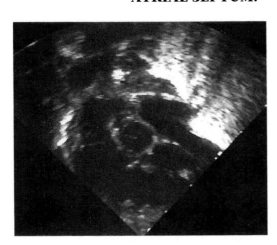
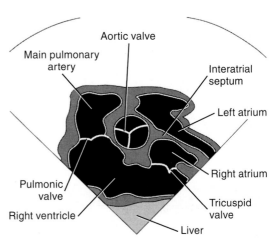

NOTE: A small angulation may be needed to fully visualize the inter-atrial septum.

7. Short axis of the **MITRAL VALVE.**

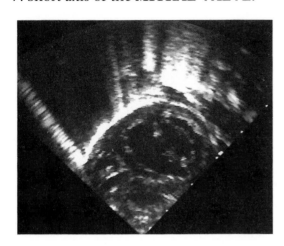
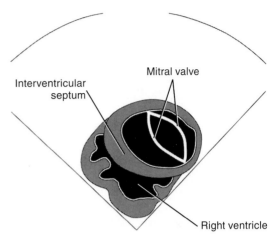

8. Short axis of the **LEFT AND RIGHT VENTRICLES.**

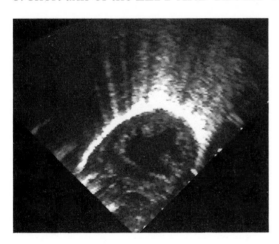
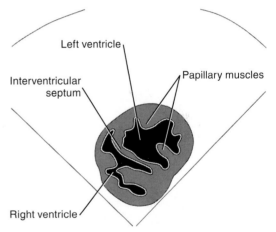

Apical Views

9. Apical **4-CHAMBER** view.

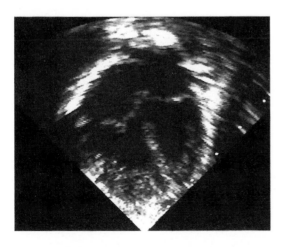
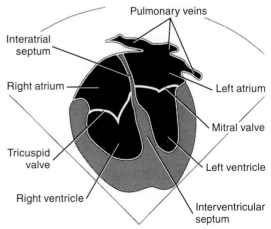

10. Long axis with **LVOT.**

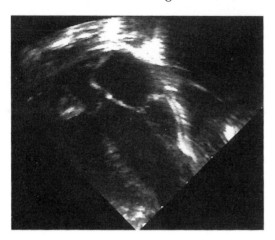

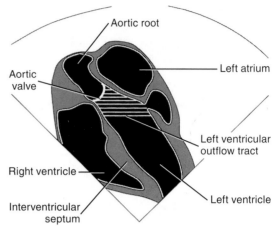

Parasternal Views
11. LONG AXIS.

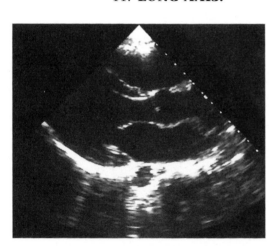

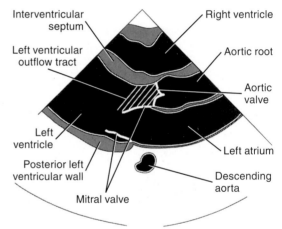

12. RIGHT VENTRICULAR INFLOW VIEW.

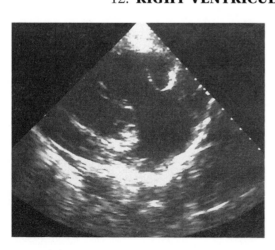

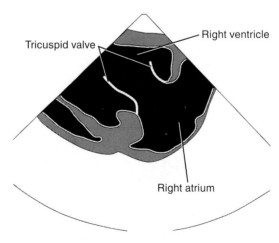

13. **RIGHT VENTRICULAR OUTFLOW VIEW.**

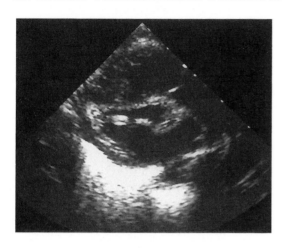
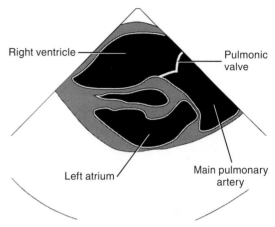

14. Short axis at **AORTIC VALVE LEVEL** with orientation of great vessels.

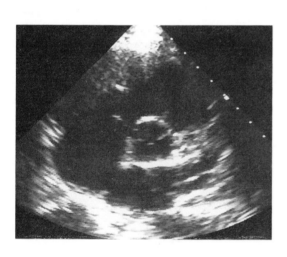
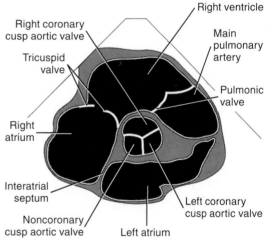

15. Short axis **LEFT CORONARY ARTERY.**

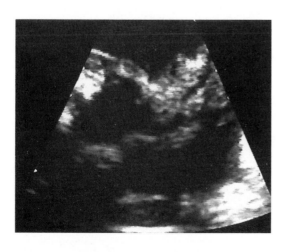
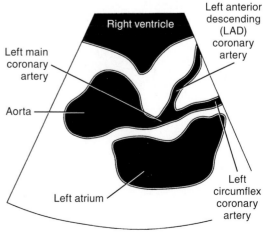

NOTE: Angle slightly above the aortic valve leaflets and zoom in on the region to simplify coronary evaluation.

16. Short axis **RIGHT CORONARY ARTERY**.

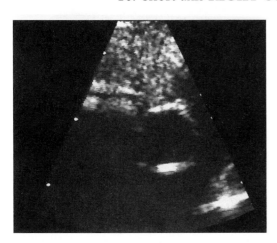
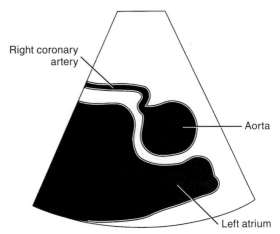

17. Short axis **RIGHT** and **LEFT PULMONARY BRANCHES** and presence/absence of **PATENT DUCTUS ARTERIOSUS**.

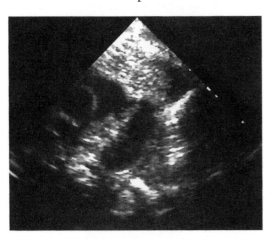
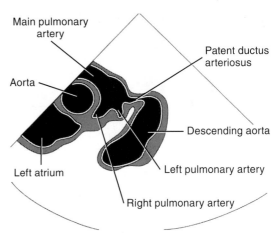

NOTE: If a ductus is present, demonstrate its connection to the aorta.

18. Short axis at **MITRAL VALVE LEVEL** with **LEAFLET MOTION** and **THICKNESS.**

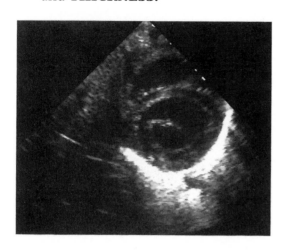 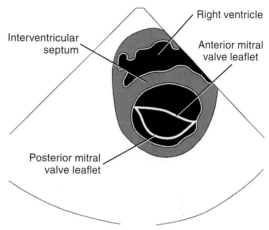

19. Short axis at **PAPILLARY MUSCLES LEVEL.**

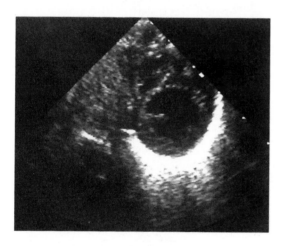 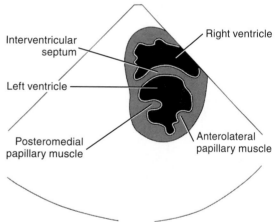

Suprasternal Notch Views

20. **AORTIC ARCH AND ITS BRANCHES.**

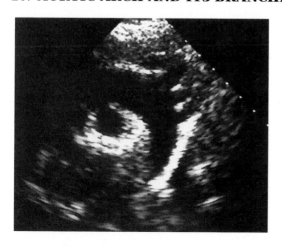 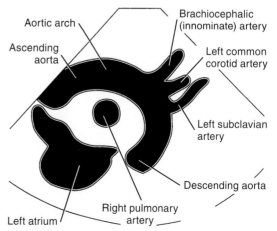

21. **BRANCH PULMONARY ARTERIES** and **SHORT AXIS OF THE AORTA**.

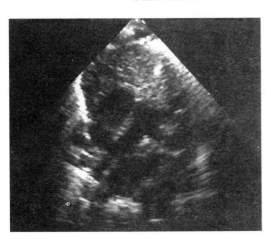

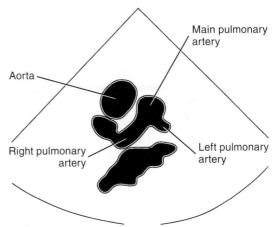

Required M-Mode Images

An M-Mode scan should be performed from either the parasternal long axis or the parasternal short axis by placing the cursor through the following 3 levels:

1. Aortic valve level.

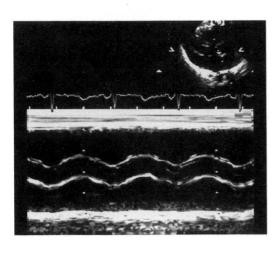

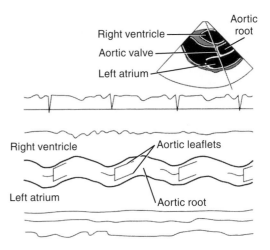

2. Mitral valve level.

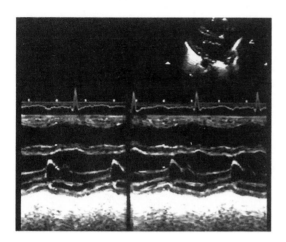

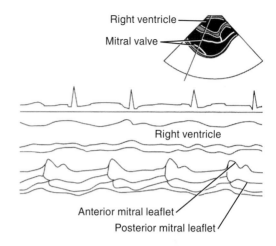

3. Left ventricular level.

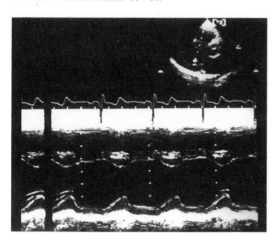

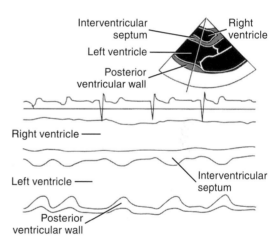

Attention should be given to the sizes of the chambers, motion of the valves, ventricular contractility, and structural continuity.

NOTE: Sweep speed of the M-Mode is increased to 100% to accommodate the increased heart rate of neonates.

Review Questions

Answers on page 631.

1. The thin area in the midportion of the interatrial septum is the
   a) sinus of Valsalva.
   b) annulus fibrosis.
   c) chordae tendineae.
   d) fossa ovalis.

2. The sonographic appearance of the pericardium is
   a) hyperechoic relative to adjacent structures.
   b) medium gray with heterogeneous echo texture.
   c) anechoic.
   d) medium gray with homogeneous echo texture.

3. The sonographic appearance of the myocardium is
   a) hyperechoic relative to adjacent structures.
   b) medium gray with heterogeneous echo texture.
   c) anechoic.
   d) medium gray with homogeneous echo texture.

4. During fetal circulation, the _____ serves as a passage to the left heart.
   a) sinus of Valsalva
   b) annulus fibrosis
   c) chordae tendineae
   d) fossa ovalis

5. The sonographic appearance of the area within the heart chambers is
   a) hyperechoic relative to adjacent structures.
   b) medium gray with heterogeneous echo texture.
   c) anechoic.
   d) medium gray with homogeneous echo texture.

6. Images are obtained from which windows?
   a) Parasternal, suprasternal
   b) Parasternal, suprasternal, apical, subcostal
   c) Parasternal, subcostal
   d) Suprasternal, apical, subcostal

AIUM: American Institute of Ultrasound in Medicine

ALARA: As low as reasonably acceptable

ANT: Anterior

ART: Artery

AV: Atrioventricular

AV: Atrioventricular valves

BIF: Bifurcation

CBD: Common bile duct

cc: Cubic centimeter

CD: Common duct

CERX: Cervix

CFA: Common femoral artery

CFV: Common femoral vein

CHD: Common hepatic duct

cm: Centimeter

COR: Coronal

CRL: Crown rump length

C-SPINE: Cervical spine

CW: Continuous-wave Doppler

DECUB: Decubitus

DP: Dorsalis pedis artery

ECG: Electrocardiogram

ER: Endorectal

EV: Endovaginal

Fd: Doppler shift frequency

Fo: Operating frequency

GB: Gallbladder

GS: Gestational sac

Hz: Hertz

IN: Inches

INF: Inferior

IVC: Inferior vena cava

IVS: Interventricular septum

kHz: Kilohertz

KID: Kidney

LA: Left atrium

LAD: Left anterior descending

LAT: Lateral

LLD: Left lateral decubitus

LPO: Left posterior oblique

L-SPINE: Lumbar spine

LT: Left

LV: Left ventricular

LVOT: Left ventricular outflow tract

MED: Medical

MHz: Megahertz

ML: Midline

mm: Millimeter

MV: Mitral valve

NIP: Nipple

OBL: Oblique

OV: Ovary

PA: Pulmonary artery

PDA: Patent ductus arteriosus

PFV: Profunda femoris vein

POP: Popliteal artery

POST: Posterior

PRF: Time and depth limitations

PROX: Proximal

PTA: Posterior tibial artery

PV: Pulmonic valve

PW: Pulsed-wave Doppler

RA: Right atrium

RCA: Right coronary artery

RI: Resistive indices

RLD: Right lateral decubitus

RPO: Right posterior oblique

RT: Right

RV: Right ventricle

SA: Sinoatrial node

SAG: Sagittal

SEM V: Seminal vesicles

SFA: Superficial femoral artery

SFV: Superficial femoral vein

SMA: Superior mesenteric artery

SUP: Superior

SVC: Superior vena cava

TGC: Time-gain compensation

TRV: Transverse

T-SPINE: Thoracic spine

TV: Tricuspid valve

UT: Uterus

VAG: Vagina

Answers to Review Questions

Chapter 1
1. d
2. a
3. b
4. d
5. c
6. a
7. b
8. b
9. c
10. c
11. c
12. d
13. d
14. c
15. b

Chapter 2
1. anterior and posterior
2. d
3. superior and inferior
4. a
5. right and left
6. a
7. two
8. c
9. c
10. b
11. how the structure of interest lies in the body.
12. the greatest margins of structures.
13. depth
14. focal zone

Chapter 3
1. b
2. b
3. c
4. a
5. b
6. d
7. d
8. c
9. d
10. (1) origin, (2) size, (3) composition, (4) number, and (5) any associated complications with adjacent structures or body systems.
11. The findings in the image can be described as: "Anechoic, intrahepatic mass just superior to the right kidney. Walls appear thin and well-defined. Increased posterior through transmission is present."
12. The findings in this image can be described as: "Heterogeneous mass in the inferior portion of the head of the pancreas (arrow). Mass appears hypoechoic relative to the pancreas. Multiple small anechoic areas scattered throughout mass."
13. The findings in this image can be described as: "Multiple echogenic foci within the gallbladder. Distal shadowing is noted."
14. The findings in this image can be described as: "Intrahepatic right lobe mass. Mass appears hyperechoic compared to the liver. Contour is smooth and defined. Mass appears confined to one area."
15. The findings in this image can be described as: "Intrahepatic right upper quadrant mass compressing the superior pole of the right kidney inferiorly. Mass appears slightly hyperechoic compared to the liver and kidney. Contour is smooth and well defined. No calcifications or anechoic areas seen in the mass. 2.7 cm anteroposteriorly, 2.6 cm long."

Chapter 4
1. b
2. a
3. b
4. b
5. b
6. a
7. a
8. b
9. b
10. b
11. d
12. b
13. d
14. c
15. b

Chapter 5
1. b
2. a
3. b
4. a
5. d
6. a
7. a
8. c
9. b
10. b
11. d
12. c
13. c
14. a
15. b
16. a

17. b
18. b
19. c
20. b
21. b
22. c
23. b
24. d
25. b
26. b
27. d

Chapter 6
1. c
2. d
3. a
4. a
5. c
6. c
7. b
8. b
9. c
10. c
11. b
12. b
13. a (right, left, caudate)
14. b
15. a

Chapter 7
1. b
2. a
3. b
4. a
5. d
6. a
7. c
8. b
9. c
10. c
11. c
12. a
13. a, True
14. a, True
15. b
16. c
17. b
18. d
19. a, True
20. a, True
21. a, True
22. a, True

Chapter 8
1. d
2. b
3. a
4. a
5. c
6. c
7. b
8. b
9. d
10. d
11. c
12. d
13. b
14. a
15. d

Chapter 9
1. d
2. b
3. c
4. d
5. c
6. c
7. b
8. d
9. a
10. c
11. c
12. a
13. d
14. b
15. Answers within Chapter 9.
16. Answers within Chapter 9.
17. Answers within Chapter 9.

Chapter 10
1. b
2. c
3. b
4. c
5. b
6. a
7. d
8. c
9. a
10. a
11. c
12. a
13. c

14. Answers within Chapter 10.
15. Answers within Chapter 10.
16. Answers within Chapter 10.

Chapter 11
1. d
2. d
3. a
4. b
5. a
6. c
7. a
8. d
9. a
10. c
11. b
12. a
13. d
14. a
15. c
16. c
17. c
18. Answer within Chapter 11.
19. Answer within Chapter 11.
20. Answer within Chapter 11.

Chapter 12
1. c
2. c
3. d
4. d
5. d
6. a
7. c
8. a
9. d
10. False
11. False
12. False
13. False

Chapter 13
1. b
2. c
3. d
4. c
5. d

6. b
7. b
8. c
9. c
10. c
11. c
12. d
13. b
14. c
15. b
16. b
17. a
18. a
19. b
20. c

Chapter 14
1. a
2. c
3. c
4. d
5. a
6. a
7. b
8. b
9. c
10. c
11. b
12. a
13. d
14. a
15. d
16. c
17. c
18. b
19. c
20. a

Chapter 15
Rotator Cuff
1. b
2. d
3. c
4. b
5. a
6. d
7. c
8. d
9. b
10. b
Carpal Tunnel
11. d
12. b

13. b
14. a
15. d
16. c
17. a
18. c
19. a
20. c
Achilles Tendon
21. c
22. e
23. d
24. a
25. a
26. d
27. b
28. b
29. c
30. a
31. d
32. c
33. b
34. a
35. a

Chapter 16
1. c
2. c
3. a
4. b
5. b
6. a
7. c
8. a
9. d
10. d
11. b
12. c
13. b
14. b
15. a
16. a
17. b
18. b
19. d
20. d

Chapter 17
1. c
2. a
3. d
4. d
5. b

6. b
7. a
8. a
9. b
10. a

Chapter 18
1. d
2. c
3. a
4. b
5. d
6. b
7. d
8. c
9. c
10. a
11. a
12. b
13. d
14. a
15. c

Chapter 19
1. c
2. b
3. a
4. d
5. a
6. d
7. c
8. b
9. c
10. a
11. d
12. c

Chapter 20
1. c
2. b
3. d
4. b
5. c
6. a
7. d
8. b
9. d
10. d

Chapter 21
1. c
2. a
3. c
4. c

5. b
6. d
7. c
8. a
9. c
10. c

Chapter 22
1. c
2. a
3. d
4. c

5. b
6. a
7. d
8. d
9. c
10. a
11. d
12. c
13. c
14. d
15. a

16. a
17. b
18. a

Chapter 23
1. d
2. a
3. d
4. d
5. c
6. b

Guidelines for Performance of the Abdominal and Retroperitoneal Ultrasound Examination

The following are proposed guidelines for ultrasound evaluation of the upper abdomen. The document consists of 2 parts:

Part I: Equipment and Documentation Guidelines
Part II: Guidelines for a General Examination of the Abdomen and Retroperitoneum

These guidelines have been developed to provide assistance to practitioners performing ultrasound studies in the abdomen and retroperitoneum. In some cases additional and/or specialized examinations may be necessary. Although it is not possible to detect every abnormality, adherence to the following guidelines will maximize the probability of detecting most of the abnormalities that occur in the abdomen and retroperitoneum.

Part I: Guidelines for Equipment and Documentation

Equipment

Abdominal and retroperitoneal studies should be conducted with a real-time scanner, preferably using sector or curved linear transducers. Static B-scan images may be obtained as a supplement to the real-time images when indicated. The transducer or scanner should be adjusted to operate at the highest clinically appropriate frequency, realizing that there is a trade-off between resolution and beam penetration. With modern equipment, these frequencies are usually between 2.25 MHz and 5.0 MHz.

Documentation

Adequate documentation is essential for high-quality patient care. This should be a permanent record of the ultrasound examination

From American Institute of Ultrasound in Medicine. Additional copies of guidelines can be ordered from the AIUM at the cost of $6.00 for AIUM members and $20.00 for nonmembers. Mail orders to AIUM Publications Department, 11200 Rockville Pike, Suite 205, Rockville, MD 20852-3139.

and its interpretation. Images of all appropriate areas, both normal and abnormal, should be recorded in appropriate imaging or storage format. Variations from normal size should be accompanied by measurements. Images are to be appropriately labeled with the examination date, patient identification, and image orientation. A report of the ultrasound findings should be included in the patient's medical record, regardless of where the study is performed. Retention of the ultrasound examination should be consistent both with clinical needs and with relevant legal and local health-care facility requirements.

Part II: Guidelines for the Abdomen and Retroperitoneum Ultrasound Examination

The following guidelines describe the examination to be performed for each organ and anatomical region in the abdomen and retroperitoneum. A complete examination would include all of the following. A limited examination would include one or more of these areas, but not all of them.

Liver

The liver survey should include both long axis (coronal or sagittal) and transverse views. If possible, views comparing the echogenicity of the liver to the right kidney should be performed. The major vessels (aorta, inferior vena cava) in the region of the liver should be imaged, including the position of the inferior vena cava where it passes through the liver. The regions of the ligamentum teres on the left and of the dome of the right lobe with the right hemidiaphragm and right pleural space should be imaged. The main lobar fissure should be demonstrated.

Survey of right and left lobes should include visualization of the hepatic veins. The right and left branches of the portal vein should be identified. The intrahepatic bile ducts should be evaluated for possible dilatation.

Gallbladder and Biliary Tract

The gallbladder evaluation should include long axis (coronal or sagittal) and transverse views obtained in the supine position. Left lateral decubitus (left side down), erect, or prone positions may also be necessary to allow a complete evaluation of the gallbladder and its surrounding area.

The intrahepatic ducts can be evaluated, as described under the liver, by obtaining a view of the liver demonstrating the right and left hepatic branches of the portal vein. The extrahepatic ducts can be evaluated in supine, left lateral decubitus, and/or semierect positions. The size of the intrahepatic and extrahepatic ducts should be assessed. With these views the relationship among the bile ducts, hepatic artery, and portal vein can be shown. When possible, the common bile duct in the pancreatic head should be visualized.

Pancreas

The pancreatic head, uncinate process, and body should be identified in transverse, and when possible, long axis (coronal or sagittal) projections. If possible, the pancreatic tail should also be imaged, and the pancreatic duct demonstrated. The peripancreatic region should be assessed for adenopathy.

Spleen

Representative views of the spleen in long axis (coronal or sagittal), and in transverse projection should be performed. An attempt should be made to demonstrate the left pleural space. When possible, the echogenicity of the upper pole of the left kidney should be compared to that of the spleen.

Kidneys

Representative long axis (coronal or sagittal) view of each kidney should be obtained, visualizing the cortex and the renal pelvis. Transverse views of both the left and right kidney should include the upper pole, middle section at the renal pelvis, and the lower pole. When possible, comparison of renal echogenicity with the adjacent liver and spleen should be performed. The perirenal regions should be assessed for possible abnormality.

Aorta and Inferior Vena Cava

The aorta and inferior vena cava should be imaged in long axis (coronal or sagittal) and transverse planes. Scans of both vessels should be attempted from the diaphragm to the bifurcation (usually at the level of the umbilicus). If possible, images should also include the adjacent common iliac vessels.

Abnormalities should be assessed. The surrounding soft tissues should be evaluated for adenopathy.

Guidelines for Performance of the Scrotal Ultrasound Examination

The following are proposed guidelines for ultrasound evaluation of the scrotum. The document consists of 2 parts:

Part I: Equipment and Documentation Guidelines
Part II: Guidelines for a General Examination of the Scrotum

These guidelines have been developed to provide assistance to practitioners performing ultrasound studies of the scrotum. In some cases, additional and/or specialized examinations may be necessary. Although it is not possible to detect every abnormality, adherence to the following guidelines will maximize the probability of detecting most of the abnormalities that occur in the scrotum.

Part I: Guidelines for Equipment and Documentation

Equipment

Scrotal studies should be conducted with a real-time scanner, preferably using sector or curved linear transducers. Static B-scan images may be obtained as a supplement to the real-time images when indicated. The transducer or scanner should be adjusted to operate at the highest clinically appropriate frequency, realizing that there is a trade-off between resolution and beam penetration. With modern equipment, these frequencies are usually between 2.25 MHz and 5.0 MHz or greater.

> **COMMENT:** Resolution should be of sufficient quality to routinely differentiate small cystic lesions from solid lesions.

Documentation

Adequate documentation is essential for high-quality patient care. This should be a permanent record of the ultrasound examination

From American Institute of Ultrasound in Medicine. Additional copies of guidelines can be ordered from the AIUM at the cost of $6.00 for AIUM members and $20.00 for nonmembers. Mail orders to AIUM Publications Department, 11200 Rockville Pike, Suite 205, Rockville, MD 20852-3139.

and its interpretation. Images of all appropriate areas, both normal and abnormal, should be recorded in any appropriate image or storage format. Variations from normal size should be accompanied by measurements. Images are to be appropriately labeled with the examination date, patient identification, and image orientation. A report of the ultrasound findings should be included in the patient's medical record, regardless of where the study is performed. Retention of the ultrasound examination should be consistent both with clinical needs and with relevant legal and local health care facility requirements.

Part II: Guidelines for the Scrotal Ultrasound Examination

The testes should be studied in at least two projections: long axis and transverse. Views of each testicle should include the superior, mid, and inferior portions as well as its medial and lateral borders. The adjacent epididymis should be evaluated. The size and echogenicity of each testicle and epididymis should be compared to its opposite side.

Any abnormality should be documented and all extratesticular structures evaluated. Additional techniques, such as Valsalva maneuver or upright positioning can be used as needed.

Guidelines for Performance of the Antepartum Obstetrical Ultrasound Examination

These guidelines have been developed for use by practitioners performing obstetrical ultrasound studies. The document consists of 2 parts:

Part I: Equipment and Documentation Guidelines
Part II: Guidelines for a General Antepartum Obstetrical Ultrasound Examination

A limited examination may be performed in clinical emergencies or if used as a follow-up to a complete examination. In some cases, an additional and/or specialized examination may be necessary. Although it is not possible to detect all structural congenital anomalies with diagnostic ultrasound, adherence to the following guidelines will maximize the possibility of detecting many fetal abnormalities.

Part I: Guidelines for Equipment and Documentation

Equipment

These studies should be conducted with real-time scanners, using an abdominal and/or vaginal approach. A transducer of appropriate frequency (3 MHz or higher abdominally, 5 MHz or higher vaginally) should be used. A static scanner (3 MHz to 5 MHz) may be used, but should not be the sole method of examination. The lowest possible ultrasonic exposure settings should be used to gain the necessary diagnostic information.

From American Institute of Ultrasound in Medicine. Additional copies of guidelines can be ordered from the AIUM at the cost of $6.00 for AIUM members and $20.00 for nonmembers. Mail orders to AIUM Publications Department, 11200 Rockville Pike, Suite 205, Rockville, MD 20852-3139.

COMMENT: Real-time observation is necessary to reliably confirm the presence of fetal life through observation of cardiac activity, respiration, and active movement. Real-time studies simplify evaluation of fetal anatomy as well as the task of obtaining fetal measurements. The choice of frequency is a trade-off between beam penetration and resolution. With modern equipment, 3-MHz to 5-MHz abdominal transducers allow sufficient penetration in nearly all patients while providing adequate resolution. During early pregnancy, a 5-MHz abdominal or a 5-MHz to 7-MHz vaginal transducer may provide adequate penetration and produce superior resolution.

Care of the Equipment

Vaginal probes should be covered by a protective sheath prior to insertion. Following the examination, the sheath should be disposed and the probe cleaned in an antimicrobial solution. The type of solution and amount of time for cleaning depends on manufacturer and infectious disease recommendations.

Documentation

Adequate documentation of the study is essential for high-quality patient care. This should include a permanent record of the ultrasound images, incorporating whenever possible the measurement parameters and anatomical findings proposed here. Images are to be appropriately labeled with the examination date, patient identification, and if appropriate, image orientation. A report of the ultrasound findings should be included in the patient's medical record, regardless of where the study is performed. Retention of the ultrasound examination should be consistent both with clinical needs and with relevant legal and local health-care facility requirements.

Part II: Guidelines for First Trimester Sonography

Scanning in the first trimester may be performed either abdominally or vaginally. If an abdominal scan is performed and fails to provide definitive information concerning any of the following guidelines, a vaginal scan should be performed whenever possible.

1. The location of the gestational sac should be documented. The embryo should be identified and the crown rump length recorded.

COMMENT: The crown rump length is an accurate indicator of fetal age. Comparison should be made to standard tables. If the embryo is not identified, characteristics of the gestational sac, including mean diameter of the anechoic space to determine fetal age and analysis of the hyperechoic rim, should be noted. During the late first trimester, biparietal diameter and other fetal measurements may also be used to establish fetal age.

2. Presence or absence of fetal life should be reported.

> **COMMENT:** Real-time observation is critical in this diagnosis. It should be noted that fetal cardiac activity may not be visible before 7 GA weeks abdominally and frequently at least 1 week earlier vaginally as determined by crown rump length. Thus, confirmation of fetal life may require follow-up evaluation.

3. Fetal number should be documented.

> **COMMENT:** Multiple pregnancies should be reported only in those instances where multiple embryos are actually seen. Because of variability in fusion between the amnion and the chorion, the appearance of more than one sac-like structure in early pregnancy is often noted and may be confused with multiple gestation or amniotic band.

4. Evaluation of the uterus (including cervix) and adnexal structures should be performed.

> **COMMENT:** This will allow recognition of incidental findings of potential clinical significance. The presence, location, and size of myomas and adnexal masses should be recorded.

Guidelines for Sonography in the Second and Third Trimester

1. Fetal life, number, and presentation should be documented.

> **COMMENT:** Abnormal heart rate and/or rhythm should be reported. Multiple pregnancies require the reporting of additional information: placental number, sac number, comparison of fetal size, and when visualized, fetal genitalia, and presence or absence of an interposed membrane.

2. An estimate of the amount of amniotic fluid (increased, decreased, normal) should be reported.

> **COMMENT:** Although this evaluation is subjective, there is little difficulty in recognizing extremes of amniotic fluid volume. Physiological variation with stage of pregnancy must be taken into account.

3. The placental location, appearance, and its relationship to the internal cervical os should be recorded.

> **COMMENT:** It is recognized that placental position early in pregnancy may not correlate well with its location at the time of delivery.

4. Assessment of gestational age should be accomplished using combination of biparietal diameter (or head circumference) and femur length. Fetal growth and weight (as opposed to age) should be assessed in the third trimester and requires the addition of abdominal diameters or circumferences. If previous studies have been performed, an estimate of the appropriateness of interval change should be given.

> **COMMENT:** Third trimester measurements may not accurately reflect gestational age. Initial determination of gestational age should therefore be performed prior to the third trimester whenever possible. If one or more previous studies have been performed, the gestational age at the time of the current examination should be based on the earliest examination that permits measurement of crown rump length, biparietal diameter, head circumference, and/or femur length by the following equation:
>
> *Current fetal age = Initial embryo/fetal age + Number of weeks from first study*
>
> The current measurements should be compared with norms for the gestational age based on standard tables. If previous studies have been performed, interval change in the measurements should be assessed.

4A. Biparietal diameter at a standard reference level (which should include the cavum septi pellucidi and the thalamus) should be measured and recorded.

> **COMMENT:** If the fetal head is dolichocephalic or brachycephalic, the biparietal diameter alone may be misleading. On occasion, the computation of the cephalic index, a ratio of the biparietal diameter to fronto-occipital diameter, is needed to make this determination. In such situations, the head circumference or corrected biparietal diameter is required.

4B. Head circumference is measured at the same level as the biparietal diameter.

4C. Femur length should be measured routinely and recorded after GA week 14.

> **COMMENT:** As with biparietal diameter, considerable biological variation is present late in pregnancy.

4D. Abdominal circumference should be determined at the level of the junction of the umbilical vein and portal sinus.

COMMENT: Abdominal circumference measurement may allow detection of growth retardation and macrosomia—conditions of the late second and third trimester. Comparison of the abdominal circumference with the head circumference should be made. If the abdominal measurement is below or above that expected for a stated gestation, it is recommended that circumferences of the head and body be measured and the head circumference/abdominal circumference ratio be reported. The use of circumferences is also suggested in those instances where the shape of either the head or body is different from that normally encountered.

5. Evaluation of the uterus and adnexal structures should be performed.

COMMENT: This will allow recognition of incidental findings of potential clinical significance. The presence, location, and size of myomas and adnexal masses should be recorded.

6. The study should include, but not necessarily be limited to, the following fetal anatomy: cerebral ventricles, 4-chamber view of the heart (including its position within the thorax), spine, stomach, urinary bladder, umbilical cord insertion site on the anterior abdominal wall, and renal region.

COMMENT: It is recognized that not all malformations of the above-mentioned organ systems such as the spine can be detected using ultrasonography. Nevertheless, a careful anatomical survey may allow diagnosis of certain birth defects that would otherwise go unrecognized. Suspected abnormalities may require a specialized evaluation.

Guidelines for Performance of the Ultrasound Examination of the Female Pelvis

The following are proposed guidelines for ultrasound evaluation of the female pelvis. The document consists of 2 parts:

Part I: Equipment and Documentation Guidelines
Part II: Guidelines for the General Examination of the Female Pelvis

These guidelines have been developed to provide assistance to practitioners performing ultrasound studies of the female pelvis. In some cases, additional and/or specialized examinations may be necessary. Although it is not possible to detect every abnormality, adherence to the following guidelines will maximize the probability of detecting most of the abnormalities that occur.

Part I: Guidelines for Equipment and Documentation

Equipment

Ultrasound examination of the female pelvis should be conducted with a real-time scanner, preferably using sector or curved linear transducers. Static B-scan images may be obtained as a supplement to the real-time images when indicated. The transducer or scanner should be adjusted to operate at the highest clinically appropriate frequency, realizing that there is a trade-off between resolution and beam penetration. With modern equipment, studies performed from the anterior abdominal wall can usually use frequencies of 3.5 MHz or higher, whereas scans performed from the vagina should use frequencies of 5 MHz or higher.

Care of the Equipment

Vaginal probes should be covered by a protective sheath before insertion. Following the examination, the sheath should be disposed and

From American Institute of Ultrasound in Medicine. Additional copies of guidelines can be ordered from the AIUM at the cost of $6.00 for AIUM members and $20.00 for nonmembers. Mail orders to AIUM Publications Department, 11200 Rockville Pike, Suite 205, Rockville, MD 20852-3139.

the probe cleaned in an antimicrobial solution. The type of solution and amount of time for cleaning depends on manufacturer and infectious disease recommendations.

Documentation

Adequate documentation is essential for high-quality patient care. There should be a permanent record of the ultrasound examination and its interpretation. Images of all appropriate areas, both normal and abnormal, should be recorded in an imaging or storage format. Variations from normal size should be accompanied by measurements. Images are to be appropriately labeled with the examination date, patient identification, and image orientation. A report of the ultrasound findings should be included in the patient's medical record. Retention of the permanent record of the ultrasound examination should be consistent both with clinical need and with the relevant legal and local health care facility requirements.

Part II: Guidelines for Performance of the Ultrasound Examination of the Female Pelvis

The following guidelines describe the examination to be performed for each organ and anatomic region in the female pelvis. All relevant structures should be identified by the abdominal or vaginal approach; in some cases, both will be necessary.

General Pelvic Preparation

For a pelvic sonogram performed from the abdominal wall, the patient's urinary bladder should be full. For a vaginal sonogram, the urinary bladder is usually empty. The vaginal transducer may be introduced by the patient, the sonographer, or the sonologist. It is recommended that a woman should be present in the examining room at all times during a vaginal sonogram, either as an examiner or a chaperone.

Uterus

The vagina and uterus provide anatomic landmarks that can be utilized as reference points for the remaining normal and abnormal pelvic structures. In evaluating the uterus, the following should be documented: (1) the uterine size, shape, and orientation; (2) the endometrium; (3) the myometrium; and (4) the cervix. The vagina should be imaged as a landmark for the cervix and lower uterine segment.

Uterine size can be determined as follows. Uterine length is evaluated in long axis from the fundus to the cervix (the external os, if it can be identified). The depth of the uterus (anteroposterior dimension) is measured in the same long-axis view from its anterior to posterior walls, perpendicular to the length. The width is measured from the transaxial or coronal view. Cervical diameters can be similarly determined.

Abnormalities of the uterus should be documented. The endometrium should be analyzed for thickness, echogenicity, and its position within the uterus. The myometrium and cervix should be evaluated for contour changes, echogenicity, and masses.

Adnexa (Ovaries and Fallopian Tubes)

When evaluating the adnexa, an attempt should be made to identify the ovaries first since they can serve as the major point of reference for adnexal structures. Frequently the ovaries are situated anterior to the internal iliac (hypogastric) vessels, which serve as a landmark for their identification. The following ovarian findings should be documented: (1) size, shape, contour, and echogenicity and (2) position relative to the uterus. The ovarian size can be determined by measuring the length in long axis, usually along the axis of the hypogastric (internal iliac) vessels, with the anteroposterior dimension measured perpendicular to the length. The ovarian width is measured in the transaxial or coronal view. A volume can be calculated.

The normal fallopian tubes are not commonly identified. This region should be surveyed for abnormalities, particularly dilated tubular structures.

If an adnexal mass is noted, its relationship to the ovaries and uterus should be documented. Its size and echopattern (cystic, solid, or mixed) should be determined.

Cul-de-sac

The cul-de-sac and bowel posterior to the uterus may not be clearly defined. This area should be evaluated for the presence of free fluid or mass. If a mass is detected, its size, position, shape, echopattern (cystic, solid, or complex), and its relationship to the ovaries and uterus should be documented. Differentiation of normal loops of bowel from a mass may be difficult if only an abdominal examination is performed. If a suspected mass is imaged that might represent fluid and feces within normal rectosigmoid colon and a vaginal scan is not performed, an ultrasound water enema study or a repeat examination after a cleansing enema may be indicated.

Guidelines for Performance of the Ultrasound Examination of the Prostate (and Surrounding Structures)

The following are proposed guidelines for the ultrasound evaluation of the prostate and surrounding structures. The document consists of 2 parts:

Part I: Equipment and Documentation
Part II: Ultrasound Examination of the Prostate and Surrounding Structures

These guidelines have been developed to provide assistance to practitioners performing an ultrasound study of the prostate. In some cases, an additional and/or specialized examination may be necessary. Although it is not possible to detect every abnormality, adherence to the following will maximize the detection of most abnormalities.

Part I

Guidelines for Equipment and Documentation

Equipment
A prostate study should be conducted with a real-time transrectal (also termed *endorectal*) transducer using the highest clinically appropriate frequency, realizing that there is a trade-off between resolution and beam penetration. With modern equipment, these frequencies are usually 5 MHz or higher.

Documentation
Adequate documentation is essential for high-quality patient care. There should be a permanent record of the ultrasound examination

From American Institute of Ultrasound in Medicine. Additional copies of guidelines can be ordered from AIUM at the cost of $6.00 for AIUM members and $20.00 for nonmembers. Mail orders to AIUM Publications Department, 11200 Rockville Pike, Suite 205, Rockville, MD 20852-3139.

and its interpretation. Images of all appropriate areas, both normal and abnormal, should be accompanied by measurements. Images are to be appropriately labeled with the examination date, patient identification, and image orientation. A report of the ultrasound findings should be included in the patient's medical record. Retention of the permanent record of the ultrasound examination should be consistent both with clinical need and with the relevant legal and local health care facility requirements.

Care of the Equipment

Transrectal probes should be covered by a disposable sheath prior to insertion. Following the examination, the sheath should be disposed of and the probe soaked in an antimicrobial solution. The type of solution and amount of time for soaking depends on manufacturer and infectious disease recommendations. Following the examination, if there is a gross tear in the sheath, the fluid channels in the probe should be thoroughly flushed with the antimicrobial solution. Tubing and stopcocks should be disposed after each examination.

Part II: Ultrasound Examination of the Prostate and Surrounding Structures

The following guidelines describe the examination to be performed for the prostate and surrounding structures.

Prostate

The prostate should be imaged in its entirety in at least 2 orthogonal planes, sagittal and axial or sagittal and coronal, from the apex to the base of the gland. In particular, the peripheral zone should be thoroughly imaged. The gland should be evaluated for size, echogenicity, symmetry, and continuity of margins. The periprostatic fat and vessels should be evaluated for asymmetry and disruption in echogenicity.

Seminal Vesicles and Vas Deferens

The seminal vesicles should be examined in 2 planes from their insertion into the prostate via the ejaculatory ducts to their cranial and lateral extents. They should be evaluated for size, shape, position, symmetry, and echogenicity. Both vas deferentia should be evaluated.

Perirectal Space

Evaluation of the perirectal space, in particular the region that abuts the prostate and perirectal tissues, should be performed. If a pathological condition of the rectum is clinically suspected, the rectal wall and lumen should be studied.

Index

Page numbers followed by f indicate figures; t, tables; b, boxes.

647